Integrating Lifestyle Medicine in Cardiovascular Health and Disease Prevention

Cardiovascular disease (CVD) is the leading cause of morbidity and mortality in the United States and around the world. Major risk factors for CVD result from poor lifestyle habits and practices, but the area of lifestyle medicine has emerged to help clinicians and their patients understand the power of positive lifestyle habits and actions.

Written by cardiologist and lifestyle medicine pioneer Dr. James M. Rippe, *Integrating Lifestyle Medicine in Cardiovascular Health and Disease Prevention* introduces the principles of lifestyle medicine with the practice of cardiology to help lower the risk of heart disease and, if already present, assist in its treatment. This book provides evidence-based information on both the prevention and treatment of CVD through lifestyle measures such as regular physical activity, sound nutrition, weight management and avoidance of tobacco products. This information aids physicians and patients to better understand multiple linkages between poor habits and practices, employing them with associated behavioral techniques to lessen the likelihood of developing CVD.

FEATURES

- Summarizes major issues in CVD including heart attack, stroke, atrial fibrillation, high blood pressure, lipid abnormalities and obesity.
- Provides protocols for overcoming a sedentary lifestyle and using lifestyle medicine techniques to optimize brain health.
- Empowers clinicians with vital information for consultations on the power of lifestyle medicine practices, to treat symptoms if already present or to prevent major components of CVD from developing in the future.

Written for practitioners at all levels, this user-friendly volume in the Lifestyle Medicine series is valuable to practitioners in general medicine or subspecialty practices including lifestyle medicine and cardiology.

Lifestyle Medicine

Series Editor

James M. Rippe, MD

Professor of Medicine, UMass Chan Medical School

Led by James M. Rippe, MD, founder of the Rippe Lifestyle Institute, this series is directed to a broad range of researchers and professionals consisting of topical books with clinical applications in nutrition and health, physical activity, obesity management and applicable subjects in lifestyle medicine.

Increasing Physical Activity: A Practical Guide, *James M. Rippe*

Manual of Lifestyle Medicine, *James M. Rippe*

Obesity Prevention and Treatment: A Practical Guide, *James M. Rippe and John P. Foreyt*

Improving Women's Health Across the Lifespan, *Michelle Tollefson, Nancy Eriksen, Neha Pathak*

Lifestyle Principles and Nursing Practice *Gia Merlo, Kathy Berra*

Integrating Lifestyle Medicine in Cardiovascular Health and Disease Prevention, *James M. Rippe*

For more information, please visit: www.routledge.com/Lifestyle-Medicine/book-series/CRCLM

Integrating Lifestyle Medicine in Cardiovascular Health and Disease Prevention

James M. Rippe, MD

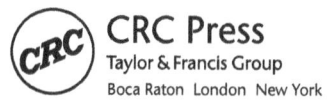

CRC Press
Taylor & Francis Group
Boca Raton London New York

CRC Press is an imprint of the
Taylor & Francis Group, an **informa** business

First edition published 2023
by CRC Press
6000 Broken Sound Parkway NW, Suite 300, Boca Raton, FL 33487–2742

and by CRC Press
4 Park Square, Milton Park, Abingdon, Oxon, OX14 4RN

CRC Press is an imprint of Taylor & Francis Group, LLC

© 2023 Taylor & Francis Group, LLC

ISBN: 978-1-032-21386-6 (hbk)
ISBN: 978-1-032-21384-2 (pbk)
ISBN: 978-1-003-26814-7 (ebk)

DOI: 10.1201/b23245

Typeset in Times
by Apex CoVantage, LLC

To my beautiful wife, Stephanie Hart Rippe, and our wonderful children, Hart, Jaelin, Devon, and Jamie who inspire me and make it all worthwhile

Contents

PART III   Specialized Topics

Preface

Cardiovascular disease (CVD) remains the leading cause of morbidity and mortality in the United States and around the world. Over 37% of deaths each year in the United States are attributed to cardiovascular disease (1). Many components of lifestyle practices and habits significantly impact risk factors for CVD disease. For example, the Nurses Health Trial reported that 80%–91% of all incident CVD and diabetes, respectively, could be eliminated if women would follow five simple lifestyle practices (2). These include

- Participate in regular physical activity (≥30 minutes of moderate-intensity physical activity each day);
- Maintain a healthy body weight (body mass index between ≥19 and ≤25);
- Follow healthy nutritional practices (more whole grains, fruits and vegetables);
- Do not smoke cigarettes; and
- If drinking alcohol, consume only one alcoholic beverage/day.

Similar findings were observed in the U.S. Male Professional Health Study (3). In fact, if only one of these positive health practices were followed, the risk of CVD was reduced by up to 50%.

More recently, researchers analyzed data from these two major ongoing cohort studies to estimate the impact of these five lifestyle practices on life expectancy in the U.S. population. During up to 34 years of follow-up, adherence to all five lifestyle-related factors significantly increased lifestyle expectancy at age 50 years for "most men and women by 12.2 and 14.0 years, respectively." The most physically active cohorts of men and women demonstrated a 78% gain in life expectancy. These investigators concluded that prevention should be a top priority in the U.S. healthcare system.

The American Heart Association (AHA) and American College of Cardiology (ACC) have been leading professional organizations emphasizing the profound importance of lifestyle habits and actions on cardiovascular health. Clearly, lifestyle factors modulate multiple risk factors for CVD including abnormal lipids, high blood pressure, diabetes mellitus, body weight and fat storage.

Recognition of the profound impact of lifestyle medicine on CVD has been increasingly embraced by the medical community. For example, one Council of the AHA in 2013 changed its name from the "Council on Nutrition, Physical Activity and Metabolism" to the "Council on Lifestyle and Cardiometabolic Health (4)." The most recent Physical Activity Guidelines for Americans (2018) demonstrated significant reductions in the risk of CVD and total mortality for individuals who engaged in ≥150 minutes of moderate-intensity physical activity and two musculoskeletal training sessions each week (5). In fact, individuals who participated in as little as 30 minutes of moderate-intensity physical activity per week reduced their risk of CVD by 20%. Moreover, it was concluded that being unfit warrants consideration as an independent risk factor, and that a low level of cardiorespiratory fitness increases the risk of CVD to a greater extent than merely being physically inactive (6).

Only 25% of U.S. adults meet the Centers for Disease Control and Prevention (CDC) guidelines for physical activity (5). When sedentary individuals are compared to individuals who engage in regular physical activity, they have a 150%–240% increased likelihood of developing CVD (7). Thus, individuals who choose to lead sedentary lifestyles double their risk of heart disease. To put this in perspective, this is the same increased risk of CVD that individuals accept who smoke a pack of cigarettes a day. Thus, physical inactivity represents a lifestyle factor that appears as dangerous as smoking a pack of cigarettes per day with regard to CVD and is four to five times as prevalent.

Despite the established links between lifestyle and CVD, few physicians (<40%) regularly counsel their patients on such issues as nutrition, physical activity, weight management, smoking cessation, and the avoidance of secondhand smoke (8). This is a wasted opportunity since over 70% of individuals in the United States see their primary care physician on at least a yearly basis.

A healthy lifestyle also plays an important role in the primary and secondary prevention of CVD, even among those taking medications for high blood pressure or elevated blood cholesterol (9). Moreover, effect estimates show convincingly the health benefits of adjunctive lifestyle changes in patients with known heart disease, the magnitude of which are similar to those conferred by cardioprotective drugs after acute myocardial infarction. Collectively, these findings and other data suggest that the effects of lifestyle change and combination drug therapy on cardiovascular risk reduction appear to be independent and additive.

The American public has also been reluctant to embrace positive lifestyle measures in their daily lives. As already indicated, the CDC estimates that only 25% of individuals meet their guidelines for regular physical activity. Less than 15% of individuals consume the recommended level of fruits and vegetables on a daily basis (10). Over 70% of the U.S. population is overweight or obese (11), and ~15% continue to smoke cigarettes (12).

The importance of lifestyle practices is relevant to all aspects of medicine, but particularly in cardiovascular medicine, where it is increasingly being recognized. In addition, the American College of Lifestyle Medicine (ACLM) now has over 8,000 members. Its membership has grown over 1,200% since 2003 (13).

The lifestyle medicine movement has also emerged in over 40 countries around the world (14). The World Health Organization recognizes lifestyle factors in their initiative to reduce noncommunicable diseases and singles out that reducing the risk of heart disease and its risk factors is a high priority around the world (15). Similarly, the AHA in its 2020 Strategic Plan emphasized that lowering the risk of heart disease and improving cardiovascular health represent top priorities (16).

Finally, failure of the client/patient to take responsibility for their own health represents the single most important factor affecting the prevention of and recovery from CVD. Clearly, a greater emphasis needs to be placed on what happens between an individual's visits to the physician. Indeed, it is estimated that patients spend more than 5,000 hours each year outside of healthcare appointments. Accordingly, self-responsibility (e.g., meeting certain basic health metrics) will become a greater priority in the contemporary healthcare environment. For example, completing health habit surveys and/or serial risk factor profiles and attaining certain risk factor goals will be increasingly mandated by insurers and employers, orchestrated in part by financial and other incentives.

With this as background, I felt there was an urgent need to provide an evidence-based book strongly linking lifestyle habits and practices not only to CVD, but also cardiovascular health. I am not aware of any other book that specifically links the independent and added benefits of lifestyle modifications to reduction in risk of CVD. I hope that this book will be valuable in helping physicians to better understand these multiple linkages and employ them in associated behavioral counseling techniques (e.g., readiness to change, motivational interviewing, etc.) with more consistency in the daily practice of medicine.

I also hope that this book will be highly beneficial to nurses who assist in the practice of cardiovascular medicine as well as nutritionists and exercise physiologists. These are professions that have an enormous number of members that far exceed the size of the physician community. For example, there are three times as many nurses in the United States as there are physicians. I hope and anticipate that all of these individuals will benefit from an evidence-based compilation of lifestyle practices that impact cardiovascular health and disease. I hope this book will help accomplish our goal of strongly linking lifestyle medicine to cardiovascular health and disease.

This book is divided into three parts. Part I provides a general framework for the components of lifestyle medicine that are useful in helping to lower the risk of cardiovascular disease and improve cardiovascular health. These include regular physical activity, proper nutrition, weight management, tobacco cessation, stress reduction and healthy sleep.

In Part II, I then move on to specific ways of addressing and treating cardiovascular disease risk factors. These include atherosclerosis, dyslipidemias, hypertension, arrhythmias, coronary artery disease, myocardial infarction, stroke, diabetes and obesity. Chapters are also devoted to overcoming a sedentary lifestyle and using lifestyle medicine techniques to optimize brain health.

Part III concludes the book with specialized topics including heart disease in women, stress reduction in children, emerging evidence in genetics and epigenetics, available data on reversing heart disease, future directions in research and applications linking lifestyle medicine to cardiovascular disease risk factor reduction and prevention.

There is no longer any serious doubt that what each of use does in our daily lives profoundly impacts our short- and long-term health and quality of life. I hope that this book will encourage practitioners at all levels to emphasize the profound linkages between lifestyle and cardiovascular health. This is clearly the future of not only cardiovascular medicine but also medicine and health, in general. The linkages between lifestyle medicine and cardiovascular health and disease prevention are profound. It will be essential for all individuals who treat aspects of CVD and its prevention to continue to educate themselves on the linkages between lifestyle habits and actions to reduce the great burden of CVD around the world. I hope that this book will assist individuals to continue to gain knowledge and clinical expertise in the vitally important area of lifestyle medicine and cardiovascular disease.

James M. Rippe, MD
Founder and Director
Rippe Lifestyle Institute
Professor of Medicine (Cardiology)
UMass Chan Medical School
Shrewsbury, Massachusetts

REFERENCES

1. Virani SS, Alonso A, Benjamin EJ, et al. Heart disease and stroke statistics—2021 update: A report from the American Heart Association. Circulation. 2021;143:e254–e743.
2. Bassuk SS, Manon JE. Lifestyle and risk of cardiovascular disease and type 2 diabetes in women: A review of the epidemiologic evidence. Am J Lifestyle Med. 2008;2(3).
3. Manson JE, Nathan DM, Krolewski AS, Stampfer MJ, Willett WC, Hennekens CH. A prospective study of exercise and incidence of diabetes among US male physicians. JAMA. 1992;268:63–67.
4. American Heart Association. Council on Lifestyle and Cardiometabolic Health. https://professional.heart.org/professional/MembershipCouncils/ScientificCouncils/UCM_322856_Council-on-Lifestyle-and-Cardiometabolic-Health.jsp. Accessed August 10, 2021.
5. 2018 Physical Activity Guidelines Advisory Committee. 2018 Physical Activity Guidelines Advisory Committee Scientific Report. Washington, DC: U.S. Department of Health and Human Services; 2018.
6. Myers J, Kaykha A, George S, Lear S, Yamazaki T, et al. Fitness versus physical activity patterns in predicting mortality in men. Am J Med. 2004;117:912–18.
7. Moore SC, Patel AV, Matthews CE, Berrington de Gonzalez A, Park Y, et al. Leisure time physical activity of moderate to vigorous intensity and mortality: A large pooled cohort analysis. PLoS Med. 2012;9(11):e1001335.
8. Rippe JM. Lifestyle Medicine (3rd edition): Physician Health Practices and Lifestyle Medicine. Boca Raton, FL: CRC Press; 2019.
9. Whelton PK, Carey RM, Aronow WS, Casey DE, Collins KJ, et al. ACC/AHA/AAPA/ABC/ACPM/AGS/AphA/ASH/ASPC/NMA/PCNA guideline for the prevention, detection, evaluation, and management of high blood pressure in adults: A report of the American College of Cardiology/American Heart Association Task Force on Clinical Practice Guidelines. Hypertension. 2018;71(6):e13–e115.
10. Rippe JM. Lifestyle Medicine (4th edition): Nutrition and Cardiovascular Disease. Boca Raton, FL: CRC Press; 2023.
11. Kuczmarski RJ, Flegal KM, Campbell SM, Johnson CL. Increasing prevalence of overweight among US adults. The national health and nutrition examination surveys, 1960 to 1991. JAMA. 1994;272(3):205–11.
12. National Center for Health Statistics, Health, United States, 2016: With Chart Book on Long Term Trends in Health. Hyattsville, MD; 2017.
13. American College of Lifestyle Medicine. www.lifestylemedicine.org/. Accessed August 10, 2021.

14. Lifestyle Medicine Global Alliance. https://lifestylemedicineglobal.org/. Accessed August 10, 2021.
15. Centers for Disease Control and Prevention. Global Noncommunicable Disease Programs. Division of Global Health Protection (DGHP). www.cdc.gov/globalhealth/healthprotection/ncd/about.html#:~:text=CDC%20collaborates%20with%20partners%20to,improve%20surveillance%20and%20evaluation%20systems. Accessed August 10, 2021.
16. Lloyd-Jones DM, Hong Y, Labarthe D, et al. American Heart Association Strategic Planning Task Force and Statistics Committee. Defining and setting national goals for cardiovascular health promotion and disease reduction: The American Heart Association's strategic Impact Goal through 2020 and beyond. Circulation. 2010; 121(4):586–613.

Acknowledgments

Textbook writing and editing are collaborative efforts that involve hard work, skill, and passion of numerous contributors. I am grateful to the many individuals who over my 30-plus years as a cardiologist have stimulated and influenced my thinking about the interaction between lifestyle and health and the specific interactions between lifestyle habits and practices and their role in both preventing and treating cardiovascular disease.

Numerous individuals have helped guide my thinking and are too many to acknowledge by name. I would like to particularly thank, however, a few individuals who have made substantial contributions to the current book and my career in cardiology.

First, my long-term editorial director, Beth Grady, who plays a critically important role in all of the major writing and editing projects that emerge from my research organization, deserves special thanks. This book is one of over 53 books that Beth has managed which have been generated through my organization. In addition to the current textbook, Beth provides editorial direction to two academic journals that I edit as well as my major *Lifestyle Medicine* textbook (*Lifestyle Medicine*, third edition, James M. Rippe [editor], CRC Press, 2019) and our major intensive care textbook (*Irwin and Rippe's Intensive Care Medicine*, ninth edition, Wolters Kluwer, 2022). Beth possesses not only superb editorial skills but also an exceptional work ethic and unfailing good humor to make all of these complex and difficult projects possible.

I would also like to express my appreciation to my office support staff, including my executive assistant, Carol Moreau, who seamlessly coordinates my schedule and travel plans to free up the time necessary for such large writing and publishing projects and also word-processed many of the chapters in this book. Our editorial office assistant, Deb Adamonis, assists all of us in the multiple daily tasks required to expedite diverse projects in our office. In addition, she tracked down hundreds of academic references for the current book. Our chief financial officer, Connie Martell, make sure that the financial processes are in place so that all of our projects move forward smoothly. The research team at Rippe Lifestyle Institute has always contributed important insights to clarify my thinking on a number of aspects of preventive cardiology and lifestyle medicine.

I would also like to acknowledge with gratitude some cardiologists who early in my career guided me and inspired me initially in invasive cardiology, coronary care and preventive cardiology. Chief among those is Dr. Joseph Alpert who served as a mentor and supporter of my career both as a medical student at Harvard Medical School and subsequently in my faculty career as a cardiologist, both at Umass Chan Medical School and Tufts Medical School. Also, Dr. Eugene Braunwald supported and guided my aspirations at Harvard Medical School to not only pursue cardiology but also establish a research career in this area.

I would like to thank the outstanding editorial team at Taylor & Francis Group/ CRC Press. Randy Brehm, senior editor, has been a key supporter of the multiple textbooks I have published with CRC Press, including the second, third, and fourth editions of my major academic textbook *Lifestyle Medicine*. Randy also has been a strong supporter of the Lifestyle Medicine Series in which this current volume resides.

Tom Connelly coordinated all aspects of the publication process and provided important day-to-day leadership and invaluable assistance on multiple issues related to manuscripts. Venkatesh Sundaram at Apex managed the editing, design and typesetting of the book with great skill.

Finally, as always, I am grateful to my family, including my loving wife Stephanie Hart Rippe and our four beautiful daughters Hart, Jaelin, Devon and Jamie who continue to love and support me through the arduous process of writing and editing many major textbooks, journal editing and the other diverse professional responsibilities that I juggle, along with my family life.

If there are errors or omissions in *Integrating Lifestyle Medicine in Cardiovascular Health and Disease Prevention*, the responsibility is mine. If there is credit due for this project, it belongs to the numerous people who have made substantial contributions to my knowledge and performance along the way.

James M. Rippe, MD
Boston, Massachusetts

Author

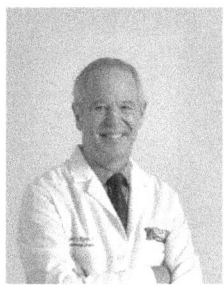

James M. Rippe, MD, is a graduate of Harvard College and Harvard Medical School with postgraduate training at Massachusetts General Hospital. He is currently the Founder and Director of the Rippe Lifestyle Institute and Professor of Medicine (Cardiology) at the University of Massachusetts Chan Medical School.

Over the past 25 years, Dr. Rippe has established and run the largest research organization in the world exploring how daily habits and actions impact short- and long-term health and quality of life. This organization, Rippe Lifestyle Institute (RLI), has published hundreds of papers that form the scientific basis for the fields of lifestyle medicine and high-performance health. RLI also conducts numerous studies every year on physical activity, nutrition, and healthy weight management. A lifelong and avid athlete, Dr. Rippe maintains his personal fitness with a regular walk, jog, swimming, and weight training program. He holds a black belt in karate and is an avid wind surfer, skier and tennis player. He lives outside of Boston with his wife, Stephanie Hart—television news anchor—and their four children, Hart, Jaelin, Devon and Jamie.

Part I

Lifestyle Medicine as an Approach to Cardiovascular Disease

1 Overview of Lifestyle Medicine and Cardiovascular Health and Disease

KEY POINTS

- Cardiovascular disease remains the leading cause of morbidity and mortality in the United States and worldwide.
- Despite abundant knowledge of how lifestyle factors impact the risk of cardiovascular disease, fewer than 40% of physicians discuss these lifestyle factors in patient encounters.
- Lifestyle measures include increased physical activity, proper nutrition, weight management, avoidance of tobacco products, stress reduction and healthy sleep, all of which powerfully lower risk for cardiovascular disease.
- It is incumbent on physicians to emphasize these lifestyle factors as an important way of lowering the leading cause of morbidity and mortality in the United States.

1.1 INTRODUCTION

What each individual does in their daily life profoundly affects numerous metabolic diseases including cardiovascular disease (CVD) (1). In particular, thousands of studies support the idea that such practices as getting regular physical activity, maintaining a proper body weight, following sound nutritional practices, avoiding tobacco products, reducing stress, and obtaining adequate sleep all significantly reduce the risk of CVD (2–10). The strength of this literature has been underscored by the inclusion of these principles in numerous documents and guidelines from the American Heart Association (AHA) (3,8,10), the American College of Cardiology (ACC) (9), the Physical Activity Guidelines for Americans 2018 (PAGA 2018) (11) and numerous other evidence-based professional recommendations.

Despite overwhelming evidence that positive lifestyle measures reduce the risk of CVD, it has been difficult to translate this information into habits and actions of individuals. For example, while improvements in lifestyle measures have been cited as the major reason for reduction of CVD in the past 30 years, major challenges remain. Between 1980 and 2000, mortality rates from coronary heart disease (CHD) in the United States fell by 40% (12). Approximately half of the reduction in CHD during this time period was attributed to improvement in lifestyle factors such as

DOI: 10.1201/b23245-2

smoking cessation, increased physical activity and better control of cholesterol and blood pressure. However, it should be noted that increases in obesity and diabetes, which continue to the present time, have moved in the opposite direction and have the potential to wipe out the gains achieved in other lifestyle risk factors, unless progress can be made in these negative trends.

Despite significant progress in lifestyle measures, CVD remains the leading cause of mortality in the United States and around the world. For example, in the United States, 37% of annual deaths result from CVD. Worldwide, over 40% of deaths result from CVD, and this number has grown precipitously over the past two decades. Thus, there are enormous challenges remaining when linking lifestyle measures to the risk of CVD.

Perhaps the biggest challenge remaining is to help individuals incorporate current knowledge into their daily lives. This is the largest gap when it comes to reducing CVD, in general, and coronary heart disease (CHD), in particular. The AHA Strategic Plan 2020 noted that only 5% of individuals achieve what was termed "ideal cardiovascular health," which encompasses lifestyle factors such as regular physical activity, sound nutrition, weight management and avoidance of tobacco, as well as other health-related factors such as control of cholesterol, blood pressure and glucose (3).

The AHA and ACC have been particularly prominent in promoting the power of lifestyle habits to lower risk of CVD. For example, the AHA Strategic Plan 2020 introduced the concept of "primordial" prevention that was defined as preventing risk factors from occurring in the first place. In addition, this Strategic Plan added and defined the concept of "ideal cardiovascular health" to the health-related lexicon.

During the same period of time, a rapidly emerging literature related to lifestyle factors and health has been published. It is now clear this discipline will coalesce under the concept of "lifestyle medicine." For example, the AHA and ACC in 2013 issued "Guideline on Lifestyle Management to Reduce Cardiovascular Risk" (9). Positive lifestyle was also listed as the leading therapeutic factor in the Joint Recommendations for Blood Pressure Control issued by the AHA, ACC and multiple other groups. Various lifestyle measures were also listed as key components for controlling blood pressure in the ACC/AHA "2017 Guideline for the Prevention, Detetion, Evaluation and Management of High Blood Pressure in Adults" (13). In addition, the council within the AHA that had previously been called the "Council of Nutrition, Physical Activity and Metabolism" (8) in 2013 changed its name to the "Council on Lifestyle and Cardiometabolic Health" (8). All these initiatives underscore the increased recognition of the power of utilizing multiple lifestyle factors and practices to lower the risk of heart disease.

The Dietary Guidelines for Americans 2020–2025 (14) and the PAGA 2018 also focus on key lifestyle issues not only for reducing the risk of cardiovascular disease but also for living with multiple other metabolic-related diseases. Thus, the role of positive lifestyle habits and practices is continuing to emerge as a cornerstone of the prevention of CVD and other metabolic diseases.

As a long-term advocate and researcher in the areas of both cardiovascular medicine and lifestyle medicine, I have found these trends to be deeply gratifying. I have authored numerous publications in the past linking cardiovascular disease prevention to daily habits and actions. For example, I named the field "lifestyle medicine" in the academic literature with the publication of the first, multi-authored textbook in this area in 1999 (*Lifestyle Medicine*, Blackwell Science, 1999) (15). The third edition of this book was published in 2019 (16), and the fourth edition will be published in 2023. This is a 1,500-page textbook with over 200 contributors who are experts in the various areas of lifestyle medicine and health.

In the current chapter, recent scientific literature related to how lifestyle habits and practices can be utilized to lower the risk of CVD is summarized. Subsequent chapters elucidate the relationship between lifestyle factors and CVD risk in greater detail. We frame this literature as a major component of "lifestyle medicine." I believe that this book is the first to strongly link the discipline of lifestyle medicine with CVD health and prevention and will encourage physicians and other healthcare providers to utilize these connections more prominently in their clinical practices.

1.2   DEFINING CARDIOVASCULAR HEALTH

Both the AHA and ACC have continued to increasingly emphasize lifestyle measures in the definition of cardiovascular health. Both organizations emphasize that daily habits and actions have a significant impact on the likelihood of developing CVD. The AHA Strategic Plan for 2020 articulated the goal that is "by 2020 to improve the cardiovascular health of all Americans by 20% by reducing deaths from CVD and stroke by 20%" (3). The AHA outlined a series of steps as key components of a strategy to reach these goals. Many of these depend on lifestyle modalities. They include

- Primordial prevention,
- Recognizing that risk factors for CVD develop early in life and
- Balancing individual risk with related population-level approaches.

The AHA Strategic Plan 2020 contained the important concept of "primordial prevention." This concept involves lowering the risk of developing cardiovascular risk factors in the first place, rather than simply treating cardiovascular risk factors once they are present. The AHA Strategic Plan 2020 also outlined the concept of "ideal cardiovascular health." This framework was defined as a series of seven health-related behaviors and health factors including not smoking, maintaining a healthy body mass index (BMI >18.5 kg/m^2 and <25 kg/m^2), achieving appropriate levels of physical activity, consuming a healthy diet, maintaining a cholesterol level of <200 mg/dL, maintaining a blood pressure <120/80 mm Hg, and maintaining a fasting glucose of <100 mg/dL. The health factors such as cholesterol, blood pressure and glucose were all defined as "untreated" values. It is clear that lifestyle factors also impact all of these parameters as well.

The AHA Policy Statement for Cardiovascular Health and Disease Surveillance for 2030 and Beyond further underscored lifestyle-related factors by focusing on healthy life expectancy (17). The concept of healthy life expectancy includes not only risk of cardiovascular mortality but also morbidity that may decrease quality of life even if an individual is free from various diseases. In essence, healthy life expectancy is defined as the average number of years a person can expect to live in "full health" by taking into account years lived in less than "full health" due to disease and/or injury.

In addition, the AHA Strategic Impact Goal provided a vision of robust development of community health platforms utilizing digital technologies, electronic health records and mobile health to reduce health disparities. The role of health disparities in overall health was starkly illustrated during the COVID-19 pandemic, when individuals who had risk factors of manifestations of chronic diseases such as CVD experienced three to four times the risk of hospitalization and mortality as a result of infection with the COVID-19 virus compared with individuals who did not have these factors.

1.3   THE CONCEPT OF RISK FACTORS

The concept of risk factors is relatively new in the history of medicine. The initial construct of risk factors was based on data from the Framingham Study, published in the 1960s. Prior to that, the concept of risk factors for CVD did not formally exist.

Framingham data clearly showed that factors such as diabetes, dyslipidemia, high blood pressure and cigarette smoking each independently and significantly increased the risk of CVD. The concept of CVD risk factors has also now been expanded by the AHA to include physical inactivity and obesity.

It should be noted that according to the Framingham data, risk factors act synergistically with each other and tend to cluster with each other. Thus, the presence of one risk factor in individuals doubles the risk of heart disease (18). The presence of two risk factors in individuals quadruples the chances of developing CVD compared to individuals with no risk factors. Individuals who have three risk factors increase their risk of developing CHD by 8- to 20-fold compared to individuals with no risk factors.

Other risk factors for CVD are currently under investigation, including inflammation as measured by elevated high-sensitivity C-reactive protein (hs-CRP). Inflammation may represent a common underlying factor that links CVD to diabetes and obesity. It is also possible that stress and other psychological factors, such as depression, may increase the risk of CVD, although less data are available in this area. We devoted an entire chapter to these latter issues.

Many of the risk factors for CVD can be modified by positive lifestyle behaviors. There are also nonmodifiable risk factors that include age, gender and family history. All of these latter risk factors may contribute in substantial ways to risk of CVD. It is important to note that even in these categories of nonmodifiable risk factors, lifestyle strategies can still significantly decrease CVD risk.

Numerous studies have demonstrated that reducing risk factors for CVD can significantly decrease its likelihood. Lifestyle measures are a particularly powerful and effective way for lowering risk factors. Furthermore, lifestyle factors are low risk, and many of them simultaneously affect multiple risk factors.

Some members of the preventive cardiology community have challenged the long-held concept of risk factors based on "one-size-fits-all" and suggested that preventive services should be allocated on the basis of proven research trial data. (This framework has been described as "what works and in whom?" rather than arbitrary scaling of goal risk.) Preventive cardiologists in the United States, Canada and Europe have listed five recommendations for simple, easily understood guidelines for use of statin therapy, for example, in the prevention of cardiovascular disease (19). They are the following:

- On the basis of high-quality, randomized, clinical trial data, statin therapy should be used as an adjunct to diet, exercise and smoking cessation in patients with previous history of myocardial infarction (MI), stroke or clinically apparent atherosclerosis.
- On the basis of high-quality, randomized, clinical trial data, statin therapy should be used as an adjunct to diet, exercise and smoking cessation in the study of primary prevention for those over age 50 years with diabetes, low HDL cholesterol, elevated hs-CRP or multiple risk factors.
- On the basis of high-quality, randomized, clinical trial data, when prescribing statin therapy, physicians should maximize the intensity of treatment and focus on compliance and long-term adherence.
- On the basis of high-quality, randomized, clinical trial data, use of non-statin-lowering agents for monotherapy or in combination with statins should be limited awaiting evidence that such an approach further reduces cardiovascular event rates in specific patients.
- Guidelines based on trial evidence are simple, practical and consistent with evidence-based principles and should, therefore, result in broad clinical acceptance.

It should be emphasized that all five of these criteria underscore the importance of lifestyle habits and actions to lower the risk of CVD.

1.4   LIFESTYLE STRATEGIES FOR CARDIOVASCULAR HEALTH

Physical Activity—Physical activity is a powerful risk factor reducer for CVD. In fact, regular physical activity is more powerful than any other lifestyle risk factors in terms of its relationship to CVD. Some studies suggested it is more powerful than either cigarette smoking or hypertension. Unfortunately, fewer than half of adults in the United States meet the minimum recommendations for physical activity, and only 25% meet the recommended criteria from the Centers for Disease Control and Prevention (CDC) and the PAGA 2018 (11). Young people are even less likely to meet recommended standards, with fewer than 20% of adolescents performing the 60 minutes or more of daily physical activity recommended by the PAGA 2018 Scientific Report.

A sedentary lifestyle is a significant risk factor for CVD. Important data have emerged in the past decade linking sedentary lifestyle to increased risk of CVD. In fact, the risk of CHD in sedentary individuals is 150%–240% higher than in those individuals who achieve physical activity levels as recommended by the CDC (20). The PAGA 2018 Scientific Report recommends 150 minutes per week of moderate-intensity physical activity or 75 minutes of vigorous physical activity and muscle-strengthening activities at least 2 days per week.

It should be emphasized that even levels of physical activity significantly lower than these recommended by PAGA 2018 yield substantial benefits. As demonstrated in Figure 1.1, the greatest benefit with regard to reduction of risk of CHD comes to those individuals engaged in 150–300 minutes per week of moderate-intensity physical activity (11).

However, as depicted in Figure 1.1, there is no lower threshold for benefits. Even individuals who engage in only 30 minutes of regular physical activity every week significantly lower their risk of all-cause mortality by approximately 20%. The data for CVD risk are virtually identical to all-cause mortality. These data strongly suggest that even small increases in physical activity could result in significant decreases in CVD for a large portion of the American population. As indicated in this figure, approximately 75% of the maximum benefit comes from meeting the guidelines from the PAGA 2018. Additional benefits come for individuals who exceed this amount of physical activity, although the reduction in the risk curve flattens out considerably at the highest levels of physical activity. These data underscore the principle articulated by both the PAGA 2018 and multiple science-based documents for the AHA that "some is better than none" when it comes to physical activity.

Both the AHA and the CDC guidelines as well as PAGA 2018 emphasize that physical activity significantly lowers the risk of adult weight gain, helps control blood pressure and lowers the risk of hypertension, in the first place. In addition, physical activity lowers the risk of stroke and heart failure in a dose-dependent relationship.

The relationship between physical activity and lipids is modest, although regular physical activity has been repeatedly shown to increase HDL cholesterol and lower triglycerides. Regular physical activity has minimal effects on LDL cholesterol.

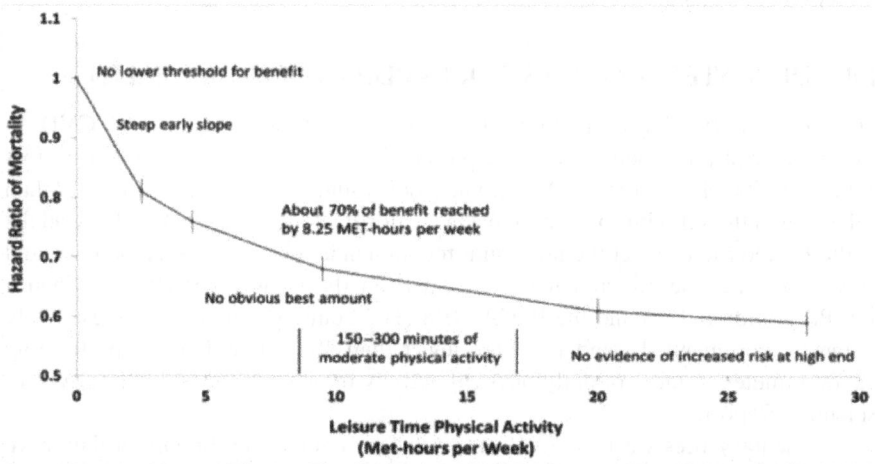

FIGURE 1.1 Relationships of moderate to vigorous physical activity to all-cause mortality, with highlighted characteristics common to studies of this type. (From the 2018 Physical Activity Guidelines Advisory Committee. 2018 Physical Activity Guidelines Advisory Committee Scientific Report. Washington, DC: U.S. Department of Health and Human Services; 2018.)

Despite the well-known benefits of physical activity, many physicians are not adequately encouraging their patients to exercise. Studies have demonstrated that less than 40% of physicians routinely recommend physical activity in patient encounters. This is a missed opportunity since over 70% of individuals see their primary care physician on at least a yearly basis. Of note, physicians who engage in regular physical activity in their own lives are more likely to counsel patients about this than those who do not.

Nutrition—Dietary factors also play an important role in multiple ways for lowering the risk of CVD and CHD. Multiple recommendations from the AHA and ACC as well as the Dietary Guidelines for Americans (DGA) 2020–2025 (14), all recommend various dietary interventions to lower the risk of CVD. These recommendations are similar and advocate diets that contain more fruits and vegetables, fish (particular oily fish), whole grains and fiber and maintenance of a caloric balance to prevent weight gain and the increased risk of obesity. All of these factors will lower the risk of CVD. These guidelines also invariably place nutrition in the context of other lifestyle factors such as regular physical activity and weight management.

The consensus documents on nutrition all now focus on overall diet patterns rather than individual foods in the diet. These dietary patterns all contain the previously referenced recommendations. In addition, nonfat dairy, seafood, legumes and nuts are included in all of the consensus statements. In addition, these guidelines recommend that those who consume alcohol (among adults) do so in moderation (no more than one alcoholic beverage/day for women and no more than two for men). All also recommend lower consumption of red and processed meats, refined grains, sugar-sweetened beverages and saturated and trans fats.

As the dietary guidelines have moved to a primary emphasis on overall dietary patterns, the following dietary patterns have been recommended to lower the risk of CVD:

- Healthy U.S.-Style Dietary Pattern (U.S. Department of Agriculture),
- Lowfat diet,
- Mediterranean diet,
- DASH (Dietary Approaches to Stop Hypertension) diet,
- Healthy vegetarian diet, and
- Healthy plant-based diet.

Recently there has been a marked increase in interest in publications concerning "plant-based" diets. These diets are defined, as the name suggests, as containing an emphasis on plants. All of the recommended diets listed earlier are, in essence, plant based and emphasize fruits, vegetables, legumes and nuts, and limit the amount of red meat, processed meat, sweets and oils.

There has been some question about what actually constitutes a "plant-based" diet. A recent publication drew a distinction between a "healthy" plant-based diet and an "unhealthy" plant-based diet. Within the healthy plant-based diet (hPBDI), emphasis was placed on whole grains, fruits, vegetables, nuts, legumes, tea and coffee. Less healthy plant foods (uPBDI) included juices/sweetened beverages, refined grains, potatoes/French fries, sweets and other animal foods that received adverse scores.

In an analysis of over 90,000 women in the U.S. Nurses' Health Study, those who scored high in the hPBDI category substantially lowered their CHD risk, whereas individuals who consumed more foods in the uPBDI experienced higher CHD risk (21). These issues are discussed in more detail in Chapter 5.

Weight Management/Obesity—Overweight and obesity are extremely prevalent in the United States and around the world. Recent data suggest that over 70% of individuals in the United States are either overweight (BMI >25 to <30 kg/m²) or obese (BMI >30 kg/m²) (22). Both overweight and obesity represent significant increased risk factors for CVD. The AHA lists obesity as a major risk factor for CVD not only because of its association with other risk factors (e.g., diabetes, dyslipidemias, elevated blood pressure, metabolic syndrome), but it also serves as an independent risk factor.

Distribution of body fat adds an additional risk since abdominal obesity is an independent risk factor for CHD. The theory for increased risk from central obesity is that the accumulation of abdominal fat preferentially promotes insulin resistance that can lead to glucose intolerance, elevated triglycerides, low HDL, as well as hypertension.

To combat overweight and obesity, the AHA, the ACC and The Obesity Society (TOS) issued guidelines in 2013 that included the five following recommendations (23):

- Use BMI as the first step in establishing criteria to judge potential health risks.
- Counsel patients that lifestyle changes can produce modest and sustained weight loss and achieve meaningful health benefits, while greater weight loss produces greater benefits.
- Multiple dietary therapy approaches for weight loss are acceptable for weight loss. However, diets should be prescribed to achieve reduced caloric intake.
- Overweight or obese patients should be enrolled in comprehensive lifestyle interventions for weight loss delivered in programs of 6 months or longer.
- Advice should be provided to patients who might be contemplating bariatric surgery (BMI ≥40 kg/m² or BMI ≥30 kg/m² with obesity-related comorbid conditions).

It is important to recognize that all five of these recommendations from the AHA/ACC/TOS carry a significant lifestyle component.

Smoking and tobacco products—Overwhelming evidence exists from multiple sources demonstrating that cigarette smoking significantly increases the risk of heart disease and stroke (24). This evidence is incorporated in virtually every risk factor reduction document from the AHA and other health organizations.

Cigarette smoking in men remains at approximately 18% and in women 14%. Thus, the overall percentage of cigarette smoking for adults over the age of 18 years is slightly more than 15%. Unfortunately, the rate of discontinuing cigarette smoking has slowed down in the past decade.

The good news is that substantial benefits accrue in terms of reduction of CVD in individuals who stop smoking. These benefits occur over a very brief period of time. Smokers lose at least one decade of life expectancy compared to never-smokers. Cessation of cigarette consumption overwhelmingly remains the single, most important intervention in preventive cardiology. Smokers who quit reduce their assessed risk of a coronary event by 50% within the first 2 years after cessation (25). Much of the benefit occurs in the first few months. CHD risk falls substantially within 1–2 years of cessation, and the risk of former smokers approaches that of never smoking after 3–5 years.

The U.S. Healthy People 2020 Initiative aimed to reduce the national problem of cigarette smoking among adults to a target of 12%. Unfortunately, the consumption of tobacco products is increasing globally. Almost 80% of the world's one billion smokers live in low- and middle-income countries. It should be noted that second-hand smoke also substantially increases the risk of CVD. These issues are discussed in more detail in Chapter 7.

Psychological factors and stress—Several different psychological factors may impact on the risk of CVD (25,26). Anxiety, with a prevalence of over 31%, is the most prevalent chronic psychological condition and increases the risk of CVD. Depression may also increase the risk of heart disease by making individuals less likely to adhere to programs to lower the risk of heart disease. Lifestyle factors can play a significant role in helping ameliorate psychological issues as well as reducing stress. (See also Chapter 8.)

Blood pressure—Elevated blood pressure represents a significant risk factor for CVD and is the leading risk factor for stroke. Using criteria from the Joint National Commission VII (JNC VII), a normal blood pressure was defined as <120 mm Hg systolic and <80 mm Hg diastolic, 120–139 mm Hg systolic and 80–89 mm Hg diastolic were defined as prehypertension, and >140 mm Hg systolic and >90 mm Hg diastolic were defined as hypertension (27). These are the criteria that were incorporated in the AHA Strategic Plan 2020.

In 2017, the ACC/AHA issued a new "Guideline for the Prevention, Detection, Evaluation and Management of High Blood Pressure in Adults." The guideline used a framework similar to the JNC VII guidelines. However, this guideline defined a normal blood pressure of systolic <120 mm Hg and diastolic <80 mm Hg. Elevated blood pressure was considered with systolic 120–129 mm Hg and diastolic <80 mm Hg. Stage one hypertension was defined as blood pressure of 130–139 mm Hg systolic or 80–89 mm Hg diastolic. Stage two hypertension was defined as blood pressure of >140 mm Hg systolic or >90 mm Hg diastolic.

These more stringent blood pressure criteria were based largely on the results of the Systolic Blood Pressure Intervention Trial (SPRINT). This study enrolled over 9,000 people at risk for CVD. It should be noted that the lower levels of blood pressure achieved in SPRINT often required utilization of three blood pressure medicines. It is difficult to imagine most people would be willing to take three antihypertensive medications. This highlights the importance of lifestyle modalities that can help lower blood pressure and act synergistically with pharmaceutical therapy.

In the 2013 AHA/ACC Lifestyle Management Guidelines for Blood Pressure Management (13), a number of lifestyle management recommendations were listed, including

- Consuming a diet high in vegetables, fruits and whole grains, low-fat dairy, poultry, fish, legumes and nontropical vegetable oils and nuts, and limiting sweets, sugar-sweetened beverages and red meat;

- Consuming no more than 2,300 milligrams of sodium per day; and
- Engaging in aerobic physical activity three to four sessions per week lasting an average of 40 minutes per session of moderate to vigorous intensity physical activity.

More information concerning the role of physical activity and diet in blood pressure control may be found in Chapters 4, 5 and 13.

Lipids—Dietary management of blood lipids, along with pharmaceutical therapy, has been a cornerstone of risk factor reduction for CVD and CHD for many years. In particular, reduction of LDL cholesterol has been demonstrated to significantly lower the risk of CHD. There is also strong evidence to demonstrate an inverse relationship between HDL cholesterol and vascular risk (2).

In general, observational data suggest that for every incremental increase in HDL cholesterol of 1 mg/dL there is a 2%–3% decrease in risk of total CVD. Pharmaceutical trials for HDL raising interventions have not only failed to find reductions in clinical events, but in some cases, they even suggested harm. However, regular physical activity has been routinely shown to raise HDL.

The issue of whether or not elevated triglycerides increase the risk of CVD has been somewhat controversial (2,9). Triglycerides tend to vary inversely with HDL. Recent genetic studies, however, have suggested that triglycerides may be a more significant risk factor for CVD than previously thought.

In the 2013 AHA/ACC Lifestyle Management Guidelines, proper nutrition is listed as an important component for managing LDL cholesterol. These guidelines, as already indicated for high blood pressure, also advocate a diet consisting of vegetables, fruits and whole grains, low-fat dairy products, poultry, fish, legumes, nontropical oils and nuts, and limited sweets, sugar-sweetened beverages and red meat as key dietary components for managing lipids.

Blood glucose, prediabetes and diabetes—Diabetes (type 2 diabetes mellitus [T2DM]) represents a significant risk factor for CHD (28). CHD is the leading cause of morbidity and mortality among individuals with diabetes. Over two-thirds of all individuals with T2DM will die of CHD. Lifestyle therapies are a cornerstone for treating diabetes, including proper nutrition, regular physical activity and weight management. Other lifestyle factors such as smoking cessation, counseling, psychosocial care and self-management education and support are also highly relevant. In addition, reducing the amount of sedentary time plays an important role in lowering the risk of diabetes. (More information on the linkage between T2DM and CVD may be found in Chapter 18.)

Metabolic syndrome—The metabolic syndrome is a clustering of metabolic abnormalities that significantly increases the risk of CVD. There are multiple different criteria for metabolic syndrome (28–30). However, the most commonly used are those found in the National Cholesterol Education Programs III and IV. Included in these criteria are the following:

- Blood pressure >130/85 mm Hg,
- Triglycerides >150 mg/dL,

- Blood glucose >100 mg/dL,
- Abdominal circumference >40 inches in men and >35 inches in women, and
- HDL <40 mg/dL.

According to National Cholesterol Education Program criteria, individuals who have at least three of these five factors are considered to have metabolic syndrome. It has been estimated that 36%–38% of the adult population in the United States have metabolic syndrome by these criteria. However, metabolic syndrome is poorly diagnosed by physicians, which is unfortunate since these individuals are at very high risk for CVD. The National Cholesterol Education Program, in fact, states that individuals who have metabolic syndrome should be treated as though they already have CVD. Therapeutic measures for treating metabolic syndrome involving lifestyle strategies are the same as for CVD, including regular physical activity, sound nutrition and weight management.

Brain health—Brain health should be considered as a key component of overall cardiovascular health. The issue of brain health has become increasingly important as the population in the United States and around the world continues to age. Many of the same strategies, in fact, employed to lower the risk of CVD are highly relevant to preserve and maintain brain health.

The AHA and the American Stroke Association (ASA) joined forces to issue a Presidential Advisory on "Optimal Brain Health" (31). This concept was designed to help physicians understand the importance of lifestyle measures that can contribute to optimizing brain health. These are the same issues that are utilized to optimize cardiovascular health.

The Optimal Brain Health Initiative utilized the seven metrics that are similar to those in the AHA Strategic Plan 2020 that have been called "life's simple seven." These metrics include nonsmoking, physical activity at goal levels, a healthy diet following current AHA guidelines, regular physical activity and a BMI of <25 kg/m^2. Ideal health measurements for untreated blood pressure, untreated cholesterol and fasting blood glucose are also included, which are identical to those listed in the AHA Strategic Plan 2020. (More information concerning CVD and optimal brain health may be found in Chapter 20.)

Inflammation—The understanding of the role of inflammation in cardiovascular risk has become increasingly prominent over the past two decades. Inflammation is involved in all phases of atherothrombosis and provides a critical link between plaque formation and acute rupture. The most well studied and clinically relevant marker of inflammation is the acute phase reactant CRP (hs-CRP). The AHA and CDC have recommended use of hs-CRP levels in clinical practices using the criteria of normal of <1, 1.3 moderate risk and higher than 3 mg/dL associated with higher relative vascular risk, when hs-CRP is considered along with traditional markers of risk (19). Many physicians now use hs-CRP and family history as components of global CVD risk prediction.

Aspirin as a primary prevention—Low-dose aspirin therapy clearly and consistently provides substantial net benefits for persons at high risk of subsequent events secondary to existing CVD. The major known liability of aspirin use is bleeding, and this should be considered when contemplating use of low-dose aspirin. Taken together, current data available show no clear benefit of low-dose aspirin in primary prevention of CVD in contrast to the established benefits/risk ratio in secondary prevention.

Direct plaque imaging—Direct vascular imaging of preclinical atherosclerosis is an alternative method to detect high-risk individuals who might benefit from early prevention. The best study data are derived from ultrasound measurements of the common carotid intima-media thickness (CIMT) test and computed tomography (CT) to detect coronary artery calcifications. These modalities have clear value in high-risk individuals. They have, however, engendered controversy in preventive practice. The difficulty with coronary calcification as a clinical biomarker is that calcification probably predicts the least likely plaques to rupture and does not detect noncalcified thin-capped lesions that are most likely to cause most clinical events. Newer modalities that are more effective in detecting plaque likely to rupture are currently under investigation.

Genetic markers for cardiovascular risk—Heritability accounts for up to one half of all susceptibility to CHD. However, genetic risk has been difficult to quantify in the past. Large-scale genome-wide association studies (GWASs) have the potential of making genetic modeling more applicable in the clinical practice of cardiovascular medicine and are currently under investigation. (More information concerning the linkages between genetics, epigenetics and CVD may be found in Chapter 23.)

1.5   BEHAVIORAL STRATEGIES AND ADHERENCE

Lifestyle factors that lower the risk of CVD require behavioral change. For this reason, it is important to adopt strategies to optimize changes in these behaviors. These are discussed in multiple subsequent chapters in this book (32).

1.6   REDUCTION OF CARDIOVASCULAR DISEASE IN CHILDREN AND ADOLESCENTS

An abundant literature supports that the roots of many CVDs and many other metabolic diseases are found in childhood (31–34). In fact, an emerging literature suggests that many of these conditions may, in fact, be found in utero. While this book does not focus on children and adolescents, there is a large body of information on such issues as physical activity and children, which can be found in the PAGA 2018. Nutritional guidance for children is also available in the Dietary Guidelines for Americans 2020–2025. Furthermore, there is a large section on various aspects of childhood health and CVD risk factor reduction found in the children's health section of Rippe's larger *Lifestyle Medicine* textbook or *Manual of Lifestyle Medicine*. (See also Chapter 22.)

1.7   PRACTICAL STRATEGIES FOR INCREASING LIFESTYLE MODALITIES IN CARDIOVASCULAR PRACTICE

We hope that healthcare providers who read this book will make an effort to reduce risk factors for CVD by counseling patients on the importance of daily habits and actions. A key way to start is simply to counsel patients that the impacts of their daily lives are profound with regard to the likelihood of developing CVD. Here are some specific suggestions for how to begin these conversations:

Physical activity—There is a wealth of information found in the Exercise is Medicine Initiative from the American College of Sports Medicine. This may be accessed by visiting their website www.exerciseismedicine.org/

Proper nutrition—Recommendations for proper nutrition are found throughout this manual and in a specific chapter on nutrition and cardiovascular health (Chapter 5). A discussion with individuals can be initiated simply by emphasizing the importance of a diet for cardiovascular health that includes increased amounts of fruits and vegetables, whole grains and fish (preferably oily fish), and proper caloric balance to prevent weight gain or help with weight loss, if that is needed.

Weight management—Less than 40% of physicians currently discuss weight with patients. A good place to start is to obtain a BMI on all patients and discuss the implications of this measurement with an emphasis on why it is important to maintain a healthy body weight for CVD risk factor reduction. The guidance from the AHA/ACC/TOS found in Chapter 6 will help frame this discussion.

Avoid tobacco products—Counseling people to avoid tobacco products or help with smoking cessation are key issues for multiple health considerations and should be discussed at every physician encounter. A discussion of avoiding secondhand smoke is also important.

(See also Chapter 7).

1.8   SUMMARY/CONCLUSIONS

An enormous literature supports the role of positive lifestyle measures in almost every metabolic disease. There are probably no stronger linkages between lifestyle habits and practices than those reducing the risk of CVD. Abundant evidence is available to show that regular physical activity, proper nutrition, weight management and avoidance of tobacco products all significantly lower the risk of CVD. Practical ways of discussing these factors are laid out in this chapter and are also discussed in subsequent chapters in such areas as counseling, physical activity, proper nutrition, weight management and smoking cessation.

Clinical Applications

- Utilize information and structures from this chapter to initiate conversations with every patient on ways that positive lifestyle factors can lower the risk for cardiovascular disease.
- Utilize materials from the Exercise is Medicine Initiative from the American College of Sports Medicine to frame a discussion on increased physical activity.

- Utilize documents from the American Heart Association or the Dietary Guidelines for Americans 2020–2025 to discuss components of a healthy diet. The specific diets to be discussed might include the DASH diet, Mediterranean diet or the Healthy U.S.-Style Dietary Pattern.
- Utilize materials available from the AHA/ACC/TOS to frame discussion of healthy weight management, particularly in individuals who are overweight or obese.

REFERENCES

1. Rippe JM. Lifestyle medicine: The health promoting power of daily habits and practices. Am J Lifestyle Med. 2018;12(6):499–512. Epub 2019/02/21.
2. Stone NJ, Robinson JG, Lichtenstein AH, et al. 2013 ACC/AHA guideline on the treatment of blood cholesterol to reduce atherosclerotic cardiovascular risk in adults: A report of the American College of Cardiology/American Heart Association Task Force on Practice Guidelines. Circulation. 2014;129(25 Suppl 2):S1–45. Epub 2013/11/14.
3. Lloyd-Jones DM, Hong Y, Labarthe D, et al. Defining and setting national goals for cardiovascular health promotion and disease reduction: The American Heart Association's strategic Impact Goal through 2020 and beyond. Circulation. 2010;121(4):586–613.
4. US Department of Health and Human Services; US Department of Agriculture. Dietary Guidelines for Americans, 2015–2020. 8th ed.; December 2015. http://health.Gov/dietaryguidelines/2015/guidelines/. Accessed December 8, 2021.
5. Mozaffarian D, Appel LJ, Van Horn L. Components of a cardioprotective diet: New insights. Circulation. 2011;123(24):2870–91. Epub 2011/06/22.
6. Estruch R, Ros E, Salas-Salvado J, et al. Primary prevention of cardiovascular disease with a Mediterranean diet. N Engl J Med. 2013;368(14):1279–90. Epub 2013/02/26.
7. Chiuve SE, McCullough ML, Sacks FM, et al. Healthy lifestyle factors in the primary prevention of coronary heart disease among men: Benefits among users and nonusers of lipid-lowering and antihypertensive medications. Circulation. 2006;114:160–7.
8. American Heart Association. Council on Lifestyle and Cardiometabolic Health. https://professional.heart.org/professional/MembershipCouncils/Scientific Councils/UCM_322856_Council-on-Lifestyle-and-Cardiometabolic-Health.jsp. Accessed December 8, 2021.
9. Eckel RH, Jakicic JM, Ard JD, et al. 2013 AHA/ACC guideline on lifestyle management to reduce cardiovascular risk. Circulation. 2014;129(25_suppl_2):S76–99.
10. American Heart Association Nutrition Committee, Lichtenstein AH, Appel LJ, et al. Diet and lifestyle recommendations revision 2006: A scientific statement from the American Heart Association Nutrition Committee. Circulation. 2006;114(1):82–96. Epub 2006/06/21.
11. Physical Activity Guidelines Advisory Committee. 2018 Physical Activity Guidelines Advisory Committee Scientific Report. Washington, DC: U.S. Department of Health and Human Services; 2018.
12. Ford ES, Ajani UA, Croft JB, et al. Explaining the decrease in U.S. deaths from coronary disease, 1980–2000. N Engl J Med. 2007;356(23):2388–98. Epub 2007/06/08.
13. Whelton PK, Carey RM, Aronow WS, et al. 2017 ACC/AHA/AAPA/ABC/ACPM/AGS/AphA/ASH/ASPC/NMA/PCNA guideline for the prevention, detection, evaluation, and management of high blood pressure in adults: A report of the American College of Cardiology/American Heart Association Task Force on clinical practice guidelines. J Am Coll Cardiol. 2018;71(19):e127–248. Epub 2017/11/18.

14. U.S. Department of Agriculture and U.S. Department of Health and Human Services. Dietary Guidelines for Americans, 2020–2025. 9th ed.; December 2020. DietaryGuidelines.gov. www.dietaryguidelines.gov/resources/2020-2025-dietary-guidelines-online-materials.

15. Rippe JM. Lifestyle Medicine. London: Blackwell Science, Inc.; 1999.

16. Rippe JM. Lifestyle Medicine. 3rd ed. Boca Raton, FL: CRC Press; 2019.

17. Angell SY, McConnell MV, Anderson CAM, et al. The American Heart Association 2030 impact goal: A presidential advisory from the American Heart Association. Circulation. 2020;141(9):e120–38. Epub 2020/01/30.

18. Hubert HB, Feinleib M, McNamara PM, et al. Obesity as an independent risk factor for cardiovascular disease: A 26-year follow-up of participants in the Framingham Heart Study. Circulation. 1983;67(5):968–77. Epub 1983/05/01.

19. Ridker PM, Libby P, Buring JE. Risk markers and the primary prevention of cardiovascular disease. In Zipes, Libby, Bonow, Mann, Tomaselli, eds. Braunwald's Heart Disease. 11th ed. Amsterdam: Elsevier; 2019. P. 876.

20. Writing Group Members, Mozaffarian D, Benjamin EJ, et al. Heart disease and stroke statistics—2016 update: A report from the American Heart Association. Circulation. 2016;133(4):e38–60. Epub 2015/12/18.

21. Satija A, Bhupathiraju SN, Spiegelman D, et al. Healthful and unhealthful plant-based diets and the risk of coronary heart disease in U.S. adults. J Am Coll Cardiol. 2017;70(4):411–22. Epub 2017/07/22.

22. National Center for Health Statistics. Health, United States, 2016: With Chartbook on Long-Term Trends in Health. Hyattsville (MD): National Center for Health Statistics; 2017 May. Report No.: 2017–1232. PMID: 28910066.

23. Jensen MD, Ryan DH, Apovian CM, et al. 2013 AHA/ACC/TOS guideline for the management of overweight and obesity in adults: A report of the American College of Cardiology/American Heart Association Task Force on Practice Guidelines and The Obesity Society. J Am Coll Cardiol. 2014;63(25 Pt B):2985–3023. Epub 2013/11/19.

24. U.S. Centers for Disease Control and Prevention. The Health Consequences of Smoking: A Report of the Surgeon General. Atlanta, GA: U.S. Department of Health and Human Services, Centers for Disease Control and Prevention, National Center for Chronic Disease Prevention and Health Promotion, Office on Smoking and Health; 2004.

25. Jha P, Ramasundarahettige C, Landsman V, et al. 21st-century hazards of smoking and benefits of cessation in the United States. N Engl J Med. 2013;368(4):341–50. Epub 2013/01/25.

26. Mittleman MA, Mostofsky E. Physical, psychological and chemical triggers of acute cardiovascular events: preventive strategies. Circulation. 2011;124(3):346–54. Epub 2011/07/20.

27. Chobanian AV, Bakris GL, Black HR, et al. The seventh report of the Joint National Committee on Prevention, Detection, Evaluation, and Treatment of High Blood Pressure: The JNC 7 report. JAMA. 2003;289(19):2560–72. Epub 2003/05/16.

28. American Diabetes Association. 9. Cardiovascular disease and risk management. Diabetes Care. 2017;40(Suppl 1):S75–87. Epub 2016/12/17.

29. Grundy SM, Cleeman JI, Daniels SR, et al. Diagnosis and management of the metabolic syndrome: An American Heart Association/National Heart, Lung, and Blood Institute scientific statement. Curr Opin Cardiol. 2006;21(1):1–6. Epub 2005/12/16.

30. Ford ES, Giles WH, Dietz WH. Prevalence of the metabolic syndrome among U.S. adults: Findings from the third National Health and Nutrition Examination Survey. JAMA. 2002;287(3):356–9. Epub 2002/01/16.

31. Gorelick PB, Furie KL, Iadecola C, et al. Defining optimal brain health in adults: A presidential advisory from the American Heart Association/American Stroke Association. Stroke. 2017;48(10):e284–e303. Epub 2017/09/09.

32. Linke SE, Robinson CJ, Pekmezi D. Applying psychological theories to promote healthy lifestyles. Am J Lifestyle Med. 2013;8(1):4–14.

33. Kavey RE, Daniels SR, Lauer RM, et al. American Heart Association guidelines for primary prevention of atherosclerotic cardiovascular disease beginning in childhood. J Pediatr. 2003;142(4):368–72. Epub 2003/04/25.

34. Kavey RE, Allada V, Daniels SR, et al. Cardiovascular risk reduction in high-risk pediatric patients: A scientific statement from the American Heart Association Expert Panel on Population and Prevention Science; the Councils on Cardiovascular Disease in the Young, Epidemiology and Prevention, Nutrition, Physical Activity and Metabolism, High Blood Pressure Research, Cardiovascular Nursing, and the Kidney in Heart Disease; and the Interdisciplinary Working Group on Quality of Care and Outcomes Research. J Cardiovasc Nurs. 2007;22(3):218–53. Epub 2007/06/05.

2 Epidemiology of Cardiovascular Disease

KEY POINTS

- Cardiovascular disease (CVD) is a worldwide pandemic.
- While some decreases in CVD have occurred in high-income countries, the prevalence of CVD in low- and middle-income countries has risen from 26% to 32% of deaths.
- Lifestyle strategies such as increased physical activity, reduction of smoking and exposure to tobacco products, control of overweight and obesity and improved diet (e.g., more fruits and vegetables), and lower salt and saturated fat all can play important roles in lowering the global burden of CVD.
- The World Health Organization has listed reduction of cardiovascular disease and its risk factors as key components of its global initiative to combat noncommunicable diseases.

2.1 INTRODUCTION

Cardiovascular disease (CVD) is the leading cause of death worldwide. CVD also is the leading cause of noncommunicable diseases (NCDs), which is the major reason for the World Health Organization (WHO) initiative to combat NCDs around the world (1). It should be noted that a large percentage of NCDs in general, and CVDs specifically, are preventable through the reduction of behavior of four main behavioral risk factors, namely, tobacco use, physical inactivity, harmful use of alcohol, and unhealthy diet. Thus, lifestyle measures play a critically important role in both the prevention and treatment of CVD worldwide.

In 2013, CVD caused an estimated 17.3 million deaths worldwide. This represents approximately 32% of all deaths (2). It is important to understand that while CVD was a major concern in high-income countries (HICs) in the past century, it is now more prevalent in low- and middle-income countries (LMICs) and is accelerating at an alarming rate.

Between 1990 and 2013, deaths from CVD increased from 26% to 32% of all deaths globally (3). This has been attributed to a rapid epidemiologic transition, particularly in LMICs (4). At the same time that deaths from CVD have increased in LMICs, there has been a decline in CVD deaths in HICs. The burden of CVD varies dramatically among various areas in the world. For example, CVD deaths are as high as 59% in Eastern Europe and as low as 12% in sub-Saharan South Africa. In the United States, CVD mortality is 37%.

With all this as background, it is important to understand that CVD is a worldwide pandemic. Importantly, lifestyle medicine interventions can play a critically

DOI: 10.1201/b23245-3

important role in lowering the risk of CVD and serving as an important component of its treatment where it is already present.

2.2   EPIDEMIOLOGIC TRANSITIONS

It has been argued that the overall increase in the global burden of CVD is a result of an "epidemiologic transition" (4). This framework is based on four basic epidemiologic stages: pestilence and famine, receding pandemics, degenerative and manmade diseases, and delayed degenerative diseases. Each of these epidemiologic stages has its own set of defining characteristics. For example, the stage of pestilence and famine is largely based on epidemics of infectious disease and hunger that were the main causes of mortality before 1900.

The next phase, receding pandemics, resulted from the emergence of public health systems, which resulted in lower death rates from infectious disease and malnutrition. In this stage, CVD accounted for 10%–35% of deaths. In the stage of degenerative and manmade diseases, continued economic improvements around the world resulted in a dramatic increase in life expectancy to almost 70 years. "Delayed degenerative diseases," the final of the four stages, was characterized by CVD and cancer as the major causes of morbidity and mortality. However, age-adjusted declines were found in both occurrences.

Within the framework of epidemiologic transitions, it has been hypothesized that we may now be entering a fifth epidemiologic transition, called the "age of inactivity and obesity" (5). This phase is characterized by worldwide decreases in physical activity and increases in caloric intake that, in combination, contribute to an epidemic of overweight and obesity and increased rates of type 2 diabetes mellitus (T2DM), hypertension, and lipid abnormalities. All of these factors contribute to the increased likelihood of developing CVD, and the increased aging of populations around the world contributes to make individuals more susceptible to CVD and its risk factors.

These underlying conditions stimulated the rise in all NCDs, but principally CVD, although increases have occurred also in diabetes (T2DM), cancers, and chronic respiratory diseases. It should be noted that while in previous epidemiologic transitions, lifestyle-related increases in CVD and T2DM occurred largely in HICs, now over 80% of cardiovascular and diabetes deaths and almost 90% of from chronic obstructive pulmonary disease occur in LMICs. As emphasized by the WHO initiative to combat NCDs, a large percentage of NCDs are preventable through reduction of lifestyle factors such as tobacco use, physical inactivity, harmful use of alcohol and an unhealthy diet.

2.3   VARIATIONS IN THE GLOBAL BURDEN
OF CARDIOVASCULAR DISEASE

A number of different factors impact the burden of CVD. First, population growth increases the number of deaths caused from CVD globally. Second, aging of the population increases the portion of death caused by CVD in many regions as does better control of communicable diseases. These factors have resulted in age-adjusted death rates from CVD decreasing by almost 22%. This reduction has been less prominent in LMICs where 85% of the world's population lives.

Income also tends to create variations in the global risk of CVD. Higher income regions had a nearly 37% rate of age-adjusted declines in CVD, while slight increases occurred in LMICs. Furthermore, CVD mortality rates declined among those in lower socioeconomic status regardless of the country that they resided in. A large percentage of NCDs in general, and CVD in particular, is preventable through modifiable risk factors such as tobacco use, physical inactivity and poor nutritional habits (diets high in fat and salt).

Hypertension and dyslipidemia are the leading causes of coronary heart disease (CHD) (6). Use of tobacco, obesity and physical inactivity are also significant risk factors. It has been estimated that high blood pressure is a factor in 54% of CVD worldwide, high cholesterol 32%, overweight and obesity 18%, poor dietary habits 67%, and smoking 18%. These factors add up to over 100% since many contribute to similar disease mechanisms.

2.4 RISK FACTORS

2.4.1 Tobacco

Almost 6 million people die from tobacco use each year—both from direct tobacco use and secondhand smoke (1). Tobacco use accounts for 10% of all deaths. According to the WHO, smoking is estimated to cause 71% of lung cancer, 42% of chronic respiratory disease and approximately 10% of CVD. More than 80% of tobacco use occurs in LMICs. If current trends continue unabated, tobacco will cause more than one billion deaths during the 21st century.

China is the largest consumer of tobacco in the world with an estimated 301 million smokers in 2010 (greater than 50% prevalence in men). Smoking rates have increased in China by 50% since 1980 (7). The rate of cigarette smoking is high in Russia, where approximately 60% of men and 25% of women smoke cigarettes. While more men than women smoke worldwide, women have a high smoking prevalence in some countries. Of note, in China, tobacco use prevalence is over 50% in men and only 2.2% in women.

Secondhand smoke also contributes to CHD risk. In 2011, approximately 600,000 nonsmokers died as a consequence of exposure to secondhand smoke.

2.4.2 Insufficient Physical Activity

According to the WHO, approximately 3.2 million individuals die each year due to physical inactivity (1). People who are insufficiently physically active have a 20%–30% increased risk of all-cause mortality. Regular physical activity has been clearly shown to reduce the risk of CVD and its risk factors such as high blood pressure, diabetes and, to some extent, dyslipidemia. Insufficient physical activity is highest in HICs, but high levels of inactivity are now increasingly seen in LMICs.

2.4.3 OVERWEIGHT AND OBESITY

According to the WHO, at least 2.8 million people die each year as a result of being overweight or obese (1). Increased body mass index (BMI) elevates risk of CVD, stroke and diabetes. The prevalence of overweight is highest in middle-income countries, but very high levels are also reported in some lower income countries.

According to the most recent Global Burden of Disease (GBD) study, there are over 1.4 billion adults in the world who are overweight, and of these, approximately 500 million are obese (8). Note that while obesity is highest in HICs, overweight and obesity are increasing faster in LMICs. The mean BMI in the United States is 28.5 kg/m^2 in men and 28.3 kg/m^2 in women. Obesity is recognized as an independent risk factor for CVD as well as a substantial contributor to other risk factors such as hypertension, diabetes and dyslipidemia.

2.4.4 UNHEALTHY DIET

Inadequate consumption of fruits and vegetables increases the risk of CVD and multiple cancers. In addition, most populations around the world consume much higher levels of salt than recommended by WHO for disease prevention. High salt consumption is an important risk factor for high blood pressure and CVD risk. High consumption of saturated fats, trans fats and fatty acids is also linked to increased risk of CVD.

Between 1970 and 2010, the average daily caloric intake in the United States increased from 2,076 to 2,534 calories (9). Worldwide, as per capita income increases, so does consumption of fat and simple carbohydrates, while consumption of plant-based foods decreases. China, again, provides a good example of how changes in nutrition are linked to socioeconomic changes. Between 1982 and 2002, calories from fat in China increased from 25% to 35% in urban areas and from 14% to 28% in rural areas (10). From 1992 to 2002 in China, the number of overweight adults increased by 41%, and the number of obese adults increased by 97%. Diets that are high in trans fats are particularly dangerous in terms of risk of CVD because trans fats both elevate LDL and reduce HDL.

2.4.5 HYPERTENSION

The GBD project estimates that 19% of deaths and 9% of all days lost globally result from elevated levels of blood pressure. Worldwide, approximately 62% of strokes and 49% of CHD are attributable to elevated systolic blood pressure (11). Age-standardized prevalence of uncontrolled high blood pressure has decreased from 33% to 29% in men and 25% to 20% in women. However, the number of people with uncontrolled hypertension defined as a systolic blood pressure (BP) ≥140 mm Hg increased to 605 million between 1980 and 2008. Multiple components of lifestyle contribute to elevated blood pressure including inactivity, cigarette smoking, a diet high in salt and saturated fat and overweight or obesity. Clearly, lifestyle measures play an important role in controlling blood pressure.

2.4.6 LIPIDS

Elevated cholesterol accounts for 56% of CHD and 18% of stroke worldwide. This risk factor accounts for over 4 million deaths annually (12). Unfortunately, cholesterol data are not available in many countries. Hence, these numbers may underestimate the amount or the degree of elevated cholesterol. Lifestyle measures such as diet high in fruits and vegetables and low in saturated fat and sodium as well as weight control, decreased cigarette smoking and increased physical activity all can assist in lowering the prevalence of dyslipidemia (see also Chapter 12).

2.4.7 DIABETES

Diabetes prevalence has grown rapidly worldwide in the last 30 years at the same time that overweight and obesity have increased. It is now estimated that over 340 million people worldwide have diabetes, and almost 50% are undiagnosed (13). The risk factors for diabetes are well known—most prevalently overweight and obesity. Lifestyle measures such as increased physical activity, weight loss, if necessary, cessation of cigarette smoking and a diet high in fruits and vegetables and low in saturated fat and salt are all known to lower the risk of diabetes. Thus, lifestyle plays a critically important role in lowering the risk of diabetes. (See also Chapter 18.)

2.4.8 AGING POPULATION

CVD is clearly associated with increased age. The average life expectancy in HICs is anticipated to reach 83 years old by 2025, and in LMIC regions the population over age 60 years will more than double from 1995 to 2025 (14). Because of the increased risk of CVD in individuals related to older age, it is particularly important for lifestyle measures to continue to be practiced for the population over the age of 65 years.

2.4.9 ENVIRONMENTAL EXPOSURE

Air pollution from a variety of sources has been clearly shown to increase mortality and morbidity from CVD (15). The increased risk of disability-adjusted life years (DALYs) from pollution shows that more than 30% of DALYs are lost because of pollution. This is approximately the same as the percentage attributable to tobacco smoking, which is a key component of environmental pollution. Air pollution is a prominent risk factor leading to approximately 7 million premature deaths annually. The majority of environmentally related premature deaths occur in LMICs, particularly in India and China.

For physicians, the message is to counsel individuals on how to avoid exposure and protect themselves from toxic environmental exposures.

2.5 LIFESTYLE MEDICINE–BASED INTERVENTIONS

Public policy interventions have reduced smoking rates and lowered BP levels as well as improved lipid profiles. Other lifestyle-related therapies such as reducing salt and cholesterol in the diet have been shown to be a cost-effective strategy to reduce stroke and myocardial infarction (MI) in HICs.

2.5.1 TOBACCO USE

Tobacco control involves strategies to reduce the supply and/or demand for tobacco. A leader in this area has been the WHO. The WHO led the creation of a global treaty against tobacco use with its Framework Convention on Tobacco Control (FCTC), which has now been ratified by 168 countries (1). This has stimulated efforts for tobacco control around the world. It has been estimated that from one component of this initiative, namely an increase in price, a reduction of between 18.9 and 56.8 million deaths in the developed world could result (16,17). In addition, nicotine replacement therapy (NRT) reduces the number of deaths to between 2.9 and 14.3 million. It is particularly important to emphasize smoking cessation for patients who have had a coronary event. One study showed that there was a 40% relative risk reduction following MI if smoking cessation occurred.

2.5.2 SALT AND LIPID REDUCTIONS

Interventions involving public education emphasize reducing saturated fat and salt in the diet and have been shown to reduce both CVD events and DALYs (18). Other cost-effective measures include increased use of statins and routine prescription of aspirin for individuals who have experienced cardiac events. The WHO has emphasized that the following public health measures would have a significant impact on NCDs in general and CVD in particular (1). WHO recommends the following:

- Protecting people from tobacco smoking and banning smoking in public places;
- Warning about the dangers of tobacco use;
- Initiating bans on tobacco advertising, promotion and sponsorship;
- Raising taxes on tobacco;
- Reducing salt intake and salt content in food;
- Replacing trans fat in food with polyunsaturated fat; and
- Promoting public awareness about diet and physical activity through mass media.

Clearly, these recommendations hinge on multiple lifestyle changes and thus, once again, emphasizing the important role of establishing strategies around the world to reduce the burden of CVD.

2.6 SUMMARY/CONCLUSIONS

CVD remains a significant global problem. This is true both of HICs and LMICs. Key factors for reducing the burden of CVD involve reducing exposure to tobacco products, improving diet (e.g., consuming more fruits and vegetables, less saturated fat and salt), increasing physical activity, and developing strategies to reduce overweight and obesity. These low-cost, preventive, and therapeutic strategies were emphasized throughout the WHO initiative to reduce the burden of CVDs.

Clinical Applications

- Lifestyle strategies such as lowering tobacco use and adopting lifestyle-related strategies to lower hypertension and diabetes are all highly relevant to lower the impact of CVD around the world.
- Lifestyle factors play a crucial role in the WHO initiative to combat communicable diseases around the world.

REFERENCES

1. World Health Organization. Global Action Plan for the Prevention and Control of Noncommunicable Diseases 2013–2020. 9789241506236_eng.pdf;jsessionid=E847CC 4CC8D8891ECA6D68C1ABFE6D1A (who.int). Accessed December 3, 2021.
2. The Global Burden of Disease; 2013. http://ghdx.healthdata.org/gbd-data-tool. Accessed December 3, 2021.
3. Omran AR. The epidemiologic transition: A theory of the epidemiology of population changes. Milbank Q. 1971;49(4):509–38, 5155251.
4. Olshansky SJ, Ault AB. The fourth stage of the epidemiologic transition: The age of delayed degenerative diseases. Milbank Q. 1986;64(3):355–91, 3762504.
5. Gaziano JM. Fifth phase of the epidemiologic transition: The age of obesity and inactivity. JAMA. 2010;303(3):275–6. Epub 2010/01/15.
6. Institute for Health Metrics and Evaluation (IHME): GBD Compare. 2020 IHME, University of Washington Seattle. Accessed December 3, 2021.
7. Eriksen MP, Mackay J, Schluger N. The Tobacco Atlas. 5th ed. Atlanta: American Cancer Society; 2015.
8. Finucane MM, Stevens GA, Cowan MJ, et al. National, regional, and global trends in body-mass index since 1980: Systematic analysis of health examination surveys and epidemiological studies with 960 country-years and 9.1 million participants. Lancet. 2011;377(9765):557–67. Epub 2011/02/08.
9. U.S. Department of Agriculture (USDA). Nutrient Content of the U.S. Food Supply: Developments between 2000 and 2006. 2011, USDA Washington, DC cover (azureedge.net). Accessed December 3, 2021.
10. China Health and Nutrition Survey (CHNS). www.cpc.unc.edu/projects/china. Accessed December 3, 2021.
11. Ogden CL, Carroll MD, Kit BK, et al. Prevalence of obesity and trends in body mass index among US children and adolescents, 1999–2010. JAMA. 2012;307(5):483. Epub 2012/01/19.
12. O'Flaherty M, Flores-Mateo G, Nnoaham K, et al. Potential cardiovascular mortality reductions with stricter food policies in the United Kingdom of Great Britain and Northern Ireland. Bull World Health Organ. 2012;90(7):522–31. Epub 2012/07/19.
13. Danaei G, Finucane MM, Lu Y, et al. National, regional, and global trends in fasting plasma glucose and diabetes prevalence since 1980: Systematic analysis of health examination surveys and epidemiological studies with 370 country-years and 2.7 million participants. Lancet. 2011;378(9785):31–40. Epub 2011/06/28.
14. United Nations Department of Economic and Social Affairs, Population Division. World Population Ageing 2013. ST/ESA/SER.A/348 World Population Ageing 2013 | Population Division (un.org). Accessed December 3, 2021.

15. Landrigan PJ, Sly JL, Ruchirawat M, et al. Health consequences of environmental exposures: Changing global patterns of exposure and disease. Ann Glob Health. 2016;82(1):10–19. Epub 2016/06/22.
16. Jha, CF, Moore J, et al. Tobacco Addiction: Disease Control Priorities in the Developing Countries. 2nd ed. New York: Oxford University Press; 2006.
17. Beaglehole R, Bonita R, Horton R, Adams C, Alleyne G, Asaria P, et al. Priority actions for the non-communicable disease crisis. Lancet. 2011;377(9775):1438–47. Epub 2011/04/09.
18. Bibbins-Domingo K, Chertow GM, Coxson PG, et al. Projected effect of dietary salt reductions on future cardiovascular disease. N Engl J Med. 2010;362(7):590–9. Epub 2010/01/22.

3 Lifestyle Medicine– Focused History and Physical Examination for Cardiovascular Disease

KEY POINTS

- There is no longer any serious doubt that what individuals do in their daily lives has profound implications for short- and long-term health and quality of life.
- An excellent place for physicians to start focusing their patients' attention on the power of lifestyle modalities is in a lifestyle medicine–focused history and physical examination for cardiovascular disease.
- Such lifestyle medicine modalities including proper nutrition, regular physical activity, weight management, stress management and healthful sleep can all be emphasized in a lifestyle medicine–focused history and physical examination and bring added value to the patient's experience and to the physician/patient interaction.

3.1 INTRODUCTION

Issues related to the interaction between daily habits and actions and their impact on short- and long-term health and quality of life are profoundly important for the prevention and treatment of many chronic diseases, perhaps none more so than cardiovascular disease (CVD) (1). Typical teachings related to history and physical examination are woefully inaccurate when they do not include significant components of the major impacts of lifestyle habits and actions on the risk of developing chronic disease in general and heart disease in particular.

A number of studies have shown, for example, that less than 40% of physicians consult patients on physical activity, weight, nutrition, or tobacco cessation (2). By not providing background and information in these areas, physicians are sending the subtle message that we do not care about them, and their patients should not care either. The purpose of the current chapter is to provide a framework for how lifestyle medicine factors should play an important role in every patient encounter, particularly in those encounters where CVD is suspected or the individual has significant risk factors for heart disease. It is hoped that this framework will encourage physicians to modify history and physical examination to be more focused on the important linkages between lifestyle factors and cardiovascular disease (CVD).

DOI: 10.1201/b23245-4

3.2 LIFESTYLE MEDICINE–FOCUSED HISTORY

A patient's history has long been understood to be critical to help narrow the fields of inquiry and also move toward accurate diagnoses. This is particularly true of lifestyle medicine issues that are often neglected in history taking. We propose that these lifestyle medicine issues should be integrated, along with standard aspects of the typical medical history, in order to gain a full understanding of the patient's current situation and their risk of chronic disease. We start with recommended aspects of the history related to six of the major pillars of lifestyle medicine. We then integrate these historical aspects related to lifestyle medicine with standard aspects of the typical medical history taken in a physician's office.

3.2.1 NUTRITION

Nutrition and alcohol consumption are factors in seven of the ten leading causes of death in the United States and worldwide. Data are now available from the American Heart Association (AHA) (3), the Dietary Guidelines for Americans 2020–2025 (DGA) (4), and numerous other organizations to guide people into healthier aspects of daily nutrition. A good way to get started might be to utilize recommended questions based on information from the AHA in their 2020 Strategic Plan (5). There are questions related to the recommendations from the AHA Plan which are consistent with the DASH (Dietary Approaches to Stop Hypertension) eating plan (6).

Here are some sample questions:

- How many fruits and vegetables do you eat on a daily basis?
  The AHA recommends ≥ 4.5 cups per day.

- How often do you eat fish meals (preferably oily fish)?
  The AHA recommends two 3.5-ounce servings per week.

- How often do you eat fiber-rich whole grains? (≥1.1 gram of fiber per 10 grams of carbohydrate).
  The AHA recommends ≥3-ounce equivalent servings per day.

- Do you take steps to reduce the amount of sodium (salt) in your diet?
  The AHA recommends less than 1,500 mg per day, although in some instances, they have recommended less than 2,300 mg per day. The current amount of sodium in the diet is 3.4 grams per day in the United States.

- How often do you consume sugar-sweetened beverages?
  The AHA recommends ≤450 kcals (36 ounces) per week. This would compute to three 12-ounce cans of sugar-sweetened soft drinks.

Of course, the AHA recognizes that nutrition is much more complicated than these simple recommendations, but this would represent a good place to start. More detail about various eating plans for lowering the risk of heart disease can be found in Chapter 5.

3.2.2 Physical Activity

A good and simple way to start the dialogue about physical activity would be to use the two-question questionnaire developed at Stanford University. You could simply ask your patient, "How often do you engage in regular physical activity on a weekly basis?" And second, "How much time do you spend each time you engage in physical activity?"

Of course, the benefits of regular physical activity are enormous. These two questions can simply lead into a broader discussion of physical activity and its multiple health benefits in general and particularly for CVD. Further information on this can be found in Chapter 4.

3.2.3 Weight

A discussion of weight might begin with "Has your weight been stable over the past 5 years?" "Have you increased your weight from over the past 20 years?" Both current weight and potential weight gain during adult years are related to cardiovascular risk. More detail in this can be found in Chapter 6.

3.2.4 Stress

"How much stress do experience in your daily life at work or at home?" Details of the relationship between stress and CVD are found in Chapter 8.

3.2.5 Sleep

"How well do you sleep?" "How often do you get at least 7 hours of sleep per night?" The patient's partner should be questioned about any signs of sleep disorder, breathing such as loud snoring or periods of apnea.

The relationship between sleep and both cardiovascular and brain health can be found in Chapter 9.

3.2.6 Emotional Well-Being

"How would you rate your emotional well-being?"

Information related to this can be found in Chapter 8. The AHA Strategic Plan 2030 elicits well-being as one of the key components of cardiovascular health.

- "Do you currently smoke or have you ever smoked cigarettes or any other form of tobacco?" Issues related to smoking cessation are discussed in detail in Chapter 7.
- "Do you consume alcohol?" "How much do you consume on a daily or weekly basis?" Levels of alcoholic consumption (up to two alcoholic drinks per day for men and no more than one alcoholic drink per day for women may improve cardiovascular health. Higher amounts might lead to cardiovascular abnormalities as well as other adverse health consequences.

3.2.7 OTHER POTENTIAL QUESTIONS

Patients may also describe their awareness of heartbeats (palpitations) using such language as "flutters," "skips" or "pounding." A history of cardiac arrhythmia is mostly appropriate with the known history of cardiac disease. An additional question might be to ask the individual if they have ever passed out suddenly with full consciousness thereafter. These may be symptoms of cardiac or noncardiac syncope. Additional questions should involve seeking information about traditional cardiovascular risk factors (e.g., blood pressure, lipids, diabetes, etc.; occupational habits; social habits; medications; drug allergies or intolerance; a family history or review of symptoms).

In addition to the lifestyle-related questions, if the individual has a high level of risk or currently is known to have CVD, then questions related to CVD are highly appropriate. Symptoms of angina included exertional shortness of breath or chest discomfort. Classic angina includes three characteristics: exertional chest discomfort initiated by exertion or stress or relieved with sublingual nitroglycerin (See also Chapters 15 and 16.)

3.3 PHYSICAL EXAM

In addition to the standard components of a physical exam that every physician learns in medical school, there are some areas that should be emphasized on physical exam in the area of lifestyle medicine. These are addressed in the sections that follow.

3.3.1 VITAL SIGNS

We recommend that in addition to weight, height should be measured and body mass index (BMI) computed. In addition, waist circumference provides useful information about body fat distribution. It is well known that increased central body fat represents an additional risk factor for CVD.

3.3.2 BLOOD PRESSURE

A very careful approach to blood pressure measure is an important component of lifestyle-related cardiovascular exam. Recommendations from the recently released AHA/American College of Cardiology (ACC) criteria for the evaluation of blood pressure (7) included the following recommendations.

The patient should be seated comfortably with back supported and legs uncrossed. The upper arm should be at the heart level. Cuff length and width should be 80% and 40% of the arm circumference, respectively. Cuff should be deflated slowly. The first audible Korotkoff sound represents systolic pressure and the last sound diastolic pressure. There should be no talking between the subject and the observer or other person. The risk of CVD doubles for every 20 mm Hg above 115 mm Hg and diastolic blood pressure >75 mm Hg. It is important that these readings be accurate (8).

The cardiovascular exam is important and should include palpation of the apical impulse that should be located at the midclavicular line of the fifth intercostal space.

In addition to the first and second heart sounds, both diastolic and systolic murmurs should be auscultated. Diastolic murmurs invariably signify cardiac disease. They include aortic regurgitation and mitral stenosis. Systolic murmurs are classified as early systolic, midsystolic or late-systolic peaking. The timing and intensity of systolic murmurs may signify the likelihood of diseases. For example, early systolic murmurs often indicate acute chronic mitral regurgitation or mitral regurgitation. Midsystolic murmurs often indicate aortic stenosis or pulmonic stenosis, whereas late-systolic more frequently indicate mitral or tricuspid valve prolapse. Additional information concerning murmurs may be obtained by ordering an echocardiogram if a murmur is appreciated on physical examination.

It is important to also evaluate the extremities for pulses and any orthopedic problems that might interfere with regular physical activity.

3.4 LABORATORY TESTS

Sequential multiple analysis 12 (SMA-12) and complete blood count (CBC) should be obtained on all patients. In addition, for patients in whom cardiovascular disease is expected or simply as a baseline, an electrocardiogram should be obtained. Additional lab tests might include hemoglobin A_{1c} if there is a history of glucose intolerance or diabetes.

3.5 SPECIALIZED TESTS

Certain specialized tests may be appropriate to pursue aspects of lifestyle medicine that may impact CVD risk. For example, the following tests may be appropriate in patients:

   3-day food records—This test would be administered by a nutritionist and allows for a detailed analysis of current nutritional habits. This would be particularly appropriate for an individual who wants to make improvements in their nutritional patterns.

   Exercise Tolerance Test—An exercise tolerance test is appropriate for an individual who has been quite sedentary or in whom the prescription for moderate-intensity physical activity (such as walking) is contemplated if the individual has not been involved in any significant level of physical activity.

   Dual-Energy X-ray Absorptiometry (DEXA) Screening—If you are fortunate to have a DEXA machine, this is a highly accurate test to determine the amount of body fat and lean muscle mass. This takes the issue of weight management a step beyond normal screening of weight, BMI and waist circumference. DEXA screening is particularly important for an individual who is contemplating weight loss, particularly if they are going to accompany it (as should be recommended) with regular physical activity. Regular physical activity should help the individual preserve lean muscle while losing body fat, which is, of course, what the overfat person should be doing.

Sleep Study—If a history of excessive snoring or periods of apnea are noted by the patient's partner, it would be appropriate to obtain a sleep study to rule out sleep apnea. Sleep apnea is associated with increased risk of hypertension and cardiovascular disease. (See also Chapter 9.)

Further cardiovascular testing such as a thallium exercise tolerance test or echocardiogram may provide additional information, particularly in individuals who have obesity.

3.6 COUNSELING AND THERAPY

A mainstay of counseling for CVD risk reduction should be the use of motivational interviewing. Motivational interviewing has been an important component of behavior change counseling for many decades. This type of counseling puts the patient at the center of the discussion and explores reasons that may serve as impediments to change from the patient's point of view. There are excellent resources to provide background on motivational interviewing. The reader is referred to these references if further information is sought on this technique.

3.6.1 NUTRITION

Physicians who feel comfortable in providing nutritional counseling may utilize a wide variety of sources. Information is available from the AHA, DGA 2020–2025 and the Academy of Nutrition and Dietetics. For those physicians who wish to make a referral to a nutritionist to assist in nutritional counseling, there are a number of resources available, including a listing of individuals through the Academy of Nutrition and Dietetics. Members of the Academy of Nutrition and Dietetics may be found in virtually every community in the United States.

3.6.2 PHYSICAL ACTIVITY

We provided a chapter giving background information on physical activity. An excellent resource that should be part of the reference library for physicians is the Physical Activity Guidelines for Americans 2018 (9). There is also an initiative from the American College of Sports Medicine entitled "Exercise is Medicine," which provides a variety of reference materials (10).

3.6.3 WEIGHT MANAGEMENT

We provide a chapter that lists the guidance on effective weight management based on a collaboration between the AHA/ACC and The Obesity Society (TOS) (11). There is also a complete book on weight management that is a volume in this Lifestyle Medicine Series (12).

3.6.4 STRESS REDUCTION

Multiple resources are available to help physicians counsel in the area of stress reduction. One key component of virtually all stress reduction programs is the advice to live in the present rather than regretting the past or fearing the future. We devote a whole chapter in this book to modern approaches to stress reduction and other psychological issues (see Chapter 8).

3.6.5 SLEEP

Both the Centers for Disease Control and Prevention and the National Institutes of Health (NIH) provide good references in the area of healthy sleep. Most recommendations for healthy sleep involve the use of techniques of "sleep hygiene." These include establishing a regular wake/sleep schedule, keeping the environment for sleep slightly cooler than the rest of the environment in the house, not using the bed for anything else other than sleep and avoiding substances that might impair sleep such as alcohol consumption. The Physical Activity Guidelines for Americans also have a section on sleep (9) (see also Chapter 9).

3.6.6 EMOTIONAL WELL-BEING

The power of connections to other people has been shown in multiple studies as a key component of emotional well-being. An important literature has arisen in the area of "positive psychology," which emphasizes using an individual's strengths to help them achieve a more positive lifestyle. The mere fact that physicians discuss these issues with patients will also underscore the importance of emotional well-being.

3.6.7 HOME BLOOD PRESSURE MONITORING

One effective way to help individuals to control their blood pressure is to utilize home blood pressure monitoring equipment. There are now multiple devices available that are highly accurate and can help the individual take their own blood pressure and report it back to their physician.

3.6.8 COUNSELING ON OTHER CARDIOVASCULAR ISSUES

Counseling on lipids and diabetes are both important. We devote separate chapters in the book to each of these issues.

3.7 REFERRALS

Multiple lifestyle medicine referrals possibilities are available. In addition to nutritionists, certified exercise physiologists through the American College of Sports Medicine (13) can be found in virtually every major city. An emerging group of individuals now are devoting their practice to advanced understandings of lifestyle medicine. These individuals may be accessed through the American College of Lifestyle Medicine (ACLM) (14). The profession of coaching has also grown exponentially in the past two decades. Certified coaches can be found through several professional organizations (15).

3.8 SUMMARY/CONCLUSIONS

The use of lifestyle medicine information and techniques as part of a focused history and physical examination for CVD offers enormous opportunities for physicians to expand their evidence-based practice and techniques. In addition to regular components of history and physical examination, lifestyle medicine modalities in such areas as nutrition, physical activity, weight management, stress, sleep and emotional well-being can all bring added value to the physician/patient relationship. At the current time, not enough physicians are making use of these modalities. We hope that information provided in this chapter and throughout the rest of this book will encourage more physicians to recognize the power of lifestyle medicine decisions to help people lower their risk of chronic disease and improve both their short- and long-term health and quality of life. There is probably no area where these issues are more important than the area of CVD.

Clinical Applications

- Physicians should utilize the power of lifestyle medicine modalities to enhance the sophistication and value of both the history and physical examination.
- Important health considerations such as nutrition, physical activity, weight management, stress reduction, smoking cessation and alcohol consumption moderation can be emphasized by the physician in a lifestyle medicine history and physical examination. A variety of specialized tests and referrals are now available to assist the physician in incorporating lifestyle medicine information and techniques in the regular history and physical examination.

REFERENCES

1. Rippe JM. Lifestyle strategies for risk factor reduction, prevention, and treatment of cardiovascular disease. [Review]. Am J Lifestyle Med. 2018;13(2):204–12. Doi:10.1177/1559827618812395.
2. Kennedy MA. What physicians need to know, do, and say to promote physical activity. In Rippe JM, ed. Lifestyle Medicine. 3rd ed. Boca Raton, FL: CRC Press; 2019.
3. Lichtenstein A, Appel L, Vadiveloo M, et al. AHA scientific statement: 2021 dietary guidance to improve cardiovascular health: A scientific statement from the American Heart Association. Circulation. 2021;144(23):e472–87.
4. American Heart Association Nutrition Committee, Lichtenstein AH, Appel LJ, et al. Diet and lifestyle recommendations revision 2006: A scientific statement from the American Heart Association Nutrition Committee. [Guideline]. Circulation. 2006;114(1):82–96. doi:10.1161/CIRCULATIONAHA.106.176158.
5. U.S. Department of Agriculture and U.S. Department of Health and Human Services. Dietary Guidelines for Americans, 2020–2025. 9th ed.; December 2020. DietaryGuidelines.gov. Accessed December 1, 2021.
6. Lloyd-Jones DM, Hong Y, Labarthe D, et al. Defining and setting national goals for cardiovascular health promotion and disease reduction: The American Heart Association's strategic Impact Goal through 2020 and beyond. [Consensus Development Conference Review]. Circulation. 2010;121(4):586–613.

7. Obarzanek E, Sacks FM, Vollmer WM, et al. Effects on blood lipids of a blood pressure-lowering diet: The Dietary Approaches to Stop Hypertension (DASH) trial. [Clinical Trial Multicenter Study Randomized Controlled Trial Research Support, U.S. Gov't, P.H.S.]. Am J Clin Nutr. 2001;74(1):80–9. doi:10.1093/ajcn/74.1.80.

8. O'Gara PT, Kushner FG, Ascheim DD, et al. ACCF/AHA guideline for the management of ST-elevation myocardial infarction: a report of the American College of Cardiology Foundation/American Heart Association Task Force on Practice Guidelines. [Practice Guideline]. J Am Coll Cardiol. 2013;61(4):e78–140. doi:10.1016/j.jacc.2012.11.019

9. Chobanian A, Bakris G, Black H, et al. The joint national committee on prevention, detection, evaluation and treatment of high blood pressure: The seventh report of the joint national committee on prevention, detection, evaluation, and treatment of high blood pressure: The JNC 7 report. JAMA. 2003;289(19):2560–72. doi:10.1001/jama.289.19.2560

10. 2018 Physical Activity Guidelines Advisory Committee. 2018 Physical Activity Guidelines Advisory Committee Scientific Report. U.S. Department of Health and Human Services. Washington, DC; 2018.

11. Exercise is Medicine—Exercise is Medicine. www.exerciseismedicine.org. Accessed December 1, 2021.

12. Jensen MD, Ryan DH, Apovian CM, et al. AHA/ACC/TOS guideline for the management of overweight and obesity in adults: A report of the American College of Cardiology/American Heart Association Task Force on Practice Guidelines and the Obesity Society. [Practice Guideline]. J Am Coll Cardiol. 2013;63(25 Pt B):2985–3023. doi:10.1016/j.jacc.2013.11.004.

13. Rippe JM, Foreyt JP. Lifestyle Medicine: Obesity Prevention and Treatment: A Practical Guide. Boca Raton, FL: CRC Press; 2021.

14. American College of Sports Medicine. ACSM | The American College of Sports Medicine. Accessed December 1, 2021.

15. American College of Lifestyle Medicine. ACLM Home. lifestylemedicine.org. Accessed December 1, 2021.

16. Wellcoaches, School of Health & Wellness Coaching. wellcoachesschool.com. Accessed December 1, 2021.

4 Lifestyle Medicine, Physical Activity and Cardiovascular Disease

KEY POINTS

- Cardiovascular disease (CVD) is the leading cause of morbidity and mortality in the United States and around the world.
- Lifestyle interventions are key components of recommendations from prestigious organizations such as the American Heart Association and other professional organizations to lower the risk of CVD.
- Regular physical activity has been repeatedly shown to lower the risk of CVD, coronary heart disease, hypertension, heart failure and type 2 diabetes.
- Assessment of levels of physical activity and recommendations for appropriate increases, if necessary, should be part of every patient encounter by physicians.

4.1 INTRODUCTION

Cardiovascular disease (CVD), as defined by the Centers for Disease Control and Prevention (CDC), encompasses coronary heart disease (CHD), stroke, hypertension and heart failure. CVD accounts for over one in three deaths in the United States each year. Approximately 2,150 Americans die from some manifestation of CVD every day—roughly one every 40 seconds (1). CVD has been the leading cause of death in the United States and worldwide and remains so despite decades-long decline in CVD mortality. In addition, over the past two decades, CVD has also become the leading cause of death worldwide.

In 2013 CVD caused an estimated 17.3 deaths and led to 330 million disability-adjusted life years (DALYs) lost. These figures represent about 32% of all deaths worldwide and 13% of all DALYs (2). In addition to high-income countries that have experienced this in the last century, low- and middle-income countries are now experiencing accelerating increases in CVD. Between 1990 and 2013, deaths from CVD increased from 26% to 32% of all deaths globally (2).

It is predicted over 650,000 Americans will experience their first myocardial infarction (MI; heart attack) this year, and 300,000 will be victims of a reinfarction (1). In addition, it is estimated that another 155,000 infarctions will be "silent" with no symptoms other than angina, which are missed or ignored. This means that an American experiences a coronary event every 34 seconds. Compared to those who are very physically active, the risk of coronary heart disease (CHD) in sedentary individuals is 150%–240% higher (1). Unfortunately, only one quarter of all Americans

DOI: 10.1201/b23245-5

engage in enough exercise to meet the minimum standards for the Centers for Disease Control and Prevention (CDC) and the Physical Activity Guidelines for Americans 2018 (PAGA 2018) (3) (at least 150 minutes per week of moderate-intensity aerobic exercise or at least 75 minutes of vigorous exercise and muscle-strengthening activities at least 2 days per week).

It is clear that the greatest reduction in risk for CHD appears to be for those engaging in even modest amounts of physical activity compared to the most physically inactive. Thus, even relatively small increases in physical activity could potentially result in a significant decrease in CHD for a large portion of the population. Epidemiologic data have suggested a 2.3% decline in physical inactivity between 1980 and 2000 prevented at least 17,445 deaths from CHD in the United States.

Despite the overwhelming evidence that inactivity is an important and significant risk factor for CHD and that physical activity substantially lowers the risk of CHD, fewer than half of adults meet even the minimum recommendations for aerobic exercise. Statistics for young people are even more disheartening, with fewer than 20% of adolescents performing the recommended 60 minutes or more of daily physical activity (3).

Despite the demonstrated benefits of physical activity, many physicians are not encouraging their patients to exercise. Of equal importance, many physicians do not appear to be adequately prepared to provide recommendations for exercise and physical activity. In one survey of 175 primary care physicians, only 12% were aware of the recommendations of the American College of Sports Medicine (ACSM) for physical activity.

There is also potential good news related to physical activity and reduction of risk of heart disease. As illustrated in Figure 4.1, the steepest part of reduction of risk

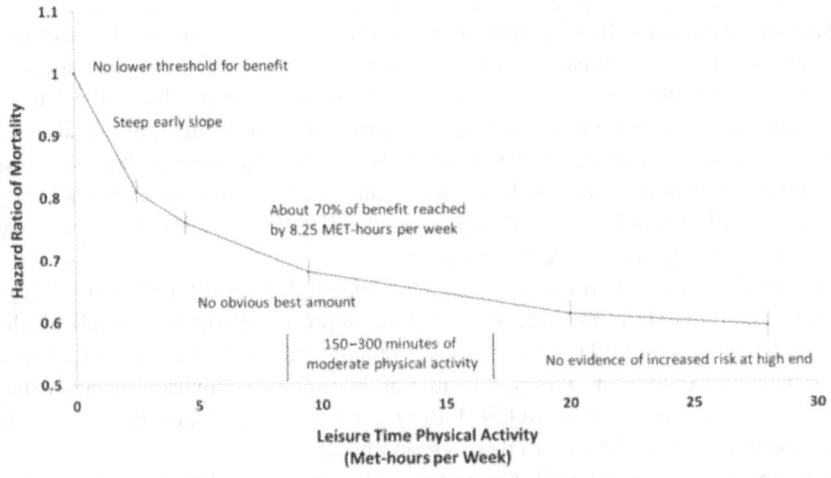

FIGURE 4.1   Relationship of moderate to vigorous physical activity to all-cause mortality, with highlighted characteristics common to studies of this type. (From the 2018 Physical Activity Guidelines Advisory Committee. 2018 Physical Activity Guidelines Advisory Committee Scientific Report. Washington, DC: U.S. Department of Health and Human Services; 2018.)

occurs in individuals who were previously sedentary and begin to engage in physical activity for as little as 30 minutes per week.

Also emphasized in Figure 4.1, which is taken from the PAGA 2018, there seems to be no lower threshold for benefit. Increasing benefits occur for individuals who engage in approximately 150 minutes of regular weekly physical activity, although meaningful benefits occur in individuals who engage in physical activity even substantially less than this. As illustrated in this figure, 70% of the benefit is achieved by individuals who engage in moderate physical activity such as walking 30 minutes five times a week. However, 20% of the benefits occurs in individuals who accumulate only 30 minutes per week.

The PAGA 2018 summarizes these findings by saying "some is better than none."

4.2 PHYSICAL FITNESS VERSUS PHYSICAL ACTIVITY

Physical fitness, specifically cardiorespiratory fitness, is defined as the ability to deliver and utilize oxygen during sustained activity and is typically quantified as maximal oxygen uptake (VO_{2max}). This measurement, however, requires sophisticated equipment to measure respiratory gases and has been shown in many studies to be valid and reliable. There are submaximal tests available such as those relying on indirect measures such as time to exhaustion during increasing levels of physical activity, but these are subject to considerable error.

Measures of physical activity, on the other hand, usually rely on retrospective self-reported data such as that available from questionnaires. The definitions of physical activity vary greatly from study to study since components of physical activity such as intensity, duration and frequency are often not reported or inadequately assessed.

Moreover, the categorization of physical activity (i.e., low, moderate, or high) varies from study to study. An example of this is that the perceived intensity of walking or brisk walking that is often used to meet the criteria for moderate physical activity, varies considerably according to the individual's age, physical condition and fitness level. Brisk walking may not be sufficiently intense to meet minimum criteria for moderate physical activity in a healthy college-aged individual, while brisk walking may be considered vigorous activity for someone over the age of 65 years.

Surprisingly, physical fitness has only modest correlations with physical activity with correlations ranging from 0.09 to 0.60. There is a higher correlation of physical fitness with a risk of CHD than for physical activity. This is illustrated in Figure 4.2 (4).

This is not to say that physical activity is not significantly important particularly given that 40% of the reduction in mortality occurs between the least active and fit and the next category of fitness or physical activity. Thus, even modest increases of physical activity or fitness, particularly those who are sedentary result in a significant reduction in mortality.

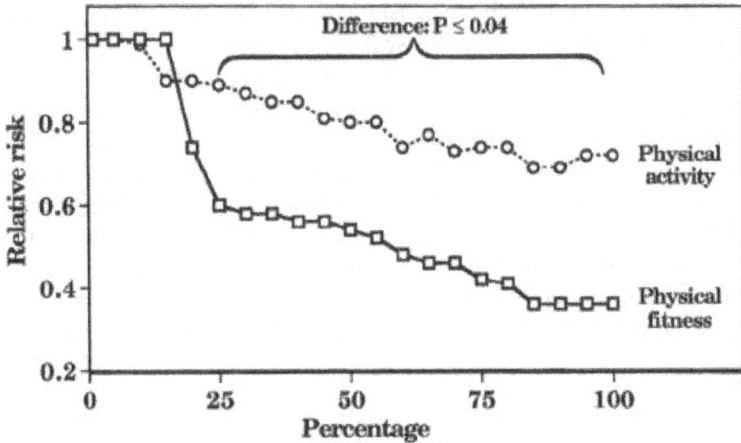

FIGURE 4.2 Estimated dose-response curve for the relative risk of either CHD or CVD by sample percentages of fitness and physical activity. Studies weighted by person-years of experience. (Zoeller R. Physical activity and fitness in the prevention of cardiovascular disease. In: Rippe JM, ed. *Lifestyle Medicine*. 3rd ed. CRC Press; 2019.)

4.3   GENERAL RECOMMENDATIONS FOR PHYSICAL ACTIVITY

The recommendations for physical activity have evolved over the past two decades. In 1996, the Surgeon General's Report on Physical Activity and Health recommended "people of all ages to include a minimum of 30 minutes of physical activity of moderate intensity (such as brisk walking) on most, if not all, days of the week" (5). It is acknowledged that for most people, greater health benefits can be obtained by engaging in physical activity of more vigorous intensity or longer duration (6). More recently, in 2018, the PAGA provided updated and more specific recommendations for different age groups and clinical populations (3). Following is a brief summary of their recommendations.

4.3.1   ADULTS

- All adults should avoid inactivity. Some physical activity is better than none, and adults who participate in any amount of physical activity gain some health benefits.
- For substantial health benefits, adults should perform at least 150 minutes a week of moderate-intensity, or 75 minutes a week of vigorous-intensity aerobic physical activity, or the equivalent combination of moderate- and vigorous-intensity aerobic activity.
- Adults should also perform muscle-strengthening activities that are appropriate or high intensity and involve all major muscle groups on two or more days per week, as those activities provide additional health benefits.

4.3.2 Older Adults

- When older adults cannot perform 150 minutes of moderate-intensity aerobic activity a week because of chronic conditions, they should be as physically active as their abilities and conditions allow.
- Older adults should perform exercises that maintain or improve balance if they are at risk of falling.
- Older adults should determine their level of effort for physical activity relative to their level of fitness.
- Older adults with chronic conditions should understand whether and how their conditions affect their ability to do regular physical activity safely.

4.4 PHYSICAL ACTIVITY AND CVD IN WOMEN

One in three women have some form of CVD, and of these, 6.6 million are diagnosed with CHD. In 2013 alone, 398,086 women died of CVD (1). This represents the equivalent of about one death every 80 seconds. Just over 40% of these deaths were attributable to CHD, including 50,742 from MI. On average, new and recurrent MIs as well as fatal CHD impact 405,000 women each year. Because women typically have heart attacks at older ages than men do, they are more likely to die from them within a few weeks. This topic is so important that an entire chapter is devoted to it (see Chapter 21).

4.5 PHYSICAL ACTIVITY AND STROKE

It is estimated that 795,000 individuals in the United States experience a new (approximately 610,000) or recurrent (approximately 185,000) stroke each year (1). Of these, a large majority are ischemic (87%), and the remainder are hemorrhagic in nature.

The risk of stroke in African Americans is nearly double that for Caucasians and tends to occur at a younger age. Hispanic people, particularly Mexican Americans, have significantly higher rates of ischemic stroke and at a younger age. Annually, 55,000 more women than men have a stroke with the incidence in women aged 45–54 years especially high.

Stroke is one of the major issues dealt with in the Presidential Advisory, which was jointly issued by the AHA and the American Stroke Association (ASA) as part of their "Optimal Brain Health." These issues are dealt with in more detail in Chapters 17 and 20.

A key understanding is that the risk factors for stroke and dementia are similar to those for CVD; in fact, the major recommendation of this Presidential Advisory was that individuals follow the Seven Simple Steps from AHA to lower the risk of CVD and maintain brain health.

Meta-analyses have shown that reduction in the risk of stroke associated with physical activity ranges between 20% and 40% depending on the type of stroke and study design.

4.6 HYPERTENSION

According to data from the National Health and Nutrition Examination Survey (NHANES), it is estimated that over 80 million adults (almost one in three American

TABLE 4.1
Classification of Blood Pressure for Adults

Blood Pressure Classification	SBP (mm Hg)	OBP (mm Hg)
Normal	<120	and <80
Prehypertension	120–139	or 80–89
Stage 1 hypertension	140–159	or 90–99
Stage 2 hypertension	>160	or >100

Source: Adapted from 2017 ACC/AHA Blood Pressure Guidelines.
Note: SBP, systolic blood pressure; DBP, diastolic blood pressure.

adults) have hypertension when it is defined as systolic blood pressure (SBP) ≥140 mm Hg and diastolic blood pressure (DBP) ≥90 mm Hg (1). The prevalence of high blood pressure in African American adults is among the highest in the world. Overall, 82.7% of individuals are aware of high blood pressure and 76.5% are being treated, but only 54.1% have their blood pressure under control. A meta-analysis of 61 studies reported in the Joint National Committee (JNC-7) guidelines showed that both CHD and stroke increase linearly from levels as low as 115 mm Hg systolic and 75 mm Hg diastolic blood pressure. For every 20 mm Hg systolic or 10 mm Hg diastolic increase in blood pressure, there is a doubling of mortality from both CHD and stroke (7).

Regular physical activity has been shown in numerous studies to be an effective way to lower blood pressure in the majority of people (75%) with hypertension. When comparing physically active to sedentary individuals, the physically active people have a lower incidence of hypertension and blood pressures that average 5 mm Hg lower than comparably aged sedentary individuals.

In 2017, ACC/AHA guidelines established a lower classification and treatment threshold for blood pressure. These Guidelines are found in Table 4.1.

As was the case in JNC-7 (7), these guidelines also recommend a variety of non-pharmacologic interventions and prominently featured physical activity consisting of 120–150 minutes per week of aerobic physical activity and 90–120 minutes per week of dynamic resistance exercise.

These lower thresholds are based on findings from the Systolic Blood Pressure Intervention Trial (SPRINT) (8). This study was conducted on over 9,000 individuals with a mean age of 67.9 years and a systolic blood pressure of 130–180 mm Hg and at increased risk for cardiovascular events. The study compared targets of systolic blood pressure (SBP) <120 mm Hg to standard targets of SBP <140 mm Hg. The SPRINT showed a 30% decrease in the composite outcome of MI, acute coronary syndrome, stroke and heart failure or death at the lower targets compared to the standard target. It should be noted that to achieve these lower levels of blood pressure, three antihypertensive medicines were required in many participants, which may make it impractical in a normal clinical setting. It should be emphasized that lifestyle modalities such as regular physical activity, weight management (or weight loss if necessary) and proper nutrition can significantly lower blood pressure, which may make these lower thresholds more achievable with less pharmaceutical therapy.

It should also be noted that the prevalence of high blood pressure increases with age. Only approximately 10% of individuals between the ages of 20 and 34 years have high blood pressure as defined by a SBP >140 mm Hg or diastolic blood pressure (DBP) ≥90 mm Hg. This increases in a linear fashion, until after the age of 75 years almost 80% of individuals have high blood pressure. (This includes approximately 73% of males and 81% of females.) This age-related increase in the prevalence of hypertension underscores the role of continued physical activity throughout the life span as one nonpharmaceutical way of lowering the risk of high blood pressure. The topic of hypertension is so important that we devote an entire chapter to it (see Chapter 13).

4.7   HEART FAILURE

It has been estimated that 5.7 million Americans experience heart failure (HF; also known as congestive heart failure). The risk of HF increases with age—by the time an individual reaches the age of 40 years, they have a 20% risk of HF (1).

There are a few studies that examine the difference between physical activity and the prevention of heart failure. Two large longitudinal studies compared sedentary individuals to those who engaged in regular vigorous exercise and showed that those who exercise vigorously had a 15%–35% lower risk of developing HF.

Moderate-intensity physical activity has also been shown to decrease the risk of HF in individuals who participate in more than 4 hours of moderate physical activity such as walking, cycling, or swimming. These individuals have approximately 15% reduction in lifetime risk of developing HF.

4.8   DIABETES

Diabetes is a significant risk factor for CHD (1). It is estimated that as many as 55% of adult individuals with diabetes have CHD. Type 2 diabetes mellitus (T2DM) is an independent risk factor for both MI and CHD in both men and women. Compared to nondiabetics, mortality from CHD has been estimated to be two times greater in diabetic men and four to five times greater in diabetic women. Cardiovascular disease is responsible for at least two-thirds of deaths in adults with T2DM. Diabetes is an important area where physical activity plays a significant role. This topic is handled in more detail in Chapter 18.

4.9   METABOLIC SYNDROME

The fact that established risk factors for CVD tend to cluster has been recognized for decades. Most CVD occurs in people who have two or more established risk factors. Metabolic syndrome represents a clustering of risk factors and is strongly linked to CVD as well as T2DM. The most commonly utilized definition for "metabolic syndrome" that has been adapted by the AHA and the National Heart, Lung, and Blood

Institute (NHLBI) utilizes the definition of "metabolic syndrome" from the National Cholesterol Education Program (NCEP), which requires three of the following five criteria be present for diagnosis of metabolic syndrome (9):

1. Impaired fasting glucose (IFG) representing a fasting blood sugar ≥100 mg/dL,
2. High-density lipoprotein cholesterol (HDL-C) <40 mg/dL in men and <50 mg/dL in women,
3. Triglycerides ≥150 mg/dL,
4. Increased waist circumference >40 inches in men or >35 inches in women, or
5. Blood pressure >130/85 mm Hg.

It has been estimated that 36%–38% of individuals in the United States have metabolic syndrome by these criteria.

The association of physical activity and prevalence of metabolic syndrome is not completely clear; however, most of the cross-sectional studies have suggested that this practice lowers both prevalence and risk of metabolic syndrome. There are, however, a number of confounding factors such as gender, age, education, socioeconomic status, as well as other risk factors such as smoking.

Several longitudinal studies have suggested that increased physical activity (particularly vigorous intensity activity) dramatically lowers the risk of developing metabolic syndrome. For example, in one study of people participating in 20 weeks of vigorous exercise for 30 minutes three times per week, metabolic syndrome was decreased by 30%. There also appears to be a relationship between cardiorespiratory fitness and metabolic syndrome, although this has not been studied as extensively as physical activity. In one study, individuals who had a VO_{2max} of ≥35.5 mL/kg/min were seven times less likely than individuals with low fitness (VO_{2max} <29.1 mL/kg/min) to have metabolic syndrome.

4.10 OBESITY

Obesity is an independent risk factor for CHD and is also associated with multiple other risk factors for CHD, including dyslipidemia and hypertension. The overall prevalence of overweight or obesity in the United States, according to recent data, is over 70% of adults (1,10). Overweight is considered a body mass index (BMI) between 25 and 30 kg/m². Obesity is defined as a BMI greater than 30 kg/m².

Although physical activity by itself is not a powerful way to lose weight, physical activity has been clearly associated with less likelihood of gaining weight and is critically important for long-term maintenance of weight loss. These issues are discussed in more detail in Chapter 6.

4.11 "FITNESS" VERSUS "FATNESS" DEBATE

Increased body weight and low levels of physical activity or fitness are both associated with increased mortality from both CHD and T2DM (11). It has been argued, however, that individuals with overweight or obesity who have moderately high levels of fitness can ameliorate the increased risk of their excess weight by increasing their fitness level. One extensive review of this debate that has been called "Fit versus Fat" concluded that a physically active lifestyle and moderately high fitness level (not in the bottom 25% of population) reduce the risk of CHD/CVD in overweight or obese individuals such that these individuals carry comparable risk associated with lean, unfit individuals. It has also been concluded, however, that the risk for these individuals is still greater than for those who are fit and active and maintain a healthy weight.

4.12 LIPIDS

The role of abnormalities in blood lipids in the pathology of atherosclerosis is well established (12). This relationship is particularly strong in the area of low-density lipoprotein cholesterol (LDL-C) and triglycerides as well as low levels of HDL-C (see Chapter 12).

The relationship between physical activity and lipids is complex. Cross-sectional studies have established the volume and intensity of physical activity are related to increases in HDL-C and negatively associated with TG levels. The literature, however, is inconsistent on other blood lipids and physical activity. Potential confounding aspects of these findings include changes in body weight and body composition. The role of lipids in CHD is discussed in more detail in Chapter 12.

4.13 THE ROLE OF PHYSICIANS IN PROMOTING INCREASED PHYSICAL ACTIVITY

Numerous studies have shown that physician recommendation represents a powerful tool for eliciting behavior change. Physician counseling has been shown to play a particularly important role in increasing physical activity. Unfortunately, less than 40% of physicians routinely discuss physical activity with patients. It has also been shown that physicians who are involved in regular physical activity in their own lives are much more likely to discuss these issues with their patients (13). At the most fundamental level, it is important that physicians discuss the important role of increasing physical activity in every patient encounter. This will, at minimum, indicate to patients the importance of this lifestyle modality.

4.14 SUMMARY/CONCLUSIONS

It is clear that CVD is by far the leading threat to health and longevity in both men and women in the United States and around the world. Finding cost-effective ways to lower the risk of this condition is of extreme importance. Greater physical activity has been repeatedly shown to be a critically important modality in risk factor reduction for all forms of CVD. For all of these reasons, it is incumbent upon physicians to inquire about levels of physical activity and, if lower than optimal, prescribe ways of increasing it.

Clinical Applications

- Every medical encounter should include assessment and recommendations for physical activity.
- Levels of physical activity should be geared to age and current level of physical activity or fitness of each patient.
- Moderate-intensity physical activity at the level to help patients escape the bottom 20% in terms of physical activity and physical fitness results in the steepest part of the benefit curve or reduction of risk of CVD.
- Recommendations from the PAGA 2018 to achieve physical activity at the level of 150 minutes of moderate-intensity physical activity on a weekly basis plus two episodes of resistance strength training on a weekly basis reduce risk of cardiovascular disease.

REFERENCES

1. Virani SS, Alonso A, Aparicio HJ, et al. Heart disease and stroke statistics—2021 update: A report from the American Heart Association. Circulation. 2021;143(8): e254–743. doi:10.1161/CIR.0000000000000950.
2. Gaziano TA, Prabhakaran D, Gaziano JM. Global Burden of Cardiovascular Disease: Braunwald's Heart Disease. In Libby P, Zipes DP, Bonow RO, Mann DL, Tomaselli GF, ed. A Textbook of Cardiovascular Medicine, 11th ed. Amsterdam, Netherlands: Elsevier; 2019, pp. 1–18.
3. 2018 Physical Activity Guidelines Advisory Committee. 2018 Physical Activity Guidelines Advisory Committee Scientific Report. Washington, DC: U.S. Department of Health and Human Services; 2018. 2018 Physical Activity Guidelines Advisory Committee Scientific Report (health.gov). Accessed November 18, 2021.
4. Williams PT. Physical fitness and activity as separate heart disease risk factors: A meta-analysis. [Meta-Analysis Research Support, U.S. Gov't, Non-P.H.S. Research Support, U.S. Gov't, P.H.S.]. Medicine and Science in Sports and Exercise. 2001;33(5):754–61. doi:10.1097/00005768-200105000-00012.
5. Physical Activity and Health: A Report of the Surgeon General. U.S. Department of Health and Human Services. Center for Disease Control and Prevention. Accessed November 18, 2021.
6. Rippe JM. Lifestyle Medicine: Increasing Physical Activity: A Practical Guide. Boca Raton, FL: CRC Press; 2020.
7. Chobanian AV, Bakris GL, Black HR. The seventh report of the Joint National Committee on Prevention, Detection, Evaluation, and Treatment of High Blood Pressure: The JNC 7 report. [Guideline Practice Guideline Research Support, U.S. Gov't, P.H.S.]. JAMA. 2003;289(19):2560–72. doi:10.1001/jama.289.19.2560.
8. U.S. National Library of Medicine. Systolic Blood Pressure Intervention Trial (SPRINT). ClinicalTrials.gov Identifier: NCT01206062. Systolic Blood Pressure Intervention Trial-Full Text View-ClinicalTrials.gov. Accessed November 18, 2021.
9. Alexander CM, Landsman PB, Teutsch SM, Haffner SM, Third National H, Nutrition Examination S, et al. NCEP-defined metabolic syndrome, diabetes, and prevalence of coronary heart disease among NHANES III participants age 50 years and older. Diabetes. 2003;52(5):1210–14. Epub 2003/04/30.
10. Rippe J, Foreyt JP. COVID-19 and Obesity: A Pandemic Wrapped in an Epidemic. Am J Lifestyle Med. 2021;15(4):364–5. Epub 2021/08/10.

11. Barbeau P, Litaker MS, Woods KF, Lemmon CR, Humphries MC, Owens S, et al. Hemostatic and inflammatory markers in obese youths: effects of exercise and adiposity. The Journal of pediatrics. 2002;141(3):415–20. Epub 2002/09/10.
12. Grundy SM, Cleeman JI, Merz CN. Implications of recent clinical trials for the National Cholesterol Education Program Adult Treatment Panel III guidelines. [Consensus Development Conference Review]. J Am Coll Cardiol. 44(3):720–32. doi:10.1016/j. jacc.2004.07.001.
13. Kennedy M. What physicians need to know, do and say to promote physical activity. In Rippe JM, ed. Lifestyle Medicine. 3rd ed. Boca Raton, FL: CRC Press; 2019.

5 Nutrition and Cardiovascular Disease

KEY POINTS

- Proper nutrition plays a critically important role in reducing the risk of cardiovascular disease (CVD).
- CVD remains the leading killer of both men and women in the United States resulting in over 37% of annual mortality.
- Dietary patterns are consistent across various recommendations from multiple organizations including increases in fruits and vegetables, whole grains, seafood (particularly oily fish), legumes and nuts and lower or nonfat dairy products and also lowering red meats and processed meats, lowering sugar-sweetened beverages and refined grains. These patterns have been repeatedly shown to lower the risk of CVD.
- Implementation of plant-based diets such as those recommended by the American Heart Association and Dietary Guidelines for Americans 2020–2025 represent a key mandate for clinicians to employ to help their patients adopt healthier eating habits.

5.1 INTRODUCTION

Cardiovascular disease (CVD) represents the largest source of morbidity and mortality in the United States and elsewhere in the developed world (1). Thousands of studies support the concept that daily lifestyle practices and habits exert profound effects on the likelihood of developing CVD. Many lifestyle practices are associated with positive benefits in both the prevention and treatment of CVD. Nutrition clearly plays a pivotal role (2–6).

Recommendations for diets that contain more fruits and vegetables, fish (particularly oily fish), whole grains and fiber, along with remaining in caloric balance to lower the risk of CVD have been supported by multiple studies (2–7). Nutrition should be placed in the context of other positive lifestyle decisions such as maintaining a proper body weight, regular physical activity including at least 30 minutes per day of physical activity and not smoking or being exposed to tobacco products (8,9).

When taken together, studies have shown that these lifestyle practices can reduce the risk of CVD by over 80% and diabetes by over 90% in both men and women.

Lifestyle practices have made major contributions to declines in mortality. For example, between 1980 and 2000, mortality rates from CVD fell by 40% (10). Half of this reduction was attributed to improvements in major lifestyle risk factors such as increased physical activity, smoking cessation, and better control of blood pressure and cholesterol. Unfortunately, during this same period, obesity and diabetes

DOI: 10.1201/b23245-6

have moved in the opposite direction. These latter two factors have the potential to wipe out all the gains achieved by other positive lifestyle-related risk factors. Unfortunately, these trends have continued to the present time.

Between 1990 and 2013, deaths from CVD worldwide rose from 26% to 32%. This appears to be due to epidemiologic transitions that have occurred during this period. Certainly, nutritional factors are one of the components that play a significant role in either positive or negative lifestyle decisions or practices.

In this chapter, we focus on nutrition and place it in the broader context of other lifestyle factors such as physical activity and weight maintenance. This overall approach is consistent with the tenets of lifestyle medicine and is consistent with the approach taken by the American Heart Association (AHA) in multiple documents and scientific statements (3–6). The Dietary Guidelines for Americans 2020–2025 Advisory Committee Report (11) also adopt this approach as do many other documents and statements including those from the Academy of Nutrition and Dietetics (AND) (12).

Nutritional guidelines offered by the AHA are contained in evidence-based documents such as the 2013 AHA/American College of Cardiology (ACC) Guidelines for Lifestyle Management to Reduce Cardiovascular Risk (5). Nutritional guidelines play a prominent role in the 2020 Strategic Plan for Improving Cardiovascular Health and Lowering Cardiovascular Risk published by the AHA (4). The recommendations from this report and many others including the Dietary Guidelines Advisory Committee 2020–2025 are similar. All of these recommendations focus not only on nutrition but also on the broader approach to positive lifestyles to improve cardiovascular health and reduce the risk of CVD.

5.2 BACKGROUND

The various consensus statements and recommendations issued by various prestigious organizations have offered similar guidance. These recommendations have drawn upon the same database, in general, including large epidemiologic studies. Published consensus statements form the basis of the recommendations made in this chapter. These consensus statements include the following:

- Diet and Lifestyle Recommendations 2021: Advisory Committee Report (11),
- Dietary Guidelines for Americans 2020–2025 (7),
- 2014 AHA/ACC Guidelines for Lifestyle Management to Reduce Cardiovascular Risk (5),
- Diet and Lifestyle Recommendations Revision 2006: A Scientific Statement from the AHA Nutrition Committee (3), and
- Defining and Setting National Goals for Cardiovascular Health Promotion and Disease Reduction: American Heart Association Strategic Impact Goals through 2020 and beyond (4).

These consensus statements consistently recommend a dietary pattern higher in fruits and vegetables, whole grains (particularly high fiber), nonfat dairy, seafood, legumes and nuts. The guidelines recommend that those who consume alcohol (among adults) do so in moderation. The guidelines consistently recommend diets lower in red and processed meats, refined grains, sugar-sweetened foods and saturated and trans fats. All of these guidelines have emphasized the importance of balancing calories and physical activity as strategies not only for independently lowering the risk of heart disease but also maintaining a healthy body weight, thereby further reducing the risk of CVD.

The national guidelines on nutrition and cardiovascular health focus on overall dietary patterns rather than on individual foods. However, there is a large literature on individual foods which is also discussed in this chapter.

One consensus recommendation from the AHA contained in its 2020 Strategic Plan defines dietary goals as in the context of a diet that is appropriate for energy balance pursuing and overall pattern consistent with DASH (Dietary Approach to Stop Hypertension). One recommendation from the AHA in the Strategic Plan for 2020 is recognizing that nutritional guidance is complicated and made the following basic recommendations:

- Fruits and vegetables ≥4.5 cups/day;
- Fish ≥two servings/week (preferably oily fish);
- Fiber-rich/whole grains ≥1.1 g fiber/10 g carbohydrate, three 1 ounce equivalent servings/day;
- Sodium ≤1,500 mg/day; and
- Sugar-sweetened beverages ≤460 calories (36 ounces)/week.

These recommendations appear to be a reasonable starting point and have been significantly expanded upon in other guidelines and recent reviews.

Since dietary patterns form the basis for modern recommendations for nutrition and cardiovascular health, this approach is adopted in this chapter. In addition, a recent emphasis in nutrition guidelines has focused on the critical aspect of implementing the guidance.

Despite the fact that nutrition plays a key role in many aspects of CVD, only a distinct minority of Americans follow these guidelines. For example, even with individuals who have hypertension, less than 20% follow the DASH diet (13). It has also been estimated that less than 12% of adults in the United States consume the recommended number of fruits and vegetables. The issue of how to encourage people to implement heart healthy guidelines in their daily lives is an important topic that is discussed toward the end of this chapter (14). Techniques adopted from behavioral medicine have increasingly been applied to nutrition and other positive aspects of lifestyle medicine and are discussed briefly in this chapter.

5.3   DIETARY PATTERNS

The 2020–2025 Dietary Guidelines for Americans integrated a wide range of available science to develop the "Healthy U.S.-Style Eating Pattern" (7). This approach allowed the blending of the overall diet to include foods, beverages, nutrients, and health outcomes. The food pattern modeling allowed more flexibility in amounts of foods from all food groups to establish healthy eating patterns that met nutrient needs and accommodated limitations for those such as saturated fats, sugars and sodium. With this approach, the DGA 2025 indicated the following:

> Within the body of evidence higher intakes of vegetables and fruits consistently have been identified as characteristic of healthy eating patterns; whole grains have been identified as well, although with slightly less consistency. Other characteristics of healthy eating patterns have been identified with less consistency including fat-free and low-fat dairy, seafood, legumes, and nuts. Lower intakes of meats including processed meats, poultry; sugar sweetened foods, particularly beverages; and refined grains have also been identified as characteristics of healthy eating patterns.
>
> (Executive Summary of the Dietary Guidelines for Americans 2020–2025)

5.3.1 HEALTHY U.S.-STYLE EATING PATTERN

As indicated in the preceding paragraphs, the U.S. Dietary Guidelines for Americans followed this procedure to develop the Healthy U.S.-Style Eating Pattern for 2,000 calorie level daily or weekly amounts for various food groups and components. These recommendations are found in Table 5.1.

The DGA 2020–2025 guidelines emphasize that calories should be balanced to maintain a healthy weight. The Healthy U.S.-Style Eating Plan is designed to meet

TABLE 5.1

Healthy U.S.-Style Eating Pattern at the 2,000 Calorie Level, with Daily or Weekly Amounts from Food Groups, Subgroups and Components

Food Group	Amount in the 2,000-Calorie-Level Pattern
Vegetables	2½ c-eq/day
Dark green	1½ c-eq/wk
Red and orange	5½ c-eq/wk
Legumes (beans and peas)	1½ c-eq/wk
Starchy	5 c-eq/wk
Other	4 c-eq/wk
Fruits	2 c-eq/day
Grains	6 oz-eq/day
Whole grains	≥3 oz-eq/day
Refined grains	≤3 oz-eq/day
Dairy	3 c-eq/day
Protein foods	5½ oz-eq/day
Seafood	8 oz-eq/wk
Meats, poultry, eggs	26 oz-eq/wk
Nuts, seeds, soy products	5 oz-eq/wk
Oils	27 g/day

recommended daily allowances and adequate intakes of potential nutrients as well as acceptable macronutrient distribution ranges. Flexibility within the dietary pattern allows for minor modifications allowing the Mediterranean diet or the DASH diet to be followed.

5.3.2 LOW-FAT DIETS

Low-fat diet consumption has been generally accepted for the past two decades in clinical guidelines for CVD prevention (3,5). Low-fat diets are based on total fat consumption of 25%–35% of total calories from all fat, no more than 7%–10% of calories from saturated fatty acid (SFA) and less than 1% of calories from trans fatty acid (TFA). The rest of the calories from fats come mainly from monounsaturated fatty acid (MUFA) and omega-3 polyunsaturated fatty acid (N-3 PUFA). This diet also calls for dietary cholesterol of less than 300 mg/day (15,16).

These recommendations can be met by emphasizing fruits and vegetables, low-fat dairy products and low-fat meat. It should also be noted that the food matrix for SFAs has been an area of recent research. Some investigators have suggested that SFAs coming from dairy products are less likely to adversely impact risk factors for CVD compared to other sources of SFAs (17,18). The AHA/ACC Guidelines for Lifestyle Management recommend that consumption of SFAs should not exceed 6% of calories.

5.3.3 LOW-CARBOHYDRATE DIET

Low-carbohydrate diets are typically defined as containing up to or less than 25% of total calories from carbohydrates (30–130 g of carbohydrates/day). These diets have been shown to reduce triglycerides and increase HDL cholesterol.

One study that compared low-carbohydrate to low-fat and Mediterranean diets found greater weight loss in the low-carbohydrate diet over the course of 1 year. At 2- and 4-year follow-up, however, there were no significant differences among the three arms (19). Thus, there are not enough data from long-term trials to demonstrate the benefits of a low-carbohydrate diet compared to low-fat and Mediterranean diets for reduction of risk of CVD (20,21).

5.3.4 MEDITERRANEAN DIET

The Mediterranean diet was initially described as typically consumed in countries bordering the Mediterranean Sea (22,23). It is characterized by relatively high fat intake (40%–50% of total daily calories) of which SFA comprises ≤8% and MUFA of 15%–25% of calories. The Mediterranean diet also has high omega-3 fatty acids from fish and plant sources and a low omega-6 to omega-3 ratio. It features seasonal, local fresh vegetables, fruits, whole grains, legumes, nuts and olive oil. Red meat is avoided. Moderate amounts of low-fat dairy products as well as eggs, chicken and fish are allowed as are moderate quantities of wine with meals in non-Islamic countries.

In a recent, multicenter, randomized intervention trial in Spain, individuals with high cardiovascular risk but no overt evidence of cardiovascular disease were divided into three diets as follows: the Mediterranean diet supplemented with extra virgin olive oil, the Mediterranean diet supplemented with mixed nuts or a control diet (advised to reduce saturated fat). The primary endpoint was an incidence of major cardiovascular events such as myocardial infarction, stroke or death from cardiovascular causes (21).

The two Mediterranean diets resulted in a decrease of approximately 30% in major cardiovascular events compared to the control diet.

5.3.5 DASH Diet

The Dietary Approaches to Stop Hypertension (DASH) diet initially was formulated in the 1990s and has undergone several modifications and iterations since that time (13,24,25). The initial goal of this diet was to lower blood pressure and CVD incidence by nutritional means. The DASH diet features vegetables and fruits as well as low-fat dairy products, whole grains, chicken, fish and nuts. It is low in fat, red meat, sweets and soft drinks (see Table 5.2).

Some subsequent studies have substituted some of the carbohydrates with MUFAs and have further decreased sodium in the diet. All of these modified DASH diets have significantly reduced both systolic and diastolic blood pressure by 7–9 mm Hg compared to the typical Western diet.

A study has combined the DASH diet with a lifestyle program with the strategy to reduce overweight and increase physical activity. This study called the ENCORE Trial showed substantial decreases in both systolic and diastolic blood pressure, which were reduced by 14.2 mm Hg and 17.4 mm Hg, respectively, thus showing the power of combined lifestyle measures including proper nutrition, physical activity and weight loss (26).

5.3.6 Vegetarian Diet

A variety of vegetarian diets are available including vegan (consuming no animal products), lacto-ovo vegetarian (consuming milk and eggs) and pesco vegetarian (consuming fish along with a vegetarian diet).

There are no data to suggest that one form of vegetarian diet is superior to others with regard to CVD risk (27–29). Randomized controlled trials (RCTs) performed on vegetarian diets have typically been small. Some observational studies have suggested that vegetarians experience improved health outcomes compared to nonvegetarians. However, there are a variety of characteristics of vegetarian diets that could account for these findings, including fewer meats and inclusion of plant-based products. Furthermore, vegetarians are often more health conscious than other individuals, which could further confound results.

5.3.7 Japanese Diet

There has been recent interest in Japanese diets, particularly those on Okinawa, which has among the lowest CVD rates in the world (30). Traditional Japanese diets emphasize fish, soy products, seaweed, vegetables, fruits and green tea and are low

TABLE 5.2
Following the DASH Eating Plan

Food Group	Servings per Day 1,600 Calories	Servings per Day 2,000 Calories	Servings per Day 2,600 Calories	Serving Sizes	Examples and Notes	Significance of Each Food Group to the DASH Eating Plan
Grains*	6	6–8	10–11	1 slice bread 1 oz dry cereal† ½ cup cooked rice, pasta or cereal	Whole wheat bread and rolls, whole wheat pasta, English muffin, pita bread, bagel, cereals, grits, oatmeal, brown rice, unsalted pretzels and popcorn	Major sources of energy and fiber
Vegetables	3–4	4–6	5–6	1 cup raw leafy vegetable ½ cup cut-up raw or cooked vegetable ½ cup vegetable juice	Broccoli, carrots, collards, green beans, green peas, kale, lima beans, potatoes, spinach, squash, sweet potatoes, tomatoes	Rich sources of potassium, magnesium and fiber
Fruits	4	4–5	5–6	1 medium fruit ¼ cup dried fruit ½ cup fresh, frozen or canned fruit ½ cup fruit juice	Apples, apricots, bananas, dates, grapes, oranges, grapefruit, grapefruit juice, mangoes, melons, peaches, pineapples, raisins, strawberries, tangerines	Important sources of potassium, magnesium and fiber
Fat-free or low-fat milk and milk products	2–3	2–3	3	1 cup milk or yogurt 1½ oz cheese	Fat-free (skim) or low-fat (1%) milk or buttermilk; fat-free, low-fat or reduced-fat cheese; fat-free or low-fat regular or frozen yogurt	Major sources of calcium and protein
Lean meats, poultry and fish	3–6	6 or less	6	1 oz cooked meats, poultry or fish 1 egg‡	Select only lean meats; trim away visible fat; broil, roast or poach; remove skin from poultry	Rich sources of protein and magnesium
Nuts, seeds and legumes	3 per week	4–5 per week	1	⅓ cup or 1½ oz nuts 2 Tbsp peanut butter 2 Tbsp or ½ oz seeds ½ cup cooked legumes (dry beans and peas)	Almonds, hazelnuts, mixed nuts, peanuts, walnuts, sunflower seeds, peanut butter, kidney beans, lentils, split peas	Rich sources of energy, magnesium, protein and fiber

(Continued)

TABLE 5.2

Following the DASH Eating Plan (continued)

Food Group	Servings per Day			Serving Sizes	Examples and Notes	Significance of Each Food Group to the DASH Eating Plan
	1,600 Calories	2,000 Calories	2,600 Calories			
Fats and oils§	2	2–3	3	1 tsp soft margarine 1 tsp vegetable oil 1 Tbsp mayonnaise 2 Tbsp salad dressing	Soft margarine, vegetable oil (such as canola, corn, olive or safflower),. low-fat mayonnaise, light salad dressing	The DASH study had 27% of calories as fat, including fat in or added to foods
Sweets and added sugars	0	5 or less per week	≤2	1 Tbsp sugar 1 Tbsp jelly or jam ½ cup sorbet, gelatin 1 cup lemonade	Fruit-flavored gelatin, fruit punch, hard candy, jelly. maple syrup, sorbet and ices, sugar	Sweets should be low in fat

Source: In Brief: Your Guide to Lowering Your Blood Pressure with DASH (nih.gov).

Abbreviations: oz = ounce; Tbsp = tablespoon; tsp = teaspoon.

* Whole grains are recommended for most grain servings as a good source of fiber and nutrients.

† Serving sizes vary between ½ cup and 1¼ cups, depending on cereal type. Check the product's Nutrition Facts label.

‡ Because eggs are high in cholesterol, limit egg yolk intake to no more than four per week; two egg whites have the same protein content as 1 oz of meat.

§ Fat content changes serving amount for fats and oils. For example, 1 Tbsp of regular salad dressing equals one serving; 1 Tbsp of a low-fat dressing equals one-half serving; 1 Tbsp of a fat-free dressing equals zero servings.

in meat. It should be noted that Japanese diets often contain high sodium from soy sauce and have been linked to higher risk of strokes. There are very few studies of Japanese diets, so issues related to CVD prevention remain to be determined.

5.3.8 PRUDENT DIET

In a sense, the diets already discussed in this section, including a low-fat diet, Mediterranean diet, DASH diet and vegetarian diet, all would fit into what AHA has called the "Prudent diet" category. These diets have been routinely shown to lower the risk of CVD.

5.3.9 PLANT-BASED DIETS

There has been a recent increase in evidence and publications concerning "plant-based" diets. Essentially, these diets are defined by an emphasis on plants, including fruits and vegetables. Low-fat diets and low-carbohydrate diets can both be turned into plant-based diets. The Mediterranean diet, DASH diet, vegetarian and Japanese diets are all, in essence, plant-based diets. It should be noted that the health benefits of plant-based diets may vary according to the foods chosen. A recent article compared a "healthy" plant-based diet to an "unhealthy" plant-based diet. The "healthy" plant-based diet resulted in decreased risk of CVD, while the "unhealthy" plant-based diet did not (31).

5.4 INDIVIDUAL FOOD ITEMS

A number of different research studies including RCTs and prospective cohort studies have provided consistent and strong evidence for cardiovascular effects of certain food products in contrast to individual nutrients. Many foods that fit into dietary patterns that have been demonstrated to lower the risk of CVD are listed in this section.

5.4.1 FRUITS AND VEGETABLES

RCTs with diets that emphasize increased consumption of fruits and vegetables have been repeatedly shown to produce substantial improvements in risk factors for CVD, including lipid levels, blood pressure, insulin resistance, inflammatory biomarker levels and weight control (3,4,6,32). These same benefits have not been duplicated with supplements and are not dependent on the dietary macronutrient composition of the diet. These benefits appear to result from phytochemicals and fiber found in fruits and vegetables and potentially increased bioavailability of these nutrients in their natural state as well as replacement of less healthful food in the diet. This is a topic of considerable current research to determine which specific fruits and vegetables are most beneficial to lower CVD risk.

5.4.2 WHOLE GRAINS AND DIETARY FIBER

Whole grains contain the endosperm, bran (the outer layer of the whole grain) and germ in relative proportions as they exist in the intact grain. Refined grains, in contrast, retain only the endosperm (33). Dietary fiber consists of the remnants of edible plant lignin, polysaccharides and associated substances that are resistant to digestion by the human gastrointestinal tract and enzymes (34). There are several types of fiber including the following: insoluble fiber (including cellulose and lignin) which is found in some vegetables, some fruits and whole grains (including wheat germ); and soluble fiber that includes pectin, fruits, guar gum and mucilage (35). Soluble fiber also is found in oat bran and legumes. Eating whole grains decreases total cholesterol by between 7 and 8 mg/dL and low-density lipoprotein cholesterol (LDL-C) levels by 6.9 mg/dL, according to a recent Cochrane analysis.

The National Cholesterol Program (ATP III), AHA and AND all have guidelines including recommendations to increase fiber intake. Whether or not added fiber as a food supplement can similarly lower the risk factor for CVD is controversial.

The U.S. Food and Drug Administration (FDA) has approved the health claim for the soluble fiber from whole oats, whole grain barley products and barley beta fiber (36). The DGA 2020–2025 recommends 25 grams of fiber for adult women and 38 grams for adult men per day. At the current time, Americans are consuming less than half the recommended amounts of fiber.

5.4.3 FISH

Fish and other seafood contain a variety of healthful substances including unsaturated fat, vitamin D, selenium and long-chain omega-3 polyunsaturated fatty acids (PUFAs). Some studies have suggested that fish oil has direct anti-arrhythmic effects, but in individuals with preexisting arrhythmias, findings have been inconsistent (37). Fish oil has been shown to lower triglyceride levels, systolic and diastolic blood pressure, and resting heart rate. Thus, regular fish consumption is associated with lower incidence of CVD and risk of cardiac death (38). This is the reason that the AHA dietary recommendations include the consumption of two fish meals (oily fish) per week. It is not clear whether the benefits of eating fish can be reproduced by consuming fish oil supplements.

5.4.4 NUTS

Nuts, including tree nuts and peanuts, are nutrient-dense foods that are high in unsaturated fats and other bioactive compounds as well as high-quality vegetable protein, fiber, minerals, tocopherols and phytosterols and phenolic compounds. Epidemiologic studies have consistently shown a negative association between nut consumption and CVD risk (39). Numerous research studies have shown that consumption of nuts can lower LDL-C concentration by approximately 10 mg/dL, while not significantly changing high-density lipoprotein cholesterol (HDL-C) levels. Triglycerides have also been shown to be reduced by >20 mg/dL in subjects with elevated blood cholesterol.

5.4.5 MEAT/PROCESSED MEATS

Dietary patterns that include lower consumption of red meat have consistently demonstrated lower CVD risk (40,41). Processed meat consumption has been associated with higher CVD risk. Consumption of red meat and processed meat has also been associated with weight gain, which may increase the risk of CVD.

5.4.6 DAIRY PRODUCTS

Dairy products are rich in minerals such as calcium, potassium, magnesium, protein (caseine and whey) and vitamins (riboflavin and vitamin B_{12}). These products may exert potential benefits by effectively lowering risk for CVD. The presence of saturated fat in full-fat dairy products has raised concerns about potential adverse CVD effects (42). For this reason, most dietary guidelines recommend low-fat dairy products rather than full-fat dairy products.

Low-fat dairy products are also included in the DASH diet as a component to help lower blood pressure (43,44). The DGA 2020–2025 recommends adults consume 3 cups of low-fat milk or the equivalent on a daily basis. This is far greater than the average serving of 1 cup per day currently consumed by adults in the United States. Children and adolescents also consume below recommended levels.

The health effects of other dairy products such as yogurt, cheese and butter are the subjects of considerable research and require further study.

5.4.7 SOY

The protein found in soybeans is typically referred to as "soy" and is often used to replace animal protein in individual diets (44–47). Soybeans are low in saturated fat and contain considerable protein. Soy is the only vegetable to contain all eight amino acids. The effect of soy on CVD risk has been inconsistent.

5.4.8 SUGAR-SWEETENED BEVERAGES

Some epidemiologic studies have suggested that increased consumption of sugar-sweetened beverages increases the risk of heart disease, diabetes and obesity. RCTs have not supported these, however (48,49).

Thus, the effect of sugar-sweetened beverages on CVD risk is controversial. The AHA recommends that adult males consume no more than 150 kcals/day in sugar-sweetened beverages and adult females no more than 100 kcals/day in sugar-sweetened beverages (50). The 2020 Strategic Plan from the AHA recommends no more than 450 kcals/week from sugar-sweetened beverages. The DGAs 2020–2025 recommend no more than 10% of calories from added sugars. This recommendation is mirrored by the FDA. This recommendation is unfortunately exceeded by over 80% of the population in the United States (51).

It should be noted that while the consumption of added sugar has increased the past 40 years in the United States, this increase is relatively less than the increase of the consumption of fats and flour products (51). The consumption of all added sugars decreased from 19% of total calories in 1972 to 17% of total calories in 2010 (52). It should be noted that excessive sugar-sweetened beverages consumption may be an indication of an overall poor-quality diet.

5.4.9   ALCOHOL

Alcohol consumption has been demonstrated in various studies to have both beneficial and adverse cardiovascular outcomes (53–55). Heavy alcohol consumption (three alcoholic drinks/day or more for men and two or more alcoholic drinks/day for women) has been associated with increased risk of cardiomyopathy and higher risk rates of atrial fibrillation (56). Heavy alcohol consumption is also associated with a variety of noncardiac, adverse health consequences, including various abnormalities of the gastrointestinal tract as well as motor vehicle accidents (57). Moderate alcohol consumption in contrast (up to two alcoholic drinks/per day for men and one drink/day for women), has been shown to result in a lower incidence of CVD and diabetes. These effects may be the result of moderate alcohol consumption raising HDL-C or reducing systematic inflammation or, perhaps, improving insulin resistance.

5.4.10   COFFEE AND CAFFEINE

Coffee is consumed throughout the world and is the leading source of caffeine. Other sources of caffeine include tea, cocoa products, cola beverages and "energy drinks" (58). It has been estimated that 80%–90% of adults regularly consume caffeine-containing beverages and food. Coffee consumption has long been suspected of being a contributing factor to development of CVD. However, accumulating data over the past years have suggested no harm, possibly even a protective association, between moderate coffee drinking and CVD mortality (59). A recent study found that individuals with the risk of type 2 diabetes mellitus (T2DM) who consumed four or more cups of coffee a day lowered their risk compared to those who drank less than two cups per day (60).

5.4.11   TEA

Tea is also widely consumed throughout the world. Numerous varieties of teas are available. Most of the tea consumed in Western countries (78%) is black tea and 20% is green tea, which is the most commonly consumed tea in Asian countries, and oolong tea (2%) which is mainly consumed in southern China. Several studies have suggested that tea consumption may protect against the incidence and progression of CVD (61,62).

It has been suggested that tea results in improvement of endothelial function, which results from the interaction between tea components and nitric oxide (NO) (63). This interaction may be a result of polyphenol-like flavonoids known as catechins in the tea, which results in the increased bioavailability of NO that, in turn, plays a significant role in endothelial function and arterial dilation.

5.4.12   EGGS

Over many years, the AHA and other organizations have advised the public to limit egg consumption due to high cholesterol content of egg yolks and the potential association with CVD (64). Subsequent research, however, has demonstrated that dietary cholesterol, in general, and cholesterol in eggs, in particular, have minimal effects on blood cholesterol (65). The DGA Guidelines 2020–2025 have, nonetheless, continued to recommend restriction of dietary cholesterol to less than 300 mg/day (7).

5.4.13 GARLIC

Garlic preparations have been investigated for both prevention and treatment of cardiovascular disease. Long-term observational studies for garlic are not available. The short-term trials on the effect of garlic on risk factors for CVD have shown modest effects appearing to be due from reduction of platelet aggregation (66). The effect on other CVD risk factors is controversial.

5.4.14 CHOCOLATE

Cocoa is similar to green teas with regard to the content of polyphenols. It is, however, important to recognize that chocolate and cocoa are not the same thing (67). While cocoa powder is used in the production of chocolate, fat and sugar are the major components of chocolate, creating a higher caloric content. With the goal of reducing risk factors for CVD, it is more appropriate to potentially recommend cocoa rather than chocolate due to the increased calories from sugar and fat in chocolate.

5.5 NUTRITIONAL SUPPLEMENTS

5.5.1 SALT AND SODIUM

Virtually every heart healthy dietary plan recommends a reduction in sodium (3,4,5,7). Dietary sodium may come in a variety of forms including processed food (a major source of sodium), table salt, snacks, and so on. As dietary sodium increases, so does blood pressure. A number of studies have shown that reduction in salt intake lowers the risk of CVD (68–70). For this reason, the AHA established the interim goal of 2,300 mg/day of sodium and less than 1,500 mg/day for individuals with hypertension, African Americans, and middle-aged or older adults. The current average intake of sodium in the United States is 3.4 g/day. Several studies have suggested that both lower intakes and higher intakes of sodium increase the risk of CVD compared to the current average amount being consumed by Americans (71). Thus, this is an area of controversy.

5.5.2 VITAMIN D

Vitamin D consumption is associated with decreased risk of bone disease in various well-designed studies. Vitamin D may also play a role in a variety of other health issues including lowering the risk of CVD (72). There are insufficient data to recommend increased vitamin D as a strategy for lowering the risk of heart disease.

5.5.3 ANTIOXIDANT VITAMINS E AND C

Initial observational studies suggested that antioxidant vitamins E and C were associated with lower risk of CVD. However, RCTs in this area have been disappointing.

In fact, several studies demonstrated increased mortality from increased vitamin E and C consumption in individuals with late-stage atherosclerosis (73).

5.6 AHA/ACC DIET AND LIFESTYLE RECOMMENDATIONS

In 2021, the AHA summarized diet and lifestyle recommendations in a scientific statement from the AHA Nutrition Committee (3). These recommendations were extended in 2013 with the AHA/ACC Guideline for Lifestyle Management to Reduce Cardiovascular Risk (5). Subsequent studies and research have refined these goals, but the basic framework for the two documents has stood the test of time and will be utilized here as a point of departure. Both of these documents recommend a broader approach to not just diet but also overall healthy lifestyle to reduce risk of cardiovascular disease. The combination of diet and physical activity in particular has been emphasized. The following goals are consistent between the two documents.

5.6.1 CONSUME AN OVERALL HEALTHY DIET

As already indicated in this chapter, this recommendation starts from the premise that we need to focus on overall dietary patterns and away from individual nutrients. This pattern is consistent with the Healthy U.S.-Style Eating Plan, Mediterranean diet and DASH diet, which were discussed in this chapter.

5.6.2 AIM FOR A HEALTHY BODY WEIGHT

The AHA guidelines utilize the framework from the Institute of Medicine to establish a healthy body weight defined as a body mass index (BMI) of 18.5–24.9 kg/m^2. The point of this goal is to recognize that obesity is a risk factor for CVD and is also related to multiple other risk factors for CVD (74–76).

5.6.3 AIM FOR A DESIRABLE LIPID PROFILE

As indicated earlier in this chapter, elevations in total cholesterol and LDL cholesterol are established risk factors for CVD. The following levels of LDL have been defined: optimal (less than 100 mg/dL), near or above optimal (100–129 mg/dL), borderline/high (130–159 mg/dL), high (160–189 mg/dL), and very high (>190 mg/dL) (77). Dietary changes such as following the AHA Healthy Diet Plan are foundational for nutritional approaches to managing total cholesterol and LDL cholesterol.

Triglycerides and HDL cholesterol levels are also related to CVD risk and can be affected by both diet and body weight (78).

5.6.4 AIM FOR A NORMAL BLOOD PRESSURE

As already indicated in this chapter, elevated blood pressure represents a significant risk factor for both CVD and stroke (79). Nutrition plays a significant role in blood pressure control (80). Issues related to nutrition and blood pressure control are discussed in greater detail in Chapter 13.

5.6.5 BE PHYSICALLY ACTIVE

All of the major guidelines for nutritional intervention to reduce CVD also incorporate the recommendation to increase physical activity. Guidelines such as the 2013 AHA/ACC Lifestyle Recommendations, the DGA 2020–2025 as well as the 2006 Nutrition Guidelines from AHA and the Physical Activity Guidelines for Americans (PAGA) 2018 all recommend increased physical activity in addition to heart healthy nutritional plans. These issues are discussed in a number of chapters throughout this book.

The best single source of information related to physical activity and health is found in the PAGA 2018.

5.6.6 AVOID USE AND EXPOSURE TO TOBACCO PRODUCTS

Overwhelming evidence exists from multiple sources that cigarette smoking and the use of tobacco products or exposure to cigarette smoke increase the risks for both CVD and stroke (81). This evidence has been summarized in multiple AHA documents and is discussed in detail in Chapter 7.

5.7 IMPLEMENTING HEART HEALTHY NUTRITION PLANS

A recent emphasis from multiple professional organizations including the AHA has been on developing strategies to help individuals consume a more heart healthy diet. The AHA issued a scientific statement in 2009 entitled "Implementing American Heart Association Pediatric and Adult Nutrition Guidelines" (14). This statement emphasized that nutrition is complex and offered a multilevel framework to implement these factors. This framework started with individual factors but then also moved on to family factors, environmental factors, and finally, macro factors. The goal in this whole initiative is to help with the continuing and difficult problem of encouraging individuals to implement AHA nutrition guidelines.

5.8 SUMMARY/CONCLUSIONS

There is no longer any serious doubt that nutritional practices strongly impact the likelihood of developing CVD. Recent guidelines from various prestigious organizations have all placed nutritional practices in the overall context of positive lifestyle habits and practices. Lifestyle medicine as a discipline offers a promising framework for impacting both nutritional practices and other lifestyle factors that impact the risk of developing CVD. The available nutritional guidance and recommendations are uniform in recommending dietary patterns that include more fruits and vegetables, whole grains, seafood, legumes and nuts, and nonfat dairy products and that include less alcohol (among adults), red meats, processed meats, sugar-sweetened beverages and refined grains, all of which support reduced risk of CVD.

Implementation of these scientific guidelines remains the key challenge that requires the recognition of multiple factors that influence both individual and population-wide nutritional choices.

Clinical Applications

- Plant-based diets from the AHA, the ACC and the DGAs are consistent with each other, so any of these can be followed to lower the risk of heart disease.
- The DASH diet has been shown to effectively lower blood pressure in individuals with hypertension.
- Nutrition plays a key role in lowering the risk of CVD, which should be placed in the context of an overall healthy approach to lowering the risk of CVD, including increasing physical activity, weight management and avoidance of tobacco products.
- Clinicians should routinely recommend that individuals follow diets that are high in fruits and vegetables, whole grains, seafood (particularly oily fish), legumes and nuts, and also nonfat dairy products, and that are lower in red meats, processed meats, sugar-sweetened beverages and refined grains to support reduction in risk of CVD.

REFERENCES

1. World Health Organization on Cardiovascular Disease. www.who.int/health-topics/cardiovascular-diseases#tab=tab_1. Accessed December 1, 2021.
2. Gaziano T, Prabhakaran D, Gazian J. The global burden of cardiovascular disease. In Zipes D, Libby P, Bonow R, Mann D, Tomaselli G, eds. Braunwald's Heart Disease: A Textbook of Cardiovascular Medicine. 11th ed. Amsterdam: Elsevier; 2018.
3. Lichtenstein A, Appel L, Vadiveloo M, et al. AHA scientific statement: 2021 dietary guidance to improve cardiovascular health: A scientific statement from the American Heart Association. Circulation. 2021;144(23):e472–87.
4. Lloyd-Jones DM, Hong Y, Labarthe D, et al. American Heart Association Strategic Planning Task Force and Statistics Committee: Defining and setting national goals for cardiovascular health promotion and disease reduction: The American Heart Association's strategic Impact Goal through 2020 and beyond. Circulation. 2010 February 2;121(4):586–613.
5. Eckel RH, Jakicic JM, Ard JD, et al. 2013 AHA/ACC guideline on lifestyle management to reduce cardiovascular risk: A report of the American College of Cardiology/American Heart Association Task Force on Practice Guidelines. Circulation. 2014;129:S76–99.
6. Mozaffarian D, Appel LJ, Van Horn L. Components of a cardioprotective diet: New insights. Circulation. 2011;123(24):2870–91.
7. U.S. Department of Health and Human Services and U.S. Department of Agriculture. 2020–2025 Dietary Guidelines for Americans. www.dietaryguidelines.gov/sites/default/files/2020-12/Dietary_Guidelines_for_Americans_2020-2025.pdf. Accessed December 15, 2021.
8. Rippe JM, Angelopoulos TA. The Role of Nutrition and Lifestyle in the Prevention and Treatment of Cardiovascular Disease: Nutrition in Lifestyle Medicine. New York: Humana Press; 2017.
9. McGuire S. Institute of Medicine. Accelerating progress in obesity prevention: Solving the weight of the nation. Washington, DC: The National Academies Press. Adv Nutr. 2012(3):708–9.
10. Ford ES, Ajani UA, Croft JB, et al. Explaining the decrease in US deaths from coronary disease, 1980–2000. N Engl J Med. 2007;356:2388–98.

11. Dietary Guidelines for Americans. Report of the 2020 Dietary Guidelines Advisory Committee. www.dietaryguidelines.gov/2020-advisory-committee-report. Accessed December 1, 2021.

12. Rozga M, Handu D. Current systems-level evidence on nutrition interventions to prevent and treat cardiometabolic risk in the pediatric population: An evidence analysis center scoping review. J Acad Nutr Diet. 2021;121(12):2501–23. Epub 2021/01/27.

13. Appel L, Brands M, Daniels S, et al. Dietary approaches to prevent and treat hypertension: A scientific statement from the American Heart Association. Hypertension. 2006;47(2):296–308.

14. Gidding S, Lichtenstein A, Faith M, et al. Implementing American Heart Association pediatric and adult nutrition guidelines: A scientific statement from the American Heart Association Nutrition Committee of the Council on Nutrition, Physical Activity and Metabolism, Council on Cardiovascular Disease in the Young, Council on Arteriosclerosis, Thrombosis and Vascular Biology, Council on Cardiovascular Nursing, Council on Epidemiology and Prevention, and Council for High Blood Pressure Research. Circulation. 2009;119(8):1161–75.

15. Eilat-Adar S, Sinai T, Yosefy C, et al. Nutritional recommendations for cardiovascular disease prevention. Nutrients. 2013(9):3646–83. Epub 2013/09/27.

16. Perk J, de Backer G, Gohlke H, et al. European Guidelines on cardiovascular disease prevention in clinical practice: The Fifth Joint Task Force of the European Society of Cardiology and Other Societies on Cardiovascular Disease Prevention in Clinical Practice (constituted by representatives of nine societies and by invited experts). Eur Heart J. 2012;33:1635–701.

17. de Oliveira Otto M, Mozaffarian D, Kromhout D, et al. Dietary intake of saturated fat by food source and incident cardiovascular disease: The multi-ethnic study of atherosclerosis. Am J Clin Nutr. 2012;96(2):397–404. Epub 2012/07/05.

18. Forouhi N, Koulman A, Sharp S, et al. Differences in the prospective association between individual plasma phospholipid saturated fatty acids and incident type 2 diabetes: The EPIC-InterAct case-cohort study. Lancet Diabetes Endocrinol. 2014;2(10):810–8. Epub 2014/08/12.

19. Nordmann AJ, Nordmann A, Briel M, et al. Effects of low-carbohydrate vs. low-fat diets on weight loss and cardiovascular risk factors: A meta-analysis of randomized controlled trials. Arch Intern Med. 2006;166:285–93.

20. Shai I, Schwarzfuchs D, Henkin Y, Shahar DR, Witkow S, Greenberg I, Golan R, Fraser D, Bolotin A, Vardi H, et al. Weight loss with a low-carbohydrate, Mediterranean, or low-fat diet. N Engl J Med. 2008;359:229–41.

21. Estruch R, Ros E, Salas-Salvadó J, et al. for the PREDIMED Study Investigators. Primary prevention of cardiovascular disease with a Mediterranean diet. N Engl J Med. 2013;368:1279–90.

22. Vardavas C, Linardakis M, Hatzis C, et al. Cardiovascular disease risk factors and dietary habits of farmers from Crete 45 years after the first description of the Mediterranean diet. Eur J Cardiovasc Prev Rehabil. 2010;17:440–6.

23. Sofi F, Abbate R, Gensini G, et al. Accruing evidence about benefits of adherence to the Mediterranean diet on health: An updated systematic review and meta-analysis. Am J Clin Nutr. 2010;92:1189–96, 117.

24. Sacks F, Obarzanek E, Windhauser M, et al. Rationale and design of the Dietary Approaches to Stop Hypertension trial (DASH): A multicenter controlled feeding study of dietary patterns to lower blood pressure. Ann Epidemiol. 1995;5:108–18.

25. Appel L, Champagne C, Harsha D, et al. Effects of comprehensive lifestyle modification on blood pressure control: Main results of the premier clinical trial. JAMA. 2003;289:2083–93.

26. Blumenthal J, Babyak M, Hinderliter A, et al. Effects of the DASH diet alone and in combination with exercise and weight loss on blood pressure and cardiovascular bio-markers in men and women with high blood pressure: The ENCORE study. Arch Intern Med. 2010;170:126–35.

27. Hakala P, Karvetti R. Weight reduction on lactovegetarian and mixed diets: Changes in weight, nutrient intake, skinfold thicknesses and blood pressure. Eur J Clin Nutr. 1989;43:421–30.

28. Barnard N, Cohen J, Jenkins D, et al. A low-fat vegan diet and a conventional diabetes diet in the treatment of type 2 diabetes: A randomized, controlled, 74-wk clinical trial. Am J Clin Nutr. 2009;89:1588S–96S.

29. Burke L, Styn M, Steenkiste A, et al. A randomized clinical trial testing treatment preference and two dietary options in behavioral weight management: preliminary results of the impact of diet at 6 months: PREFER study. Obesity (Silver Spring). 2006;14:2007–17.

30. Key T, Fraser G, Thorogood M, et al. Mortality in vegetarians and non-vegetarians: A collaborative analysis of 8300 deaths among 76,000 men and women in five prospective studies. Public Health Nutr. 1998;1:33–41.

31. Satija A, Bhupathiraju S, Spiegelman D, et al. Healthful and unhealthful plant-based diets and the risk of coronary heart disease in U.S. adults. J Am Coll Cardiol. 2017(4):411–22.

32. Dauchet L, Amouyel P, Hercberg S, et al. Fruit and vegetable consumption and risk of coronary heart disease: A meta-analysis of cohort studies. J Nutr. 2006;136:2588–93.

33. De Moura F, Lewis K, Falk M. Applying the FDA definition of whole grains to the evidence for cardiovascular disease health claims. J Nutr. 2009;139:2220S–6S.

34. Prosky L. When is dietary fiber considered a functional food? Biofactors. 2000;12:289–97.

35. Slavin JL. Position of the American Dietetic Association: Health implications of dietary fiber. J Am Diet Assoc. 2008;108:1716–31.

36. U.S. Food and Drug Administration, H.H.S. Food labeling: Health claims; soluble fiber from certain foods and risk of coronary heart disease: Interim final rule. Fed Regist. 2008;73(37):9938–47. Epub 2008/04/09.

37. Leaf A, Kang JX, Xiao YF, et al. Clinical prevention of sudden cardiac death by n-3 polyunsaturated fatty acids and mechanism of prevention of arrhythmias by n-3 fish oils. Circulation. 2003;107:2646–52.

38. Wang C, Harris W, Chung M, et al. Omega-3 fatty acids from fish or fish-oil supple-ments, but not α-linolenic acid, benefit cardiovascular disease outcomes in primary- and secondary-prevention studies: A systematic review. Am J Clin Nutr. 2006;84:5–17.

39. Sabaté J, Ang Y. Nuts and health outcomes: New epidemiologic evidence. Am J Clin Nutr. 2009;89:1643S–8S.

40. Mente A, de Koning L, Shannon HS, et al. A systematic review of the evidence support-ing a causal link between dietary factors and coronary heart disease. Arch Intern Med. 2009;169:659–69.

41. Micha R, Wallace S, Mozaffarian D. Red and processed meat consumption and risk of incident coronary heart disease, stroke, and diabetes: A systematic review and meta-analysis. Circulation. 2010;121:2271–83.

42. Jakobsen M, O'Reilly E, Heitmann B, et al. Major types of dietary fat and risk of coronary heart disease: A pooled analysis of 11 cohort studies. Am J Clin Nutr. 2009;89:1425–32.

43. Miller E, Erlinger T, Appel L. The effects of macronutrients on blood pressure and lipids: An overview of the DASH and OmniHeart Trials. Curr Atheroscler Rep. 2006;8:460–5.

44. Al-Solaiman Y, Jesri A, Mountford W, et al. DASH lowers blood pressure in obese hypertensives beyond potassium, magnesium and fibre. J Hum Hypertens. 2009;24:237–46.

45. Mozaffarian D, Hao T, Rimm E, et al. Changes in diet and lifestyle and long-term weight gain in women and men. N Engl J Med. 2011;364(25):2392–404.

46. Teff K, Grudziak J, Townsend R, et al. Endocrine and metabolic effects of consuming fructose- and glucose-sweetened beverages with meals in obese men and women: Influence of insulin resistance on plasma triglyceride responses. J Clin Endocrinol Metab. 2009;94(5):1562–69. Epub 2009/02/12.

47. Antar M, Little J, Lucas C, et al. Interrelationship between the kinds of dietary carbohydrate and fat in hyperlipoproteinemic patients. 3. Synergistic effect of sucrose and animal fat on serum lipids. Atherosclerosis. 1970;11(2):191–201. Epub 1970/03/01.

48. Sievenpiper JL, Tappy L, Brouns F. Fructose as a driver of diabetes: An incomplete view of the evidence. Mayo Clin Proc. 2015;90(7):984–8.

49. Kaiser K, Shikany J, Keating K, et al. Will reducing sugar-sweetened beverage consumption reduce obesity? Evidence supporting conjecture is strong, but evidence when testing effect is weak. Obes Rev. 2013;14(8):620–33.

50. Johnson R, Appel L, Brands M, et al. American Heart Association Nutrition Committee of the Council on Nutrition, Physical Activity, and Metabolism and the Council on Epidemiology and Prevention: Dietary sugars intake and cardiovascular health: A scientific statement from the American Heart Association. Circulation. 2009;120:1011–20.

51. Rippe J, Sievenpiper J, Le K-A, et al. What is the appropriate upper limit for sugars consumption? Nutr Rev. 2017;75(1):18–36.

52. US Department of Agriculture, Economic Research Service. Calories average daily per capita calories from the US food supply, adjusted for spoilage and other waste. Loss-Adjusted Food Availability Documentation. www.ers.usda.gov/data-products/food-availability-(per-capita)-data-system/loss-adjusted-foodavailability-documentation.aspx. Updated August 24, 2016. Accessed December 1, 2021.

53. Marmoy M, Brunner E. Alcohol and cardiovascular disease: The status of the U-shaped curve. BMJ. 1991;303:565–8.

54. Ronksley P, Brien S, Turner B, et al. Association of alcohol consumption with selected cardiovascular disease outcomes: A systematic review and meta-analysis. BMJ. 2011;342:d671.

55. Mukamal K, Maclure M, Muller J, et al. Binge drinking and mortality after acute myocardial infarction. Circulation. 2005;112:3839–45.

56. Costanzo S, di Castelnuovo A, Donati MB, et al Cardiovascular and overall mortality risk in relation to alcohol consumption in patients with cardiovascular disease. Circulation. 2010;4:1951–9.

57. Corrao G, Bagnardi V, Zambon A, et al. A meta-analysis of alcohol consumption and the risk of 15 diseases. Prev Med. 2004;38:613–19.

58. Cornelis M, El-Sohemy A. Coffee, caffeine, and coronary heart disease. Curr Opin Lipidol. 2007;18:13–19.

59. De Koning Gans J, Uiterwaal C, van der Schouw Y, et al. Tea and coffee consumption and cardiovascular morbidity and mortality. Arterioscler Thromb Vasc Biol. 2010;30:1665–71.

60. Muley A, Muley P, Shah M. Coffee to reduce risk of type 2 diabetes? A systematic review. Curr Diabetes Rev. 2012;8:162–8.

61. Kuriyama S. The relation between green tea consumption and cardiovascular disease as evidenced by epidemiological studies. J Nutr. 2008;138:1548S–53S.
62. Wang Z, Zhou B, Wang Y, et al. Black and green tea consumption and the risk of coronary artery disease: A meta-analysis. Am J Clin Nutr. 2011;93:506–15.
63. Deka A, Vita J. Tea and cardiovascular disease. Pharmacol Res. 2011;64:36–145. doi:10.1016/j.phrs.2011.02.008.
64. Kritchevsky SB, Kritchevsky D. Egg consumption and coronary heart disease: An epidemiologic overview. J Am Coll Nutr. 2000;19:549S–55S.
65. Jones P. Dietary cholesterol and the risk of cardiovascular disease in patients: A review of the Harvard egg study and other data. Int J Clin Pract. Suppl. 2009;63:28–36.
66. Ackermann R, Mulrow C, Ramirez G, et al. Garlic shows promise for improving some cardiovascular risk factors. Arch Intern Med. 2001;161:813–24.
67. Ding EL, Hutfless SM, Ding X, Girotra S. Chocolate and prevention of cardiovascular disease: A systematic review. Nutr Metab. (Lond.). 2006;3–2.
68. He F, MacGregor G. Effect of modest salt reduction on blood pressure: A meta-analysis of randomized trials: Implications for public health. J Hum Hypertens. 2002;16:761–70.
69. Taylor R, Ashton K, Moxham T, et al. Reduced dietary salt for the prevention of cardiovascular disease. Cochrane Database Syst Rev. 2011;7:CD009217.
70. IOM Committee Report on Sodium Intake in Populations. www.iom.edu/Reports/2013/Sodium-Intake-in-Populations-Assessment-of-Evidence.aspx. Accessed December 1, 2021.
71. O'Donnell M, Mente A, Yusuf S. Sodium and cardiovascular disease. N Engl J Med. 2014;371(22):2137–8. Epub 2014/11/27.
72. Holick M. Evidence-based D-bate on health benefits of Vitamin D revisited. Dermato-Endocrinology. 2012;4:83–90.
73. Bjelakovic G, Nikolova D, Gluud L, et al. Antioxidant supplements for prevention of mortality in healthy participants and patients with various diseases. Cochrane Database Syst Rev. 2012;3:CD007176.
74. Rippe J. Obesity and cardiovascular disease. In Rippe JM, Foreyt JP, eds. Obesity Prevention and Treatment. Boca Raton, FL: CRC Press; 2021.
75. Rippe J, Angelopoulos T. Obesity and heart disease. In Rippe JM, Angelopoulos TA, eds. Obesity: Prevention and Treatment. Boca Raton, FL: CRC Press; 2012.
76. Rashid M, Fuentes F, Touchon R, et al. Obesity and the risk for cardiovascular disease. Prev Cardiol. 2003;6:42–7.
77. Stone N, Robinson J, Lichtenstein A, et al. 2013 ACC/AHA guideline on the treatment of blood cholesterol to reduce atherosclerotic cardiovascular risk in adults: A report of the American College of Cardiology/American Heart Association Task Force on Practice Guidelines. Circulation. 2014;129(25 Suppl 2):S1–45. Epub 2013/11/14.
78. Miller M, Stone N, Ballantyne C, et al. on behalf of the American Heart Association Clinical Lipidology, Thrombosis, and Prevention Committee of the Council on Nutrition, Physical Activity, and Metabolism, Council on Arteriosclerosis, Thrombosis and Vascular Biology, Council on Cardiovascular Nursing, and Council on the Kidney in Cardiovascular Disease. Triglycerides and cardiovascular disease: A scientific statement from the American Heart Association. Circulation. 2011;123:2292–333.
79. Chobanian A, Bakris G, Black H, et al. The seventh report of the Joint National Committee on Prevention, Detection, Evaluation, and Treatment of High Blood Pressure: The JNC 7 Report. JAMA. 2003;289(19):2560–72. Epub 2003/05/16.
80. Whelton PK, Carey RM, et al. 2017 ACC/AHA/AAPA/ABC/ACPM/AGS/APhA/ASH/ASPC/NMA/PCNA guideline for the prevention, detection, evaluation, and

management of high blood pressure in adults: A report of the American College of Cardiology/American Heart Association Task Force on Clinical Practice Guidelines. J Am Coll Cardiol. 2018:71(19):e127–248.

81. The Health Consequences of Smoking: A Report of the Surgeon General. Atlanta, GA. US Department of Health and Human Services, Centers for Disease Control and Prevention, National Center for Chronic Disease Prevention and Health Promotion, Office on Smoking and Health; 2004.

6 Weight Management and Obesity and Cardiovascular Disease

KEY POINTS

- There are multiple, strong linkages between overweight and obesity and risk factors for cardiovascular disease (CVD), in general, and coronary heart disease (CHD), in particular. In addition, obesity is strongly associated with other risk factors for heart disease.
- Obesity is also an independent risk factor for heart disease.
- Obesity is very common in both men and women in the United States.
- A significant weight gain in adult years also increases the risk of CVD.
- Physicians should counsel individuals who are overweight or obese concerning the links between excess weight and risk of CVD.
- Physicians should counsel individuals who are currently at a healthy weight range about the importance of not gaining weight during adult years in order to not increase the risk of CHD.

6.1 INTRODUCTION

Both overweight and obesity are significant risk factors for cardiovascular disease (CVD) (1–10). The American Heart Association (AHA) lists obesity as a major risk factor for CVD because of its association with other risk factors (e.g., diabetes, dyslipidemias, elevated blood pressure, metabolic syndrome, inflammation) and because obesity itself is an independent risk factor.

In addition to the overall increased risk of obesity, distribution of body fat carries additional risk and represents an independent risk factor for coronary heart disease (CHD) over and above obesity (11). The accumulation of intra-abdominal fat appears to produce insulin resistance that can contribute to glucose intolerance, elevated triglycerides, and low HDL as well as high blood pressure.

Recent estimates indicate that the prevalence of overweight and obesity in the United States is over 73%. Estimates of overweight, body mass index (BMI) ≥ 25 to ≥ 30 kg/m², in the United States for adult women is 30% and for adult men is approximately 40%. Estimates for obesity (BMI ≥ 30 kg/m²) are currently 40% for women and approximately 35% for men. The prevalence of severe obesity BMI ≥ 35 kg/m² is approximately 16% (12). The high prevalence of obesity and overweight constitutes a major public health concern because of the relationship of excess body fat to multiple chronic diseases, in general, and CVD, in particular.

DOI: 10.1201/b23245-7   71

Guidelines were published in 2013 by the AHA, American College of Cardiology (ACC) and The Obesity Society (TOS) to help physicians manage obesity (13). These guidelines incorporate five major recommendations including the following:

- Use BMI as a first step in establishing criteria to judge potential health risks.
- Counsel patients that lifestyle changes can produce modest and sustained weight loss and achieve meaningful health benefits, while greater weight loss produces greater benefits.
- Let patients know that multiple dietary therapy approaches to weight loss are acceptable for weight loss. However, the diet should be prescribed to achieve reduced caloric intake.
- Patients who are overweight or obese should be enrolled in comprehensive lifestyle interventions for weight loss delivered in programs of 6 months or longer.
- Advice should be provided to patients who might be contemplating bariatric surgery (BMI $\geq$40 kg/m^2 or BMI $\geq$30 kg/m^2 with obesity-related comorbid conditions).

It should be noted that the key therapeutic modalities to treat weight gain and obesity are uniformly lifestyle based, featuring increased physical activity and sound nutrition. Physicians are often concerned that achieving lasting weight loss is very difficult. There are data, however, to suggest that it is possible. For example, the large National Institute of Diabetes and Digestive and Kidney Diseases–funded Look AHEAD (Action for Health and Diabetes) study showed that individuals who lost 7% of body weight significantly lowered cardiovascular risk factors, except for LDL, and were able to maintain these weight losses for 4 years (14).

6.2 HEMODYNAMICS OF ADIPOSE TISSUE

Research over the past two decades has shown that adipocytes, particularly those in the abdominal region, are highly metabolically active and supplied by an extensive capillary network. While resting blood flow in adipose tissue is considerably less than skeletal muscle, it can increase dramatically after a meal. For example, resting blood flow in adipose tissue is usually on the order of 2–3 mL/minute/hundred grams but may increase up to tenfold after a meal (15,16).

Adipose tissue is a complex endocrine organ that secretes a variety of compounds into the bloodstream that can interact with the cardiovascular system. For example, adipose tissue is a significant source of leptin, adiponectin, insulin-like growth factor-1 (IGF-1), tumor necrosis factor alpha (TNFα), plasminogen activating factor inhibitor-1, lipoprotein lipase and interleukin-6 (IL-6) (17–22).

Studies have shown that approximately 30% of the circulating concentrations of IL-6 originate in adipose tissue (23). This is significant in cardiovascular disease since IL-6 is involved in the modulation of C-reactive protein (CRP) production in the liver, and CRP is a recognized marker for chronic inflammation that can trigger acute coronary syndromes.

6.3 HEMODYNAMIC EFFECTS OF OBESITY

Obesity generates high output or volume overload in the cardiovascular system. Thus, left ventricular filling pressures and volume are higher in individuals who are obese than in lean individuals (24). The total blood volume and cardiac output are also increased (25). The combination of higher loading pressures and increased cardiac output may result in left ventricular dilatation and, ultimately, congestive heart failure. Left atrial enlargement may also occur as a result of left ventricular diastolic dysfunction. Atrial enlargement may also contribute to excess risk of atrial fibrillation in obese individuals (26). Left ventricular hypertrophy is common in long-standing obesity and may contribute to both systemic volume overload and hypertension (27). Many of these hemodynamic issues can be partially ameliorated by weight loss.

6.4 EFFECTS ON LEFT VENTRICULAR FUNCTION

Long-standing obesity increases the risk of left ventricular systolic dysfunction and impaired left ventricular diastolic function (28). Fatty infiltration of the cardiac muscle may further occur and compound these problems.

6.5 OBESITY AND CORONARY HEART DISEASE

Multiple studies have established that obesity correlates with established risk factors for CHD as well as constituting an independent risk. There are well-established relationships between obesity, type 2 diabetes (T2DM), hypertension, and dyslipidemias (particularly elevated triglycerides and diminished HDL) (29). Figure 6.1 shows that the relative risk of all of these relationships increases as BMI increases.

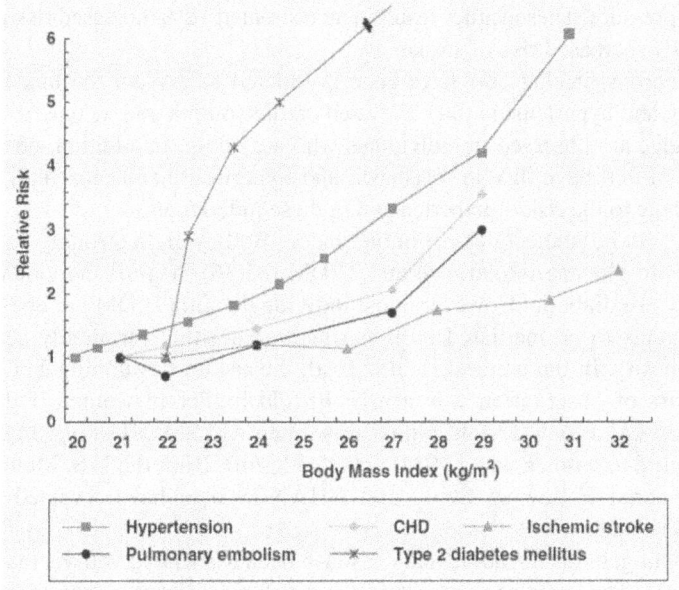

FIGURE 6.1 Relationships between obesity and various chronic conditions and diseases.

In addition to its association with other increased risk factors for CHD, obesity independently increases the risk of CHD. There appears to be a linear relationship over a wide range of BMI values suggesting that individuals, even at average weight at midlife, are at increased risk for CHD compared to leaner individuals. As already indicated, increased abdominal fat ("central obesity") yields an increased risk of CHD that appears to be based on metabolic consequences of the highly metabolically active adipocytes in the abdominal region.

There appears to be a linkage between obesity and the process of atherosclerosis. A number of studies have shown that atherosclerotic processes can be manifest in children as early as 5–10 years old. The process starts with fatty streaks and may result in endothelial cell dysfunction in the vessel wall (30,31). These changes become more complicated as an individual ages. Both fatty streaks and more advanced lesions in one study of individuals 15–30 years old who died from suicide were found in the coronary arteries and were associated with obesity.

6.6   OBESITY AND RISK FACTORS FOR CORONARY HEART DISEASE

- Obesity and hypertension—Observational studies have consistently demonstrated a direct association between weight and blood pressure. The prevalence of hypertension is increased by two to four times in individuals who are obese compared to individuals in the healthy weight range (32,33). It has been estimated that more than one-third of cases of hypertension in the United States are associated with obesity. In addition, weight gain is associated with an increased risk of developing hypertension. A 20-pound weight gain in adulthood is associated with an average 3 mm Hg higher systolic and 2.3 mm Hg higher diastolic blood pressure. These values result in an estimated 12% increased risk of CHD and 24% increased risk of stroke.

   Numerous mechanisms have been postulated to explain the link between obesity and hypertension (34). Elevated cardiac output and increased vascular resistance are observed in individuals who are obese. In addition, obese individuals often have insulin resistance and hyperinsulinemia that may further contribute to the risk of hypertension in these individuals.
- Obesity and diabetes/glucose intolerance—Body weight strongly correlates with both glucose intolerance and T2DM (35,36). Not all individuals with obesity are diabetic. However, most individuals with T2DM are obese. This link seems to be mediated by hyperinsulinemia that frequently accompanies obesity. In the Nurses' Health Trial, the risk of developing T2DM over 16 years of observation was nearly 40-fold higher in women if the BMI was ≥35 kg/m^2 and 20-fold higher in women with a BMI of 30–34.9 kg/m^2 compared to women whose BMI was ≤23 kg/m^2. Both the U.S. Male Health Professional Follow-up Study and NHANES data have revealed similar trends in males.

   Weight gain during adult years has also been associated with increased risk of T2DM. The increase in prevalence of developing diabetes varies from study to study with a 4- to 12-fold increase in individuals who gain 5–20 kg during the adult years. Since approximately 75% of individuals with T2DM die of CHD, the links between obesity and diabetes are particularly worrisome for the development of CHD.

- Obesity and dyslipidemias—A variety of lipid abnormalities are associated with obesity (37,38). These include higher triglyceride levels and lower HDL cholesterol which are related to BMI in both men and women in all age groups. In addition, total cholesterol and LDL cholesterol in both men and women between the ages of 20 and 40 years correlate with BMI. The etiology of these dyslipidemias is complex but may result from the lipolytic nature of the adipocytes, particularly in the abdominal area. Abdominal adipocytes may contribute to higher levels of free fatty acids that are released into the portal circulation and thereby contribute to a wide range of metabolic derangements and hepatic dysfunction leading to a variety of dyslipidemias.

- Obesity and metabolic syndrome—The prevalence of the metabolic syndrome (MetS) has increased dramatically in the United States in the past 30 years. It is now estimated that between 36% and 38% of the adults in the United States have MetS. MetS is a clustering of abnormalities, particularly elevated triglycerides and depressed HDL, glucose intolerance, hypertension and abdominal obesity. MetS represents a significant risk factor for both diabetes and CHD. The NCEP-ATP III Guidelines, in fact, recommend that individuals with metabolic syndrome be treated as though they already have CHD.

- Obesity and vascular disease—A variety of vascular diseases and/or conditions are frequently present in obesity. Pedal edema is common in obesity and may be related to volume overload or elevated left and right ventricular pressures (39). Venous thromboembolism is more common in obese individuals than normal weight individuals, and this may contribute to an increased risk of pulmonary embolism in women with obesity (40).

- Arrhythmias—Individuals who are obese are at increased risk for arrhythmias and sudden cardiac death (41). According to Framingham data, cardiac death risks in men and women with obesity can be as much as 40 times higher than the nonobese population. A prolonged QTc interval is found in approximately 30% of individuals with glucose intolerance or obesity. A prolonged QTc interval has been associated with a variety of cardiac arrhythmias. In addition, an enlarged left atrium may contribute to increased risk of atrial fibrillation in obese individuals. Alterations in the autonomic nervous system such as increased sympathetic tone and increased heart rate have also been associated with increased body weight. Both increase the risk of CHD.

- Inflammation—There is a strong correlation between obesity and markers in inflammation including IL-6 and CRP (42). Some studies have suggested that obesity may be likened to total-body low-grade systematic inflammation. The inflammatory process may, in turn, play a role in multiple cardiac issues and may contribute to endothelial dysfunction and hypertension.

- Sleep apnea—A variety of respiratory conditions may be present in individuals with obesity (43). The most prominent among these conditions is sleep apnea. It has been estimated that 40 million individuals have sleep disorders. The prevalence of these disorders increases substantially in individuals with obesity. Sleep apnea may result in hypertension and increased levels of CRP. Both of these elevate the risk of CHD.

6.7 EFFECTS OF OBESITY TREATMENT ON RISK FACTORS FOR CORONARY HEART DISEASE

- Effects of weight loss on hypertension—Weight loss has been repeatedly demonstrated to lower both systolic and diastolic blood pressure independent of other lifestyle factors (44–46). The National High Blood Pressure Education Program Working Group on Primary Prevention of Hypertension and the Joint National Commission on Prevention, Detection, Evaluation and Treatment of High Blood Pressure (JNC VIII) have both recommended weight loss as a primary therapeutic modality for individuals with obesity and high blood pressure (47). Large, randomized controlled trials of weight reduction utilizing lifestyle measures in adults with high or normal blood pressure have consistently shown that weight loss is the most effective lifestyle modality for lowering blood pressure in individuals who are overweight or obese.

  Reductions in systolic and diastolic blood pressure with weight loss are comparable to many hypertensive agents. Weight loss may also serve as an adjunctive therapy to improve blood pressure control. Postulated mechanisms for the lowering of blood pressure through weight loss include decreased vascular tone, decreased blood volume and decreased adrenergic tone.
- Effects of weight loss on T2DM and glucose intolerance—Multiple trials with T2DM and glucose intolerance have repeatedly shown that intentional weight loss in individuals with obesity, either alone or combined with physical activity, improves both glucose levels and insulin responsiveness (48–50). The U.S. Diabetes Prevention Program (DPP), which was of study of 3,334 men and women between the ages of 25 and 85 years with baseline impaired glucose intolerance (IGT) demonstrated a 58% reduction in the progression of IGT to diabetes in the lifestyle intervention group (49). These individuals lost 5%–7% of their body weight and exercised an average of 30 minutes/day. Similar results were found in the Finnish Diabetes Prevention Study, the Swedish Obese Subject Study (SOS) and the Look AHEAD (Action for Health and Diabetes) trials.
- Effects of weight loss on dyslipidemia—Weight loss has been shown to result in a variety of beneficial effects on lipid profiles. These benefits may be somewhat confounded by nutritional components of lipid management. A meta-analysis of 70 trials utilizing diet alone showed that weight loss resulted in significant decreases in total cholesterol, triglycerides, and LDL cholesterol in individuals with dyslipidemia (51). In addition, significant improvements in HDL

cholesterol were also achieved once individuals achieved stabilized reduced weight. Clinically relevant changes in cholesterol/HDL ratio can occur with weight loss of 5%–10% of initial body weight.

- Cardiopulmonary benefits of weight loss—In addition to reducing risk factors for CHD, intentional weight loss can improve aspects of the physiology of the cardiovascular system in obese individuals. These benefits include potential improvement of left ventricular systolic and diastolic function and reduction of abnormalities of high output (decreased filling pressures in the right and left side of the heart) (52). In addition, shortened QTc intervals and increased heart rate variability have been demonstrated following weight loss in overweight or obese individuals.
- Risks of weight loss—While there are multiple benefits that typically accompany weight loss in individuals with obesity, certain weight loss approaches may result in increased cardiovascular risk (53). For example, very low-calorie diets, liquid protein diets and starvation have all been associated with prolonged QTc interval. In addition, liquid protein diets have been associated with potentially life-threatening arrhythmias based on 24-hour Holter monitoring (54). Some medications for weight loss have resulted in cardiac valve disorders and have been removed from the market, including fenfluramine and dexfenfluramine. Sibutramine has been associated with high blood pressure and should not be utilized in individuals with preexisting hypertension.

6.8 DOES TREATMENT OF OBESITY DECREASE THE RISK OF CORONARY HEART DISEASE?

There currently are less available data on long-term effects of weight loss on CHD rather than on its risk factors. For example, the Look AHEAD trial achieved a reduction in risk factors for CHD but not in CHD itself (55). The Cancer Prevention Study, which is a long-term study of over 750,000 women, demonstrated that obesity-related health conditions such as T2DM and hypertension were reduced in individuals who achieved potential weight loss resulting in a 9% reduction in CHD mortality.

There is currently controversy related to cardiovascular risk related to numerous cycles of weight loss and weight gain (weight cycling) (56). Framingham data suggested that individuals who weight cycle may increase their risk of heart disease. A meta-analysis performed by the National Task Force on Prevention and Treatment of Obesity achieved the opposite conclusion with a finding that weight cycling did not increase the risk of CHD (57).

A number of studies have suggested that abdominal obesity may be particularly affected by weight loss in a positive manner (58–62). This would convey additional decreased risks of CHD following voluntary weight loss.

6.9 THE ROLE OF WEIGHT GAIN AS A RISK FACTOR FOR CHD

As noted earlier in this chapter, adult weight gain dramatically increases the risk of T2DM for adults (63). Adult weight gain also is associated with increased CHD risk independent of obesity. In the Nurses' Health Trial, weight gain between the ages of 18 years and midlife was associated in a linear fashion with increased risk of CHD. Women who gained between 5 and 7.9 kg during this stage of life increased their risk of CHD by 1.25 times. Individuals who gained ≥20 kg increased their risk by 2.65 times. Significant weight gain after age 21 years has also been correlated with increased risk of CHD in men in the U.S. Male Professional Follow-up Study (64).

6.10   CHILDHOOD OBESITY

This chapter does not focus on childhood obesity, per se. But it should be noted that the earliest changes of atherosclerosis may be apparent as early as age 5 years in children with obesity. Moreover, the prevalence of childhood obesity has dramatically increased in the United States as well as risk factors for CHD, T2DM and MetS.

6.11   CLINICAL ASSESSMENT OF INDIVIDUALS WITH OBESITY

- History and physical examination—in addition to those issues discussed in Chapter 3, related to a general history and physical examination focused on CVD, special issues should be particularly emphasized in individuals who are overweight or obese. A weight history should be taken in any individual with obesity to determine at what stage in life weight gain occurred. Physical examination may be difficult in an individual with obesity, and manifestations of cardiovascular pathophysiology may be underestimated. However, certain tests may be particularly valuable in individuals with obesity from a CHD risk factor standpoint.
- Electrocardiogram—The electrocardiogram (ECG) in individuals with obesity may be difficult to interpret because of increased distance between the electrodes and the heart due to excessive pannus (65–66). A variety of changes may also occur in the ECG related to increased obesity. These include low voltage, left access deviation and nonspecific ST and T wave flattening, particularly in the inferior and lateral leads. Dramatic elevation of ST segments may occur because of horizontal displacement of the heart. Voltage criteria for either left atrial abnormality or left ventricular hypertrophy are common findings. False-positive criteria for inferior myocardial infarction may also be present. This is thought to be due to diagrammatic elevations (67).
- Echocardiography—Echocardiography may be useful in individuals with obesity to help ascertain cardiac status (68). Chamber size and wall thickness as well as a variety of left ventricular indices may be derived by echocardiographic means.
- Various imaging techniques to assess CHD may be valuable in patients with obesity, particularly in those who have risk factors for CHD. Due to impaired exercise tolerance, dipyridamole thallium scans may be utilized to evaluate the

presence of ischemic heart disease (69). Esophageal echocardiography may also be useful. If cardiac catheterization is contemplated, the use of a percutaneous radial approach may be most appropriate to minimize the risk of bleeding complications from a femoral approach (70).

6.12   TREATMENT OF OBESITY IN CLINICAL PRACTICE

Physician recommendations for behavioral change have been shown in a number of studies to be a powerful motivator to achieve in significant clinical improvements. In the area of obesity as a risk factor for CVD, medical involvement has been less than optimal. In a survey of 2,000 adults with a BMI ≥25, only 22% of males and 39% of females ever received counseling about their weight (71).

There are many reasons why physician involvement in this important area of risk factor reduction for CHD in individuals with obesity may be lacking. Perhaps physicians underestimate the interaction between obesity and other risk factors for heart disease. Lack of reimbursement from insurance for counseling related to obesity has often been cited as a reason physician do not perform counseling in this area. It has also been argued that physician reluctance to treat obesity results from a lack of demonstrated efficacy for the long-term treatment. Unfortunately, physicians may also share negative stereotyping of obesity as a lack of discipline or willpower. We hope that as scientific understandings for obesity as a chronic disease and a risk factor for CHD continue to evolve, more physicians will become involved in treating obesity to lower the risk of CHD. Here are some suggestions on how to start:

- Vital signs of obesity—One way to start treating obesity it to take the vital signs of obesity. Weight, of course, is important, BMI and waist circumferences, however, are also important variables. More detail on this is found in Chapter 3.
- Counseling for lifestyle management of obesity—Physicians should counsel patients concerning a variety of lifestyle modalities including improved nutrition, increased physical activity and behavioral modification (72). Caloric restriction is a mainstay for the nutritional support of weight loss. Increased physical activity has also been demonstrated to confer multiple benefits for both short- and long-term weight loss. (See Chapter 4). Physical activity is particularly important for maintenance of weight loss and may play an important role in loss of abdominal fat as well as long-term adherence to weight loss strategies.

  Behavioral strategies for weight loss have also been shown to play a positive role in the overall approach to weight loss and maintenance of weight loss. The issue of maintenance of weight loss is often misunderstood in the medical community. In the Look AHEAD and the DPP trial, both have created 90% of maintained weight loss for periods of 2.5 and 40 years. In addition, the National Weight Registry has over 5,000 individuals who have lost a significant amount of weight and kept if off for a year. All of these efforts have shown that individuals who adopt daily strategies for monitoring nutrition and participating in regular physical activity are highly successful in both short- and long-term weight loss.

- Pharmacologic therapy for obesity—A number of pharmacologic modalities are available for the treatment of obesity. A full discussion of these is beyond the scope of this chapter and may be found in multiple sources elsewhere. Pharmaceutical agents should always be used in used in conjunction with lifestyle measures and appear to have synergistic effects when used with these practices.
- Coronary artery disease revascularization procedures in individuals with obesity—Obese individuals tend to have a high percentage of multivessel coronary artery disease but no more severity of disease than normal individuals in one study of heart catheterization. It should be noted that patients with obesity have a higher incidence of multiple postoperative complications following coronary artery bypass grafting (CABG) than lower weight individuals (73). Individuals with obesity are particularly at risk for a thromboembolic disease and should be aggressively treated with venous thrombosis prophylaxis.
- Bariatric surgery—Bariatric surgery has been demonstrated to be highly efficacious for reducing risk factors for CVD and T2DM in individuals with morbid obesity. Indications for bariatric surgery vary from institution to institution but typically involve a BMI of >40 kg/m^2 or ≥ 30 kg/m^2 with other cardiovascular risk factors.

6.13   SUMMARY/CONCLUSIONS

There are multiple, strong and independent links between obesity and CHD. Obesity is also associated with multiple risk factors for CHD, including hypertension, dyslipidemias, T2DM and MetS.

The clustering of risk factors that occurs in obesity-related conditions such as MetS is common in people who develop obstructive atherosclerosis. Weight loss provides an attractive and efficacious option for simultaneously treating multiple risk factors for CHD. Physicians should be aware of the multiple links between obesity and heart disease and emphasize not only treatment itself but how this treatment is associated with reducing cardiac risk factors.

Clinical Applications

- Obesity is associated with multiple other risk factors for CHD including hypertension, dyslipidemias, T2DM and MetS.
- Obesity is an independent risk factor for CHD.
- Clinicians should emphasize to patients with obesity and overweight the linkages between excessive weight and a risk of CHD.
- Abdominal obesity is also particularly linked to increased risk of CHD.
- Clinicians should take time to counsel patients about obesity and include the vital signs of obesity that include not only weight but also BMI and waist circumference as they counsel patients about the links between obesity and heart disease.

REFERENCES

1. Rippe J. Lifestyle medicine: The health promoting power of daily habits and practices. Am J Lifestyle Med. 2018;13:6.
2. Stone N, Robinson J, Lichtenstein A, et al. 2013 ACC/AHA guideline on the treatment of blood cholesterol to reduce atherosclerotic cardiovascular risk in adults: A report of the American College of Cardiology/American Heart Association Task Force on Practice Guidelines. Circulation. 2014;129 (25 suppl 2):S1–S45.
3. Lloyd-Jones D, Hong Y, Labarthe D, et al., American Heart Association Strategic Planning Task Force and Statistics Committee. Defining and setting national goals for cardiovascular health promotion and disease reduction: The American Heart Association's strategic impact goal through 2020 and beyond. Circulation. 2010:121:586–613.
4. U.S. Department of Health and Human Services; U.S. Department of Agriculture. Dietary Guidelines for Americans, 2015–2020. 8th ed. http://health.Gov/dietaryguidelines/2015/guidelines/Published December 2015. Accessed August 26, 2020.
5. Mozaffarian D, Appel L, Van Horn L. Components of a cardioprotective diet: New insights. Circulation. 2011;123:2870–91.
6. Estruch R, Ros E, Salas-Salvadó J, et al.; PREDIMED Study Investigators. Primary prevention of cardiovascular disease with a Mediterranean diet. N Engl J Med. 2013;368:1279–90.
7. Chiuve SE, McCullough ML, Sacks FM, et al. Healthy lifestyle factors in the primary prevention of coronary heart disease among men: Benefits among users and nonusers of lipid-lowering and antihypertensive medications. Circulation. 2006;114:160–7.
8. American Heart Association. Council on Lifestyle and Cardiometabolic Health. https://professional.heart.org/professional/MembershipCouncils/ScientificCouncils/UCM_322856_Council-on-Lifestyle-and-Cardiometabolic-Health.jsp. Accessed September 19, 2018.
9. Eckel R, Jakicic J, Ard J, et al. 2013 AHA/ACC guideline on lifestyle management to reduce cardiovascular risk: A report of the American College of Cardiology/American Heart Association Task Force on Practice Guidelines. Circulation. 2014;129(25 suppl 2):S76–99.
10. Lichtenstein A, Appel L, Vadiveloo M, et al. AHA scientific statement: 2021 dietary guidance to improve cardiovascular health: A scientific statement from the American Heart Association. Circulation. 2021;144(23):e472–87.
11. Despres JP. Abdominal obesity as important component of insulin-resistance syndrome. Nutrition. 1993;9:452–9.
12. National Center for Health Statistics. United States, 2016: With Chartbook on Long-Term Trends in Health. Hyattsville, MD: National Center for Health Statistics; 2017.
13. Jensen M, Ryan D, Apovian C. 2013 AHA/ACC/TOS guideline for the management of overweight and obesity in adults: A report of the American College of Cardiology/American Heart Association Task Force on Practice Guidelines and the Obesity Society. J Am Coll Cardiol. 2014;63(25 pt B):2985–3023.
14. Look AHEAD Research Group. Wing R, Bolin, P. Cardiovascular effects of intensive lifestyle intervention in type 2 diabetes. N Engl J Med. 2013;369:145–54.
15. Lesser G, Deutsch S. Measurement of adipose tissue blood flow and perfusion in man by uptake of 85Kr. J Appl Physiol. 1967;23:621–30.
16. Oberg B, Rosell S. Sympathetic control of consecutive vascular sections in canine subcutaneous adipose tissue. Acta Physiol Scand. 1967;71:47–56.
17. Wajchenberg B. Subcutaneous and visceral adipose tissue: Their relation to the metabolic syndrome. Endocr Rev. 2000:21;697–738.

18. Hotamisligil G, Arner P, Caro J, et al. Increased adipose tissue expression of tumor necrosis factor-alpha in human obesity and insulin resistance. J Clin Invest. 1995;2409–15.
19. Lundgren C, Brown S, Nordt T, et al. Elaboration of type-1 plasminogen activator inhibitor from adipocytes: A potential pathogenetic link between obesity and cardiovascular disease. Circulation. 1996;93:106–10.
20. Yudkin J, Stehouwer C, Emeis J, et al. C-reactive protein in healthy subjects: Associations with obesity, insulin resistance, and endothelial dysfunction: A potential role for cytokines originating from adipose tissue? Arterioscler Thromb Vasc Biol. 1999;19:972–8.
21. Karpe F, Fieding V, Ilie V, et al. Monitoring adipose tissue blood flow in man: A comparison between the xenon washout method and microdialysis. Int J Obes Relat Metab Disord. 2002;(26):1–5.
22. Cigolini M, Targher G, Bergamo A, et al. Visceral fat accumulation and its relation to plasma hemostatic factors in healthy men. Arterioscler Thromb Vasc Biol. 1996;16:368–74.
23. Mohamed-Ali V, Goodrick S, Rawesh A, et al. Subcutaneous adipose tissue releases interleukin-6, but not tumor necrosis factor-alpha, in vivo. J Clin Endocrinol Metab. 1997;82:4196–200.
24. Alpert M. Obesity cardiomyopathy: Pathophysiology and evolution of the clinical syndrome. Am J Med Sci. 2001;321:225–36.
25. Kaltman A, Goldring R. Role of circulatory congestion in the cardiorespiratory failure of obesity. Am J Med. 1976;60:645–53.
26. Sasson Z, Rasooly Y, Gupta R, et al. Left atrial enlargement in healthy obese: Prevalence and relation to left ventricular mass and diastolic function. Can J Cardiol. 1996;12:257–63.
27. Alpert M, Lambert C, Panayiotou H, et al. Relation of duration of morbid obesity to left ventricular mass, systolic function, and diastolic filling, and effect of weight loss. Am J Cardiol. 1995;76:1194–7.
28. Hubert H, Feinleib M, McNamara P, et al. Obesity as an independent risk factor for cardiovascular disease: A 26-year follow-up of participants in the Framingham Heart Study. Circulation. 1983;67:968–77.
29. Bassuk S, Manson J. Lifestyle and risk of cardiovascular disease and type 2 diabetes in women: A review of the epidemiologic evidence. Am J Lifestyle Med. 2008;3:191–213.
30. McGill H Jr. Fatty streaks in the coronary arteries and aorta. Lab Invest. 1968;18:560–4.
31. Skalen K, Gustafsson M, Rydberg E, et al. Subendothelial retention of atherogenic lipoproteins in early atherosclerosis. Nature. 2002;417:750–4.
32. Stamler J. Epidemiologic findings on body mass and blood pressure in adults. Ann Epidemiol. 1999;4:347–62.
33. Fagerberg B, Berglund A, Anderson O, et al. Weight reduction versus antihypertensive drug therapy in obese men with high blood pressure: Effects upon plasma insulin levels and association with changes in blood pressure and serum lipids. J Hypertens. 1992;10:1053–61.
34. Stepniakowski K, Egan B. Additive effects of obesity and hypertension to limit venous volume. Am J Physiol. 1995;268:R562–8.
35. Mokdad A, Ford E, Bowman B, et al. Prevalence of obesity, diabetes, and obesity-related health risk factors. 2001; JAMA 2003:289(1):76–9.
36. Field A, Coakley E, Must A, et al. Impact of overweight on the risk of developing common chronic diseases during a 10-year period. Arch Intern Med. 2001;161(13):1581–6.
37. Denke M, Sempos C, Grundy S. Excess body weight: An unrecognized contribution to high blood pressure cholesterol levels in White American women. Arch Intern Med. 1993;153:1093–103.

38. Denke M, Sempos C, Grundy S. Excess body weight: An unrecognized contribution to high blood pressure cholesterol levels in White American women. Arch Intern Med. 1994;154:401–10.

39. Nakajima T, Fujioka S, Tokunaga K, et al. Correlation of intraabdominal fat accumulation and left ventricular performance in obesity. Am J Cardiol. 1989;64:369–73.

40. Hansson P, Eriksson H, Welin L, et al. Smoking and abdominal obesity: Risk factors for venous thromboembolism among middle-aged men: The study of men born in 1913. Arch Intern Med. 1999;159:1886–90.

41. Kannel W, Plehn J, Cupples L. Cardiac failure and sudden death in the Framingham Study. Am Heart J. 1988;115:869–75.

42. Peterson H, Rothschild M, Weinberg C, et al. Body fat and the activity of the autonomic nervous system. N Engl J Med. 1988;318:1077–83.

43. Strollo P, Rogers R. Obstructive sleep apnea. N Engl J Med. 1996;334:99–104.

44. Stamler R, Stamler J, Gosch F, et al. Primary prevention of hypertension by nutritional-hygienic means: Final report of a randomized, controlled trial. JAMA. 1989;262:181–1807.

45. Hypertension Prevention Trial Research Group. The hypertension prevention trial: Three year effects of dietary changes on blood pressure. Arch Intern Med. 1990;150:153–62.

46. Trials of Hypertension Prevention Collaborative Research Group. The effects of non-pharmacologic interventions on blood pressure of persons with high normal levels: Results of the trials of hypertension prevention, phase I. JAMA. 1992;267:1213–20.

47. National High Blood Pressure Education Program Working Group: National High Blood Pressure Education Program Working Group. Report on primary prevention of hypertension. Arch Intern Med. 1993;153:186–208.

48. Katzel L, Bleeker E, Colman E, et al. Effects of weight loss vs aerobic exercise training on risk factors for coronary heart disease to healthy, obese, middle-aged and older men. JAMA. 1995;274:915–1921.

49. Knowler W, Barrett-Connor E, Fowler SE, et al. Reduction in the incidence of type 2 diabetes with lifestyle intervention or metformin. N Engl J Med. 2002;346(6):393–403.

50. Tuomilehto J, Lindstrom J, Eriksson JG, et al. Prevention of type 2 diabetes mellitus by changes in lifestyle among subjects with impaired glucose tolerance. N Engl J Med. 2001;344(18):1343–50.

51. Dattilo A, Kris-Etherton P. Effects of weight reduction on blood lipids and lipoproteins: A meta-analysis. Am J Clin Nutr. 1992;56:320–8.

52. Himeno E, Nishino K, Nakashima Y, et al. Weight reduction regresses left ventricular mass regardless of blood pressure level in obese subjects. Am Heart J. 1996;131:313–19.

53. Isner J, Sours H, Paris A, et al. Sudden, unexpected death in avid dieters using the liquid-protein-modified fast diet: Observations in 17 patients and the role of the prolonged QT interval. Circulation. 1979;60:1401–12.

54. Pringle T, Scobie I, Murray R, et al. Prolongation of the QT interval during therapeutic starvation: A substrate for malignant arrhythmias. Int J Obes. 1983;7:253–61.

55. Ryan D, Espeland M, Foster G, et al. Look AHEAD (Action for Health in Diabetes): Design and methods for a clinical trial of weight loss for the prevention of cardiovascular disease in type 2 diabetes. Control Clin Trials. 2003;24(5):610–28.

56. Hamm P, Shekelle R, Stamler J. Large fluctuations in body weight during young adulthood and 25 year risk of coronary death in men. Am J Epidemiol. 1989;129:312–18.

57. National Task Force on the Prevention and Treatment of Obesity. Weight cycling. JAMA. 1994:272:1196–202.

58. Despre J. Dyslipidemia and obesity. Balliere Clin Endocrinol Met. 1994:8:629–60.

59. Despres J. Abdominal obesity as important component of insulin-resistance syndrome. Nutrition. 1993;4:452–9.

60. Ford E, Giles W, Dietz W. Prevalence of the metabolic syndrome among U.S. adults: Findings from the third National Health and Nutrition Examination Survey. JAMA. 2002;287(3):356–9.
61. Poirier P, Despres J. Waist circumference, visceral obesity, and cardiovascular risk. J Cardiopulm Rehabil. 2003;23:161–9.
62. Hansen B. The metabolic syndrome X. Ann NY Acad Sci. 1999;892:1–24.
63. Willett W, Manson J, Stampfer M, et al. Weight, weight change, and coronary heart disease in women: Risk within the "normal" weight range. JAMA. 1995;273(6):461–5.
64. Rexrode K, Hennekens C, Willett W, et al. A prospective study of body mass index, weight change, and risk of stroke in women. JAMA. 1997;227:1539–45.
65. Eisenstein I, Edelstein J, Sarma R, et al. The electrocardiogram in obesity. J Electrocardiol. 1982;15:115–18.
66. Master A, Oppenheimer E. A study of obesity: Circulatory, roentgen-ray and electro-cardiographic investigations. JAMA. 1929;92:1652–6.
67. Alpert M, Terry B, Cohen M, et al. The electrocardiogram in morbid obesity. Am J Cardiol. 2000;85:908–10.
68. Alpert M, Kelly D. Value and limitations of echocardiography assessment of obese patients. Echocardiography. 1986;3:261–72.
69. Ferraro S, Perrone-Filardi P, Desiderio A, et al. Left ventricular systolic and diastolic function in severe obesity: A radionuclide study. Cardiology. 1996;87:347–53.
70. McNulty P, Ettinger S, Field J, et al. Cardiac catheterization in morbidly obese patients. Catheter Cardiovasc Interv. 2002;56:174–7.
71. X-Factor Study. New York: Louis Harris and Associates, Inc.; 1997.
72. Lem M, Wing R, McGuire M, et al. A descriptive study of individuals successful at long-term maintenance of substantial weight loss. Am J Clin Nutr. 1997;66:239–346.
73. Gruberg L, Weissman J, Waksman R, et al. The impact of obesity on the short-term and long-term outcomes after percutaneous coronary intervention: The obesity paradox? J Am Coll Cardiol. 2002;39–578–84.

7 Lifestyle Medicine
Tobacco Cessation and Cardiovascular Disease

KEY POINTS

1. Cigarette smoking is the single most important risk factor for coronary artery disease. While cigarette smoking prevalence has decreased in the last 40 years, over 15% of individuals in the United States still smoke cigarettes.
2. A variety of counseling programs and strategies are available to help people quit smoking.
3. There are seven approved pharmaceutical therapies available to help with smoking cessation.
4. A combination of pharmaceutical therapy and counseling has been shown to be most effective in cigarette smoking cessation.
5. Other lifestyle interventions such as regular exercise may play important roles as adjuncts to therapy to begin smoking cessation.

7.1 INTRODUCTION

Smoking is the leading preventable cause of death and disease in the United States and the single most important risk factor for coronary heart disease (CHD). Over 20 million premature deaths are attributable to smoking exposure and secondhand smoke in the United States, as documented in the 2014 Surgeon General's Report (1).

Most of the deaths have occurred among those with a history of smoking, but 2.5 million are among nonsmokers who died from diseases caused from exposure to secondhand smoke (2). Despite years of decline in the prevalence of smoking, cigarette consumption still accounts for approximately 480,000 deaths from smoking-related diseases in the United States each year. Smoking causes 32% of CHD deaths. Despite the untold health misery, smoking attributable costs are also extremely high. The annual smoking attributable economic costs from 2009 to 2012 are over 300 billion dollars, including direct healthcare expenditures and loss of productivity.

More than 6 million deaths worldwide can be attributed to smoking each year. In high-income countries like the United States, significant strides have been made to reduce smoking prevalence in certain segments of the population, but there are some areas where efforts have been minimal. One area that may be particularly important is the change in the *Diagnostic and Statistical Manual of Mental Disorders–Fifth Edition (DSM-5)* that added tobacco use disorder as a psychiatric diagnosis in 2013 (2). This properly aligns cigarette smoking with other substance use disorders. Moreover, this diagnosis should help accurately identify those who are most at risk

DOI: 10.1201/b23245-8

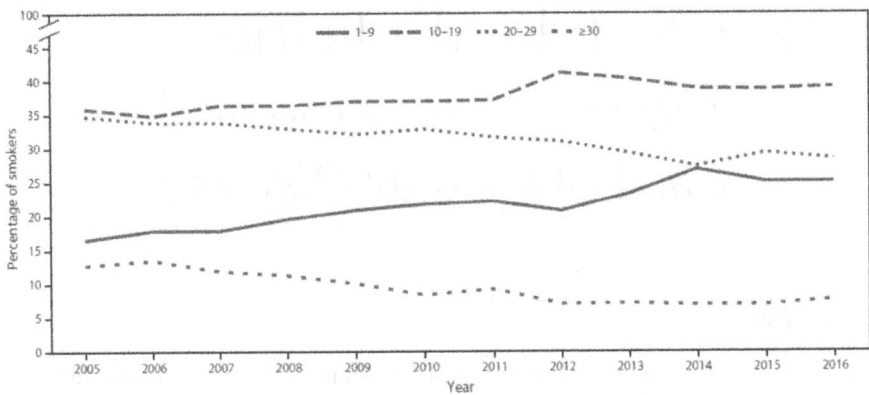

FIGURE 7.1 Percentage of daily smokers* aged ≥18 years who smoked 1–9, 10–19, 20–29, and ≥30 cigarettes per day – National Health Interview Survey, United States, 2005-2016. *Persons who had smoked ≥100 cigarettes during their lifetime and reported smoking cigarettes every day at the time of interview. (Jamal A, Phillips E, Gentzke, AS, et al. Current Cigarette Smoking Among Adults–United States, 2016. MMWR Morb Mortal Wkly Rep. 2018;67:53–59.)

for the negative consequences of use, identify those who need active intervention and inform treatment recommendations concerning what type or dose of treatment is needed.

The prevalence of adult smoking cigarettes declined to 15.5% in 2019 compared to 42% in 1965 (3). While this is good news, the decline in smoking prevalence has slowed recently. This is depicted in Figure 7.1.

Large disparities exist in tobacco use across racial and ethnic groups and also between groups defined by educational level, socioeconomic status and region. The prevalence of cigarette smoking is lowest among non-Hispanic Asians (9.5%) and highest among Hispanic American Indians and Alaskan Natives (19.2%) (4). The prevalence is much higher among those reporting a General Education Development certificate (43.0%) as well those living below the federal poverty line (26.3%) and those receiving Medicaid or who are uninsured (28%).

The U.S. Healthy People 2020 initiative aimed to reduce the national prevalence of cigarette smoking among adults to 12% (5). As already indicated, the consumption of tobacco products is high and increasing globally with almost 80% of the world's 1 billion smokers living in lower- or middle-income countries.

7.2 HEALTH CONSEQUENCES OF SMOKING

The negative health effects that result from cigarette smoking are very clear. Cigarette smoke contains more than 7,000 chemical compounds and harms nearly every organ in the body. As already indicated, smoking is a major cause of cardiovascular disease (CVD), stroke, periodontitis, aneurysms, pneumonia, chronic obstructive pulmonary disease (COPD), asthma, erectile dysfunction and low bone mineral density (6).

Cigarette smoking is also implicated in a variety of cancers including cancer of the lung, bladder, cervix, oral cavity, larynx, esophagus, stomach, kidney, uterus and pharynx. Cigarette smoking has additional adverse effects on early childhood and reproductive health.

More than 16 million Americans are living with a disease caused by smoking. In addition to the more than 480,000 deaths per year (approximately 1,300 each day) caused by cigarette smoking, it is estimated that there are 41,000 deaths each year resulting from secondhand smoke (7). Thus, cigarette smoking causes multiple adverse health consequences. Although in this chapter, we focus mostly on issues related to smoking and CVD.

7.3   SMOKING AND CVD

Landmark studies in the 1950s first reported a strong positive association between cigarette smoking exposure and CVD. These data have been consistently documented in studies since that time and are summarized in multiple Surgeon Generals' Reports. In 1989, the Surgeon General's Report showed that smoking doubles the incidence of CHD and increases CHD mortality by 50% (8). These risks increase with age and number of cigarettes smoked. In addition to myocardial infarction (MI), cigarette consumption directly relates to increased risks of sudden death, aortic aneurysm formation, symptomatic peripheral vascular disease and ischemic stroke. Continued smoking is a major risk factor for recurrent MI and adverse clinical outcomes in patients undergoing coronary artery bypass grafting (CABG) or percutaneous coronary intervention (PCI) (9). Passive smoking exposure can cause endothelial dysfunction as well as increased bronchial responsiveness and pulmonary dysfunction. There is no safe level of secondhand tobacco smoke.

Cigarette smoking causes unfavorable effects on blood pressure and a reduction in myocardial oxygen supply and also contributes to the pathogenesis of atherothrombosis by a variety of other mechanisms including compromised endothelium and impaired vasodilatation. Smoking has inflammatory effects including increasing level of C-reactive protein (CRP). There is evidence now to suggest that insulin resistance caused by cigarette smoking may also be linked to premature atherosclerosis.

Smokers lose at least one decade of life expectancy compared to never smokers. Women's risk of CVD from smoking have risen sharply over the last 50 years and are now equivalent to those of men. Smoking also acts synergistically with oral contraceptives, making young female smokers who take oral contraceptives particularly at elevated risk for premature CHD, stroke and venovenous thromboembolism. Smoking is particularly hazardous to individuals with diabetes.

7.4   RATES OF SMOKING CESSATION

The risk and severity of many diseases caused by smoking are directly related to how long the smoker has smoked and the number of cigarettes smoked per day. It is beneficial to quit smoking at any age. After quitting, the risk of heart attack drops sharply in just 1 year (6). Stroke risk can fall to about the same as that of nonsmokers after 2–5 years, and risk of cancer of the mouth, throat, esophagus and bladder are all cut in half after 5 years. The risk of dying of lung cancer drops by half after 10 years.

Recent studies have suggested that 68.0% of current smokers would like to stop smoking and 55.4% made a quit attempt in the past year. However, only 7.4% were able to quit for more than 6 months over the past year. In general, cessation rates are higher among those who participate in a smoking cessation program compared to those who try to quit without assistance. Unfortunately, between 2000 and 2015, less than one-third of U.S. smokers used evidence-based cessation methods while trying to quit smoking.

7.5 INTERVENTIONS FOR SMOKING CESSATION

7.5.1 PHARMACEUTICAL AIDS

Modern approaches to pharmaceutical therapy for smoking cessation take into account the addictive nature of this habit. The combination of behavioral counseling and medication has been shown to be more effective than either treatment modality alone (10,11). The most recent estimate shows that just about 29% of smokers attempted to quit using any kind of medication, and only 6.8% utilized counseling. It is important to recommend that smokers wishing to quit seek some kind of behavioral support and some type of medicine (unless medically contraindicated). A clarification of medications that are often utilized are listed in the next paragraph.

There are seven U.S. Food and Drug Administration (FDA) approved first-line medications shown to be helpful for increasing long-term smoking abstinence rates. These include over-the-counter (OTC) products (nicotine gum, nicotine lozenges, and the nicotine patch) and prescription-only medications (nicotine nasal spray, nicotine inhaler, sustained release bupropion and varenicline) (12). When used properly, these nicotine replacement therapies (NRTs) can significantly reduce nicotine withdrawal and have been shown to increase the rate of quitting by 50%–70%. Bupropion is an antidepressant, and it has been shown to be an effective medication for smoking cessation. It appears to reduce withdrawal symptoms and decrease nicotine's rewarding effects by blocking the reuptake of norepinephrine and dopamine in the mesolimbic system and nucleus accumbens. These are key areas for nicotine reinforcement.

Varenicline has been shown to triple abstinence rates for smokers when compared to an unassisted quit attempt. Varenicline attenuates the rewarding effects of nicotine, and it can reduce the symptoms of nicotine withdrawal. It is important to note that these medications can have side effects that range from dry mouth to more serious side effects such as lowering seizure threshold, and many of them have not been extensively studied in certain subpopulations of smokers (e.g., adolescents). More studies about how best to combine these medications with counseling strategies are urgently needed.

7.5.2 BEHAVIORAL SMOKING CESSATION STRATEGIES

A variety of scientific and community resources have been used to explore ways to reduce tobacco use and increase smoking cessation (12). Some of these strategies have been conducted at the population level (e.g., government-based initiatives and media-based campaigns). Others have targeted individual-level interventions. Regardless of their classification, the programs attempt to provide smokers with the information and behavioral skills thought to be necessary to achieve not only initial cessation but sustained abstinence.

7.5.3 COUNSELING AND THERAPY-BASED APPROACHES

7.5.3.1 Individual Counseling

Face-to-face counseling is a well-established method for delivering smoking cessation treatment. This type of intervention can be delivered by practitioners with varying levels of education and training and can be done in different formats for different lengths of time. Individual counseling has been shown to increase the likelihood of quitting smoking by 40%–60% when compared to less-intensive treatments.

7.5.3.2 Group Therapy

Smoking cessation intervention in a group format has been used for many years and remains popular. This has a special benefit of allowing individuals the unique opportunity to learn about challenges other smokers face when trying to quit.

Existing data indicate that smokers have a 50%–130% greater chance of quitting in a group when compared to just using self-help materials.

7.5.3.3 Phone Counseling

One benefit of phone counseling is that it can be used as a substitute for face-to-face contact and thereby reach a large number of smokers at a much lower cost. This can be done either proactively or reactively. Reactive phone counseling occurs when a smoker calls a quit-line such as 1–800-QUIT-NOW. When individuals call a reactive quit-line, this can then be followed up with materials being sent to the individual.

Current data suggest that individuals who call a quit-line significantly increase abstinence for up to 9 months, but long-term studies are not available.

7.5.3.4 Motivational Interviewing

Motivational interviewing has been available since the 1980s as a treatment for various substance abuse disorders. It is an individually administered, client-centered counseling approach to elicit behavior change by helping individuals explore and resolve ambivalence. The first study to use motivational interviewing for nicotine dependence was published in 1998, and since then, over 30 trials have been published. It appears to be efficacious for smoking cessation across a wide array of patients and is within the range of other behavioral treatments for nicotine dependence.

Motivational interviewing may be ideal for those with low levels of nicotine dependence, low motivation to quit, or younger smokers or those who have medical comorbidities.

7.6 SMOKING CESSATION IN MEDICAL SETTINGS

Smoking is more common in a variety of medical populations than the public at large. For example, smoking rates among patients with heart disease, COPD, and stroke are at least 10% greater than the general population. Cessation after such problems can still make a major impact on reducing morbidity and mortality. For example, stopping smoking after a myocardial infarction (MI) increases the risk of 2-year mortality by up to 46%. Thus, smoking cessation in medical populations can function as an important secondary prevention intervention.

One framework that has been effective for brief medical visits for counseling and smoking cessation utilizes the "5 As" smoking cessation framework (Ask, Advise, Assess, Assist and Arrange). This framework calls for all clinicians to assess smoking status at each visit (i.e., Ask) followed by providing strong personal advice on quitting (Advise). The discussion then moves to the patient's willingness to make a cessation attempt at this time (i.e., Assess). For individuals who are ready to quit, the clinician can "Assist" in ways such as developing a quit plan, prescribing pharmacotherapy, and so on. The final step in the "5 As" framework is "Arrange," which is utilized to reinforce cessation and encourage another quit attempt if the patient has relapsed.

7.6.1 Primary Care Visits

Over 70% of smokers see some type of a primary care provider (PCP) each year. Thus, primary care–based cessation interventions can reach most smokers. About 20% of smokers in primary care are willing to make a serious quit attempt. However, PCPs can use a targeted approach utilizing the "5 As" framework to help assist cessation. In addition, PCPs may be able to refer smokers to an in-house provider for continued services.

7.6.2 Inpatient Hospitalization

When individuals are hospitalized for another cause, this may represent a "teachable moment" when the health effects of smoking are top of mind and patients are more likely to accept cessation treatment. In addition, U.S. hospitals are now smoke-free, so regardless of whether or not an individual desires to quit, they will experience temporary abstinence. Counseling interventions described earlier in this chapter can also be used in an inpatient setting.

Recent reports have suggested that tobacco use patterns are changing, including the increasing use of other products such as electronic cigarettes and hookahs. These are typically still low in prevalence (4%–5%); however, among high school students, up to 16% use e-cigarettes. No form of smoking is safe.

Currently good data are not available to assess long-term patterns of e-cigarette smoking. The U.S. Preventive Services Task Force (PSTF) has concluded that current evidence is insufficient to recommend electronic nicotine delivery systems for tobacco cessation in adults (13). In 2016 the U.S. Food and Drug Administration extended the agency's regulatory authority to all tobacco products including e-cigarettes and hookahs (water pipes) and required manufacturers to report ingredients and undergo agency premarket review to achieve marketing authorization (14). In addition, food-flavored e-cigarettes have been banned in many locations (15).

7.7   COMMUNITY-BASED PROGRAMS

The following sections present community-based programs addressing the topic of smoking (12).

7.7.1   MASS MEDIA CAMPAIGNS

Many smokers worldwide still underestimate the full extent of the risk to themselves and others. Mass media, which includes television, film, internet, radio, newspapers, magazines, billboards and cigarette packaging, can play a key role in shaping smoking-related knowledge, attitudes and behaviors. Studies have shown that mass market attempts have yielded an increase in the number of calls to telephone quit-lines.

7.7.2   WORKSITE PROGRAMS

Nearly 25% of full-time and part-time workers smoke. These individuals generate increased healthcare costs and disability, greater absenteeism, poorer job performance and an increased risk of injury. This has led employers to become motivated to provide support for effective worksite smoking cessation programs. One advantage of such a worksite program is access to a large, stable population and potential for high participation and compliance as well as a socially reinforcing network and positive atmosphere.

7.8   TECHNOLOGY-DRIVEN APPROACHES

Individuals who use the internet in the United States may potentially be offered an emerging opportunity to participate in innovative smoking cessation programs. Approximately 88% of the population uses the internet. Internet-based services have the advantage of potentially providing smokers with an option of finding information any day or time that they choose. There is some evidence that suggests that interactive and internet-based interventions with or without behavioral support are moderately more effective than assessment-only or waitlist control conditions when compared to print-based interventions. This is an area of active research.

It is estimated that 95% of the U.S. population owns a cell phone, and 77% own a smartphone. There is currently research in progress examining the efficacy of using text message interventions on smartphones for smoking cessation. These utilize messages that are similar to face-to-face smoking cessation support. More research is needed to determine whether sustained smoking cessation effects can be achieved by utilizing this technology.

7.9   OTHER LIFESTYLE MEDICINE APPROACHES

7.9.1   EXERCISE

Other lifestyle approaches in combination with smoking cessation counseling have been utilized and appear to be effective. For example, the U.S. Department of Health and Human Services currently promotes using exercise as an aid to quit smoking, and many studies have shown that exercise is effective as an adjunct treatment. There is some evidence that exercise can reduce nicotine cravings; however, the majority of studies have not shown stronger consistent effects. Ongoing research is needed to test exercise as an explicit strategy that a smoker can use to quit.

7.9.2 ABRUPT QUITTING VERSUS GRADUAL REDUCTION

A traditional behavioral method used in smoking cessation is to determine a "quit day" and then abruptly stop using all cigarettes. An alternative approach that has gained some support is to gradually reduce the number of cigarettes smoked before quitting entirely. This latter approach could potentially reduce withdrawal symptoms and increase self-efficacy for quitting and reduce the likelihood of relapse. The value of one approach versus the other remains controversial in terms of long-term success of smoking cessation.

7.10 SUMMARY/CONCLUSIONS

Cigarette smoking remains the single most significant lifestyle risk factor for CVD. There is an urgent need to reduce cigarette smoking in the United States and around the world. A range of approaches and strategies are discussed in this chapter. Thus, smokers should be matched with a cessation program based on their individual preference and should be incorporated in medical systems and community-based organizations as well as individual counseling. Smoking cessation is the most important of all the lifestyle-related risk factors for CVD; while the others are also very important, strong attention must be paid to cigarette smoking cessation.

Clinical Applications

- Smoking is the leading preventable cause of death and disease in the United States and the single most important risk factor for CHD.
- Smoking cessation yields multiple short-term benefits.
- Smokers who quit reduce their excess risk of a coronary event by 50% within the first 2 years of cessation.
- The risk of former smokers developing CHD becomes equivalent to the risk of never-smokers after 3–5 years.
- A variety of pharmaceutical agents in combination with counseling has been shown to be highly effective for smoking cessation.
- Other lifestyle interventions such as regular exercise carry considerable promise as adjuncts to smoking cessation programs.

REFERENCES

1. U.S. Centers for Disease Control and Prevention. The Health Consequences of Smoking: 50 Years of Progress: A Report of the Surgeon General. Atlanta, GA. 2014.
2. Creamer MR, Wang TW, Babb S, et al. Tobacco product use and cessation indicators among adults: United States, 2018. MMWR Morb Mortal Wkly Rep. 2019;68:1013–19. http://dx.doi.org/10.15585/mmwr.mm6845a2external icon.

3. Jamal A, Phillips E, Gentzke AS, et al. Current cigarette smoking among adults: United States, 2016. MMWR Morb Mortal Wkly Rep. 2018;67:53–9.
4. Centers for Disease Control and Prevention. Current cigarette smoking among adults: United States, 2011. MMWR Morb Mortal Wkly Rep. 2012;61(44):889–94. Epub 2012/11/09.
5. Jamal A, Homa DM, O'Connor E, et al. Current cigarette smoking among adults: United States, 2005–2014. MMWR Morb Mortal Wkly Rep. 2015;64(44):1233–40. Epub 2015/11/13.
6. Centers for Disease Control and Prevention. Healthy People 2020. Healthy People-Healthy People; 2020. cdc.gov. Accessed December 10, 2021.
7. Jha P, Ramasundarahettige C, Landsman V, et al. 21st-century hazards of smoking and benefits of cessation in the United States. N Engl J Med. 2013;368(4):341–50.
8. Gaziano TA, Prabhakaran D, Gaziano JM. Global burden of cardiovascular disease. In Braunwald's Heart Disease. 11th ed. Zipes, Libby, Bonow, Mann, Tomaselli. Amsterdam: Elsevier; 2019.
9. Windom RE, Mason JO, Koop CE. The Surgeon General's 1989 report on reducing the health consequences of smoking: 25 years of progress: Executive summary. MMWR Morb Mortal Wkly Rep. 1989;38(S2):i-32. www.jstor.org/stable/24246143. Accessed December 15, 2021.
10. Zhang YJ, Iqbal J, van Klaveren D, et al. Smoking is associated with adverse clinical outcomes in patients undergoing revascularization with PCI or CABG: The SYNTAX trial at 5-year follow-up. J Am Coll Cardiol. 2015;65(11):1107–15. Epub 2015/03/21.
11. U.S. Centers for Disease Control and Prevention. The Guide to Community Preventive Services, Reducing Tobacco Use and Secondhand Smoke Exposure. www.cdc.gov/. Accessed December 15, 2021.
12. Stead LF, Perera R, Bullen C, et al. Nicotine replacement therapy for smoking cessation. Cochrane Database Syst Rev. 2012;11:CD000146. Epub 2012/11/16.
13. Ciccolo JT, SantaBarbara NJ, Busch AM. Behavioral approaches to enhancing smoking cessation. In Rippe JM, ed. Lifestyle Medicine. 3rd ed. Boca Raton, FL: CRC Press; 2019.
14. U.S. Preventive Services Task Force. Home page. uspreventiveservicestaskforce.org. Accessed December 15, 2021.
15. Abbasi J. FDA extends authority to e-cigarettes: Implications for smoking cessation? JAMA. 2016;316(6):572–4. Epub 2016/07/16.

8 Psychiatric and Behavioral Aspects of Cardiovascular Disease

KEY POINTS

- Both acute and chronic stress are associated with increased risk of cardiovascular disease (CVD).
- Stress reduction/mind-body techniques can be very effective in helping individuals reduce stress in their daily lives.
- A variety of psychiatric disorders are also associated with CVD, including depression, anxiety and post-traumatic stress disorder.
- Several personality traits such as anger and hostility are also associated with CVD.
- Lifestyle medicine therapies such as stress reduction and regular physical activity can play significant roles in helping individuals overcome these psychiatric and behavioral issues and reduce the risk of CVD.

8.1 INTRODUCTION

While stress reduction is one of the pillars of lifestyle medicine, the issue of psychiatric conditions (including stress) and their impact on cardiovascular disease (CVD) is broader and has an impact not only on the prevention and treatment of CVD but also on various aspects of behavior related to CVD. For this reason, this chapter takes a broader view of the relationship between lifestyle and CVD. It incorporates not only acute and chronic stress and various techniques of stress reduction but also issues related to post-traumatic stress disorder (PTSD), depression and anxiety. In addition, we focus some attention on the impact of these psychiatric conditions in both the prevention and treatment of CVD and the importance of understanding and utilizing various behavioral techniques.

8.2 THE STRESS RESPONSE

The stress response is a mechanism that allows humans to counteract potentially damaging stimuli (1). This response incorporates stimulation of the sympathetic nerve system and the hypothalamic pituitary adrenal (HPA) axis with the release of cortisol and catecholamines. While the activation of this stress system can be physiologically important to counteract stresses, if stimulation of the sympathetic nerve system is prolonged or exaggerated, it can promote or exacerbate the development of CVD (2). The mechanisms by which risk of CVD are increasing include increases in blood pressure

DOI: 10.1201/b23245-9

and heart rate, insulin resistance and other metabolic abnormalities, systemic vascular resistance, other ventricular arrhythmias and dysregulation of the inflammatory and immune systems. It is important to recognize psychological and psychiatric factors both in the prevention of CVD and the management of individuals with existing disease not only because of the physiologic issues previously listed, but also because of the relationship of these factors to health behaviors and lifestyle risk factors.

It should be noted that psychological and psychiatric conditions are significantly less likely to be recognized and managed in the current practice of medicine, particularly as related to CVD risk factors. Recent recommendations from the American Heart Association (AHA) and American College of Cardiology (ACC) have urged cardiologists to be more proactive in this area (3). This chapter focuses on psychological and psychiatric aspects of CVD and concludes with recommendations for how lifestyle modalities can play an important role in controlling these risk factors.

8.3   ACUTE STRESS

A number of studies have suggested an increase in hospital admissions for acute coronary syndromes after emotionally stressful events such as terrorist attacks or even professional football games. This is particularly true in sporting events when the team that the particular fan/or fans were cheering for loses.

In addition, acute emotional responses such as anger as well as acute negative emotion such as grief and sadness can also act as triggers for CVD events (4,5). In one study, a 21-fold increase in acute myocardial infarction was noted in the 24 hours following the death of a significant other (6). In another study, people who experienced bereavement had a doubling of the risk of cardiovascular events in the 30 days following their partner's death. Other stressful situations such as tight deadlines have also been associated with increased acute cardiovascular events. It should be noted, however, that the absolute increase that negative emotions play has been estimated to result in less than 4% of acute cardiac events.

The issue of mental stress and cardiovascular consequences has also been frequently studied. These studies have suggested that mental stress can cause ischemia in one-third to two-thirds of patients with coronary heart disease. A number of longitudinal studies with follow-up in 1–5 years have found consistent doubling in the risk of subsequent cardiac events for individuals who experience ischemia related to mental stress.

The key pathophysiologic event thought to underly an acute coronary event related to stress is progression from a stable plaque to a "vulnerable" plaque. This may be a result of increases in blood pressure and heart rate or increases in systemic vascular resistance (7,8). Acute mental stress can also induce cardiac electrical instability and lead to arrythmias. Finally, inflammation and immunity appear to be key factors in cardiovascular responses to acute psychological stress (9). Thus, there are multiple physiologic responses that occur in response to emotional stress that could trigger cardiac ischemia or sudden death. The literature conclusively demonstrating this relationship, however, is subject to considerable debate.

Whether or not therapies for CVD prevention such as aspirin, statins or angiotensin-converting enzyme (ACE) inhibitors might protect against harmful effects of emotional triggers is not known.

8.4   CHRONIC STRESS

A variety of situations can lead to chronic stress. In these situations, increased symptomatic tone may increase the likelihood of CVD. Some of these situations have to do with stress at work or at home or other circumstances that the individual finds themselves in.

- *Low Socioeconomic Status*—Socioeconomic status (SES) is typically defined by a number of factors such as occupational status, education, economic resources and social class. It has long been understood that there is a significant social gradient in health and disease (10). This is also true of CVD (11). Low SES is frequently accompanied by poor health habits and higher frequencies of standard CVD risk factors such as obesity, hypertension, smoking and an unhealthy diet, which may partially account for the CVD gradient that accompanies social class (12).

  A variety of external factors such as the neighborhood environment, lack of access to healthy foods ("food islands"), or lack of opportunities to be physically active may all contribute to chronic stress and weight gain which, in turn, may increase blood pressure and CVD risk (13,14). Thus, low SES can be viewed as compositive of chronic stresses that result in adverse physiologic and behavioral consequences.

  The adverse impact of low SES was clearly demonstrated in the response of various groups to the COVID-19 pandemic. Minority populations such as Black and Hispanics were three to four times as likely to require hospitalization and to die from COVID-19 compared to Caucasians (15). Moreover, individuals who were obese and/or had hypertension were also three to four times as likely to experience adverse health consequences.

- *Work Stress*—A number of studies have examined work stress and the potential CVD effects. A leading model in this area focuses on the issue of "job strain," which postulates that high work demands in combination with low control produce stress because workers are unable to moderate work pressure by organizing their time or other needs (12). An additional source of work stress comes from lack of support from colleagues.

  Another model suggests that work stress comes from an effort and reward imbalance. Both of these models have been linked to adverse CVD events. Recently, this model has been applied to physician burnout where additional demands such as excessive charting time, to satisfy electronic records, have led to many physicians feeling there is a significant mismatch between workload and payback in terms of professional and personal recognition.

- *Social Isolation*—The number and quality of a person's social contacts have been related to CVD and total mortality rate (16,17). Increased social support may improve health by helping people follow a healthy diet, potentially involving more physical activity and providing emotional support.

- *Marital and Caregiver Stress*—Marital stress has been studied as a component of social support in a number of studies. Being married has been related to lower risk of death from ischemic heart disease in both men and women (18). Divorce and caregiving stress have both been related to an increase in CVD risk (19). In the Caregiver Health Effects Study, caregiving was associated with a 63% higher adjusted mortality risk (20). Not all caregivers experience stress, but it occurs particularly in people who report feeling strained.

The recent COVID-19 pandemic has created a great deal of stress for both medical caregivers as well as family caregivers. To date there have been few studies incorporating measures of chronic stress on CVD risk prediction. However, there have been recent efforts to look at components of chronic stress and their effects on burnout, particularly in the physician population.

8.5   STRESS REDUCTION TECHNIQUES

Stress reduction is one of the key pillars in lifestyle medicine (21,22). Stress reduction can play a significant role in a variety of chronic conditions including CVD. Stress reduction techniques focus on adaptive responses that initiate physiological and biochemical reactions in the body. Mind-body therapies can help reduce the long-term harmful effects of chronic stress. In addition, mind-body therapies can play a role in helping individuals make positive behavioral modifications that help counteract the stress response and enhance coping mechanisms for perceived stress. A variety of mind-body therapies are available. These include meditation, body scans, relaxation response, contemplation and prayer, movement (e.g., yoga and tai chi), gratitude and various cognitive techniques such as cognitive reappraisal. These techniques are beyond the scope of this chapter and are discussed in numerous other places (21,22). The role of various mind-body techniques both in the prevention and treatment of CVD continues to be explored.

8.6   PSYCHIATRIC DISORDERS AND CVD

In addition to issues related to stress, a number of psychiatric disorders may impact both the risk of CVD and also its treatment. Conditions such as depression and anxiety are very common in the United States and merit consideration as part of the overall psychiatric evaluation of patients either with CVD or at risk for CVD. PTSD has also become quite common in a variety of settings including following military service in combat situations and should be considered as a component of the overall evaluation for people at risk for CVD or who already have CVD.

- *Depression*—Depression is very common in the United States and around the world. Depression is three times more common in cardiac patients than controls, and 15%–30% of cardiac patients have significant depression (3,23).

  There are a range of levels of depression. It has been demonstrated in individuals with the clinical diagnosis of major depression that there is significant interaction with CVD. Several studies have shown that 15%–30% of cardiac patients have significant depression.

Observational studies have routinely shown evidence for an association between clinical depression and CVD risk, both among individuals free of heart disease and a variety of patient populations with heart disease. There are a number of potential mechanisms that contribute to the relationship between depression and CVD (24). For example, depression is associated with other CVD risk factors including hypertension, smoking, sedentary lifestyle, obesity and diabetes (25). Studies have shown, however, that depression is an independent risk factor even when adjusting for these factors.

There is some evidence that depressed individuals have reduced parasympathetic flow and other indications of autonomic dysfunction that can increase the risk of CVD. There is also some evidence that depression may relate to decreased immune dysfunction and increased inflammation (26). Finally, depression can create barriers for people adhering to not only healthy lifestyles but also cardiovascular medications.

For all these reasons, lifestyle intervention in patients who are depressed can play a significant role in reducing the risk of CVD. For this reason, it is important that physicians inquire about mood states in all of their patients.

- *Anxiety*—Anxiety is the second leading psychiatric condition in the United States. As many as 18% of Americans may be affected by an anxiety disorder (2,27). It should be noted that anxiety often coexists with depression. There are a variety of anxiety disorders that may range from panic disorder, phobic anxiety and obsessive-compulsive disorder.

Various lifestyle measures can play a significant role in lessening the burden of anxiety. These include regular aerobic exercise as well as various mind-body therapies including stress reduction, as described in the previous section.

- *Post-Traumatic Stress Disorder (PTSD)*—PTSD has become more commonly described in news media, particularly as it relates to conditions found in some soldiers after returning from war zones. While this linkage is commonly depicted in the news media, it is important to note that there are more cases of PTSD in civilians who have not experienced combat than there are in those who have experienced combat. Lifestyle prevalence of PTSD in civilians has been estimated to be between 1.3% and 7.8% (28). PTSD has been associated with approximately 50% increased risk for CVD (29). In patients with already existing heart disease, PTSD contributes to at least doubling of subsequent events.

Individuals with PTSD may be less likely to engage in positive lifestyle behaviors such as physical activity and may be predisposed to cardiovascular risk factors such as hypertension, obesity and diabetes (30). For all these reasons, prescription of lifestyle modalities is particularly relevant for people with PTSD.

8.7 PERSONALITY TRAITS

- *Anger and Hostility*—The potential harmful effects of chronic feelings of anger on health, in general, and CVD, in particular, have been known for many years (27). Anger and hostility are often used interchangeably. Initially a cognitive trait characterized as "type A personality" was believed to be a risk factor for CVD. However, this relationship has not been supported by subsequent studies.

An outburst of anger has been well established to potentially trigger acute coronary events (31). Anger as a personality trait is less established as a risk factor for CVD. The risk of anger and hostility appears to be more marked in men than in woman and may be accompanied by behavioral factors such as smoking and inactivity. Potential pathophysiologic links between anger and hostility and CVD may be stimulated by exaggerated autonomic function, inflammation and platelet aggregation. Discussing with patients whether or not they are prone to angry outbursts is worthwhile for physicians practicing in lifestyle medicine since mind-body therapies and physical activity may be useful lifestyle medicine modalities in this area.

There is also a related condition that has been called "type D personality" that describes individuals who have both negative emotions (excessive tension or worry) and also are inhibited with regard to social interaction (32). There are some data to suggest that this type of personality may also contribute to increased risk for CVD.

8.8 LIFESTYLE EVALUATION AND MANAGEMENT OF MENTAL HEALTH

Because of the various mental health issues described in this chapter and their relationship with CVD, it is important to discuss these issues not only with patients with CVD but also with patients who are at increased risk for CVD. This is particularly important since lifestyle modalities such as stress reduction, other mind-body therapies and physical activity can all be helpful to help ameliorate adverse mental health conditions. In addition, since individuals with these conditions are at increased risk for CVD, all of the other lifestyle-related modalities discussed in various chapters in this book which help lower the risk of CVD are highly appropriate in these individuals.

8.9 LIFESTYLE PREVENTION AND TREATMENT OF PSYCHIATRIC CAUSES OF CVD

Multiple medicine modalities are highly relevant in the area of psychiatric and behavioral aspects of CVD. A cornerstone of lifestyle medicine is behavior change (33). There are multiple frameworks to help people make behavioral changes in their lives. This is highly relevant not only for risk factors for CVD, but also for individuals who already have established disease.

One particularly valuable counseling technique involves motivational interviewing (34). This type of interaction between physician and patient puts the patient at the center of the discussion and helps identify and overcome barriers to behavioral change. Other frameworks for enhancing behavioral change are beyond the scope of this chapter but may be found in multiple other places. As already indicated, both regular physical activity and mind-body/stress reduction techniques are highly relevant in the area of psychiatric and behavioral aspects of CVD.

8.10   SUMMARY/CONCLUSIONS

There are significant relationships between psychiatric and behavioral issues and CVD. These range from acute and chronic stress to depression and anxiety as well as a variety of personality traits. There are multiple, effective therapies in the area of lifestyle medicine which can help reduce the risk of CVD in individuals who may experience some of these psychiatric issues. In particular, regular physical activity and stress reduction/mind-body techniques can play highly relevant roles in reducing the psychiatric risk factors associated with CVD. Thus, clinicians should discuss these issues with patients in every clinical encounter and offer proven therapies to individuals who are experiencing these psychiatric conditions.

Clinical Applications

- Both acute and chronic stress are associated with an increased risk of CVD.
- Stress reduction/mind-body techniques can be extremely helpful in reducing the impact of stress on individuals' lives.
- Regular physical activity can also reduce the impact of stress as well as anxiety and depression in individuals' lives.
- Psychiatric and behavioral aspects are associated with increased risk of CVD making it important for clinicians to discuss all of these issues in every clinical encounter.

REFERENCES

1. Steptoe A, Kivimaki M. Stress and cardiovascular disease: An update on current knowledge. Annu Rev Public Health. 2013;34:337–54. Epub 2013/01/10.
2. Shah AJ, Vaccarino V. Psychosocial risk factors and coronary artery disease. In Roncella A, Pristipino C, eds. Psychotherapy for Ischemic Heart Disease: An Evidence-Based Clinical Approach. Switzerland: Springer International Publishing; 2016, pp. 29–44.
3. Lichtman JH, Froelicher ES, Blumenthal JA, et al. Depression as a risk factor for poor prognosis among patients with acute coronary syndrome: Systematic review and recommendations: A scientific statement from the American Heart Association. Circulation. 2014;129(12):1350–69. Epub 2014/02/26.
4. Mostofsky E, Maclure M, Tofler GH, et al. Relation of outbursts of anger and risk of acute myocardial infarction. Am J Cardiol. 2013;112(3):343–8. Epub 2013/05/07.
5. Mostofsky E, Penner EA, Mittleman MA. Outbursts of anger as a trigger of acute cardiovascular events: A systematic review and meta-analysis. Eur Heart J. 2014;35(21):1404–10. Epub 2014/03/05.
6. Mostofsky E, Maclure M, Sherwood JB, et al. Risk of acute myocardial infarction after the death of a significant person in one's life: The determinants of myocardial infarction onset study. Circulation. 2012;125(3):491–6. Epub 2012/01/11.
7. Vaccarino V. Mental stress-induce myocardial ischemia. In Baune BT, Tully PJ, eds. Cardiovascular Diseases and Depression: Treatment and Prevention in Psychocardiology. Switzerland: Springer International Publishing; 2016, pp. 105–121.
8. Jiang W, Samad Z, Boyle S, et al. Prevalence and clinical characteristics of mental stress-induced myocardial ischemia in patients with coronary heart disease. J Am Coll Cardiol. 2013;61(7):714–22. Epub 2013/02/16.

9. Wohleb ES, McKim DB, Sheridan JF, et al. Monocyte trafficking to the brain with stress and inflammation: A novel axis of immune-to-brain communication that influences mood and behavior. Front Neurosci. 2014;8:447. Epub 2015/02/06.

10. Backe EM, Seidler A, Latza U, et al. The role of psychosocial stress at work for the development of cardiovascular diseases: A systematic review. Int Arch Occup Environ Health. 2012;85(1):67–79. Epub 2011/05/18.

11. Vaccarino V, Bremner JD. Psychiatric and behavioral aspects of cardiovascular disease. In Mann DL, Zipes DP, Libby P, Bonow RO, eds. Braunwald's Heart Disease: A Textbook of Cardiovascular Medicine. 10th ed. Philadelphia, PA: Elsevier-Saunders; 2015.

12. Brunner EJ. Social factors and cardiovascular morbidity. Neurosci Biobehav Rev. 2017;74(Pt B):260–8. Epub 2016/05/15.

13. Wing JJ, August E, Adar SD, et al. Change in neighborhood characteristics and change in coronary artery calcium: A longitudinal investigation in the MESA (Multi-ethnic study of atherosclerosis) cohort. Circulation. 2016;134(7):504–13. Epub 2016/08/17.

14. Arcaya M, Glymour MM, Chakrabarti P, et al. Effects of proximate foreclosed properties on individuals' systolic blood pressure in Massachusetts, 1987 to 2008. Circulation. 2014;129(22):2262–8. Epub 2014/06/04.

15. Berkowitz SA, Cene CW, Chatterjee A. Covid-19 and health equity: Time to think big. N Engl J Med. 2020;383(12):e76. Epub 2020/07/25.

16. Holt-Lunstad J, Smith TB, Baker M, et al. Loneliness and social isolation as risk factors for mortality: A meta-analytic review. Perspect Psychol Sci. 2015;10(2):227–37. Epub 2015/04/25.

17. Valtorta NK, Kanaan M, Gilbody S, et al. Loneliness and social isolation as risk factors for coronary heart disease and stroke: Systematic review and meta-analysis of longitudinal observational studies. Heart. 2016;102(13):1009–16. Epub 2016/04/20.

18. Floud S, Balkwill A, Canoy D, et al. Marital status and ischemic heart disease incidence and mortality in women: A large prospective study. BMC Med. 2014;12:42. Epub 2014/03/13.

19. Dupre ME, George LK, Liu G, et al. Association between divorce and risks for acute myocardial infarction. Circ Cardiovasc Qual Outcomes. 2015;8(3):244–51. Epub 2015/04/16.

20. Bevans M, Sternberg EM. Caregiving burden, stress, and health effects among family caregivers of adult cancer patients. JAMA. 2012;307(4):398–403. Epub 2012/01/26.

21. Loiselle E, Mehta D, Proszynski J. Behavioral approaches to manage stress. In Rippe JM, ed. Lifestyle Medicine. 3rd ed. Boca Raton, FL: CRC Press; 2019.

22. Nedley N, Ramirez FE. Emotional health and stress management. In Rippe JM, ed. Lifestyle Medicine. 3rd ed. Boca Raton, FL: CRC Press; 2019.

23. Vaccarino V, Bremner JD. Behavioral, emotional and neurobiological determinants of coronary heart disease risk in women. Neurosci Biobehav Rev. 2017;74(Pt B):297–309. Epub 2016/08/09.

24. Hamer M, Steptoe A. Cortisol responses to mental stress and incident hypertension in healthy men and women. J Clin Endocrinol Metabol. 2012;97(1):E29–34. Epub 2011/10/28.

25. Penninx BW. Depression and cardiovascular disease: Epidemiological evidence on their linking mechanisms. Neurosci Biobehav Rev. 2017;74(Pt B):277–86. Epub 2016/07/28.

26. Liu Y, Ho RC, Mak A, Interleukin (IL)-6, tumour necrosis factor alpha (TNF alpha) and soluble interleukin-2 receptors (sIL-2R) are elevated in patients with major depressive disorder: A meta-analysis and meta-regression. J Affect Disord. 2012;139(3):230–9. Epub 2011/08/30.

27. Thurston RC, Rewak M, Kubzansky LD. An anxious heart: Anxiety and the onset of cardiovascular diseases. Prog Cardiovasc Dis. 2013;55(6):524–37. Epub 2013/04/30.

28. Bremner JD. Posttraumatic Stress Disorder: From Neurobiology to Treatment. Hoboken, NJ: WileyBlackwell; 2016.

29. Edmondson D, Kronish IM, Shaffer JA, et al. Posttraumatic stress disorder and risk for coronary heart disease: A meta-analytic review. Am Heart J. 2013;166(5):806–14. Epub 2013/11/02.

30. Vaccarino V, Bremner JD. Posttraumatic stress disorder and risk of cardiovascular disease. In Alvarenga M, Bryne D, eds. Handbook of Psychology. Singapore: Springer; 2015.

31. Suls J. Anger and the heart: Perspectives on cardiac risk, mechanisms and interventions. Prog Cardiovasc Dis. 2013;55(6):538–47. Epub 2013/04/30.

32. Denollet J, Pedersen SS, Vrints CJ, et al. Predictive value of social inhibition and negative affectivity for cardiovascular events and mortality in patients with coronary artery disease: The type D personality construct. Psychosomatic Med. 2013;75(9):873–81. Epub 2013/10/29.

33. Gholami M, Herman C, Ainsworth MC, et al. Applying psychological theories to promote healthy lifestyles. In Rippe JM, ed. Lifestyle Medicine. 3rd ed. Boca Raton, FL: CRC Press; 2019.

34. Fifield P, Suzuki J, Minski S, et al. Motivational interviewing and lifestyle change. In Rippe JM, ed. Lifestyle Medicine. 3rd ed. Boca Raton, FL: CRC Press; 2019.

9 Sleep and Cardiovascular Disease

KEY POINTS

- Healthy sleep is important for virtually every bodily system.
- Disordered sleep represents a significant risk factor for multiple conditions, particularly cardiovascular disease.
- Disordered sleep is a significant risk factor for hypertension.
- Individuals who are overweight or obese are at increased risk for obstructive sleep apnea that can further increase the risk of cardiovascular disease.
- Weight loss (for overweight or obese individuals), increased physical activity and nutrition are all lifestyle factors that can positively impact on sleep and improve quality of life, while reducing the risk of CVD.

9.1 INTRODUCTION

Healthy sleep is essential for life and optimal health. Sleep plays a significant role in virtually every aspect of living including metabolism, brain function, systemic physiology, appetite regulation and the function of the cardiovascular system as well as the immune system and hormonal systems (1,2). Lifestyle factors play a very important role in maintaining healthy sleep (3).

Sleep is particularly important for the normal functioning of the cardiovascular system. Conversely, disordered sleep significantly increases the risk of many aspects of cardiovascular disease (CVD). This chapter focuses on both the benefits of healthy sleep and the role that lifestyle factors play in it as well as issues related to disordered sleep and the cardiovascular system and how lifestyle issues can play a significant role in ameliorating this problem.

Normal, healthy sleep is characterized by good quality, sufficient duration, appropriate timing and regularity and the absence of sleep disorders. Despite the importance of sleep, up to 70 million people in the United States have a chronic sleep disorder that impacts daily functioning and health and increases the risk of CVD (4).

There are over 100 sleep disorder classifications. They are typically manifested by one of three of the following ways: failure to obtain necessary amount or quality of sleep (sleep deprivation) and inability to maintain sleep continuity (disrupted sleep), difficulty maintaining sleep (insomnia) and events that occur during sleep (e.g., sleep apnea, restless leg syndrome) (5). This chapter focuses first on normal sleep and subsequently on problems that can disrupt sleep and their health consequences, with a particular emphasis on disordered sleep patterns and their effect on CVD. The chapter concludes with some issues related to what has been called "sleep hygiene" and tips for healthy sleeping.

DOI: 10.1201/b23245-10

9.2   CHARACTERISTICS OF NORMAL SLEEP

Stages of sleep have historically been divided into two stages. The first rapid eye movement (REM) and then four stages of non-rapid eye movement (NREM) characterized by increasing sleep depth (6). Stages three and four have been deemed to be the most restorative type of sleep and typically occur during the first one-third of the night. In contrast, REM sleep increases as the night progresses and is longest in the last third of sleep. Both REM and NREM sleep are characterized by physiologic changes including brain activity, heart rate, blood pressure, sympathetic nervous activity and muscle tone as well as blood flow to the brain, respiration, airway resistance, renal and endocrine function, body temperature and sexual arousal. The sleep/wake cycle is controlled by daily rhythms called circadian rhythms. Both sleep and wake cycles are regulated by the hypothalamus (2). Circadian rhythms work to synchronize sleep with the external day/night cycle.

9.3   SLEEP DISRUPTION

Sleep disruption is very common. The National Sleep Foundation in a 2014 survey reported that 35% of American adults rated their sleep quality as "poor" or "only fair." Prolonged sleep at least one night per week was reported by 45% of respondents, while 53% of respondents had trouble staying asleep at least one night of the previous week, and 23% of respondents had trouble staying asleep on five or more nights (7). Snoring was also common, reported by 40% of respondents. Interestingly, 17% of respondents had been told by a physician that they had a sleep disorder. The majority of those who were told they had a sleep disorder (68%) were told they had sleep apnea.

Risk factors for sleep disruptions are numerous and include a combination of biological, psychologic, genetic and social factors (8). Lifestyle factors also play a role such as consuming excessive amounts of caffeine or drinking alcohol. Shift work is a risk for sleep disruption, as is being a college student. Excessive nighttime light pollution and underexposure to daylight/sunlight can also create a disruption in circadian rhythm. Stressful life circumstances such as serving as a caregiver for a family member with a chronic, life-threatening or terminal illness or being a parent of a young infant can also create sleep disruptions.

Sleep disruption is a broader characteristic, but it may be attributable to a sleep disorder such as obstructive sleep apnea (OSA) or restless leg syndrome (9,10,11). A major medical condition may be associated with sleep disruption, particularly those that require nighttime medical monitoring or hospitalization, particularly in intensive or critical care units (12–14).

Sleep deprivation studies and research in insomniacs have demonstrated mechanisms by which sleep disruption may result in detrimental short- or long-term health effects. These are thought to be evidenced by increased levels of catecholamines, lower epinephrine as well as increased oxygen consumption and carbon dioxide production. These findings suggest that the sympathetic nervous system is activated by sleep disruption (15–18). In addition, disrupted sleep may result in increased insulin release that may explain the increase of sleep disruption in individuals with type 2 diabetes (T2DM). Other metabolic changes include decreased leptin and increased ghrelin that may contribute to increased appetite. Sleep abnormalities may also induce inflammatory cytokines such as tumor necrosis factor alpha (TNF-α), interleukins 1 and 6 and C-reactive protein (CRP) (19,20). Studies now suggest that chronic sleep deprivation causes adverse physiologic changes on multiple body systems. In addition, insufficient sleep may contribute to alterations in the neuroendocrine stress response that can ultimately lead to stress-related disorders, mood disorders and depression.

9.4 SHORT-TERM HEALTH CONSEQUENCES OF SLEEP DISRUPTION

Numerous health consequences have been reported related to short-term sleep disruption. These include increased sympathetic activation that may be one of the reasons why sleep disruption is associated with CVD as well as psychiatric conditions (21,22). Disruptions may directly influence cognition and mood. This may increase the likelihood of depression and is often associated with increased feelings of irritability and impatience. Sleep disruption may alter cognition and cognitive performance. In one study of primary care physicians, disrupted sleep was associated with high burnout levels.

9.5 LONG-TERM HEALTH CONSEQUENCES OF SLEEP DISRUPTION

There are multiple long-term consequences of sleep disruption that impact the cardiovascular system, including increased levels of hypertension, dyslipidemia, weight-related issues, metabolic syndrome and T2DM (23–25). The negative impacts on the cardiovascular system are thought to largely result from increased activity of the sympathetic nervous system that can lead to elevated blood pressure.

Four prospective cohort studies found the relative risk of hypertension was 20% higher in individuals with sleep disruptions (23). Two large population-based studies showed an association between CVD and sleep disruption. The Atherosclerosis Risk In Communities (ARIC) study showed a 50% increase in risk of CVD for individuals who had difficulty falling asleep or nonrestorative sleep compared to individuals with healthy sleep (24). Short sleep duration was associated with increased risk of CVD in middle-aged women, who participated in the MONICA/KORA Study (26). These studies suggested that disruption of sympathetic activity, glucose metabolism and possibly inflammation may contribute to the increased likelihood of CVD adverse effects.

9.6 SLEEP-DISORDERED BREATHING AND CARDIOVASCULAR DISEASE

Sleep-disordered breathing (SDB) is a subset of the general category of sleep disruption and is prevalent in patients with cardiac diseases where it contributes to reduced quality of life. SDB can also exacerbate cardiac ischemia, reduce systolic and diastolic function, cause cardiac structural and electrical remodeling and increase the risk of cardiac arrhythmias and sudden death. Unfortunately, the SDB often goes unrecognized in cardiology practice.

SDB is a spectrum of sleep-related breathing disorders that includes OSA, central sleep apnea (CSA), Cheyne-Stokes respiration and sleep-related hypoventilation. All of these are associated with impaired ventilation during sleep and sleep disruption. OSA is characterized by episodes of either complete (apnea) or partial hypopnea or upper airway occlusion and affects 34% of middle-aged males and 17% of middle-aged females. OSA and CVD have shared risk factors (e.g., central obesity). For this reason, OSA may be found in 40%–80% of patients with hypertension, heart failure, coronary heart disease or cerebrovascular disease (27). Patients with OSA typically report loud or disruptive snoring and poor sleep quality as well as excessive daytime sleepiness, which is a cardinal symptom. People with OSA also experience impaired quality of life (28). Diagnosis of OSA is based on symptoms such as snoring or breathing pauses or daytime sleepiness or fatigue. Sleep studies are typically utilized to diagnose degree of apneas or hypopneas.

- *Pathophysiology of obstructive sleep apnea*—A number of factors increase the risk of OSA. The presence of an anatomically small airway and lying in a supine position increase the neuromuscular drive needed to maintain airway patency (29). In addition, reduced lung volume such as that found in individuals with obesity or pulmonary congestion can increase the risk of OSA. Causal conditions such as pregnancy or allergies associated with nasal swelling increase the risk of OSA. OSA can also worsen following acute ingestion of alcohol that reduces neuromuscular activation, particularly when a person is in supine position. During sleep, the blood CO_2 typically mildly increases which helps activate respiratory muscle and protect the upper airway. However, depressed sensitivity to CO_2 is common in obesity, hypoventilation and sleep hypoventilation syndromes.
- *Risk factors and recognition of sleep disorder breathing*—A variety of risk factors should increase the risk of OSA. For example, male sex and older age as well as obesity are well-recognized OSA risk factors (30). OSA is two to four times more prevalent in men than in women (8). Central obesity is more commonly found in men than women as it predisposes to OSA.

  Being overweight or obese accounts for approximately 40%–60% of cases of OSA (31). Obese middle-aged individuals are four times more likely to have OSA than normal weight individuals. Obesity is thought to contribute to OSA through effects on airway narrowing caused by fat deposition in the tongue and parapharyngeal tissues and also by reducing lung volume. Obesity-associated cytokine levels may also adversely impact on ventilatory control. Even modest weight loss or weight gain can have an impact on severity of OSA.

  A 1% increase in body mass based on body mass index (BMI) increases episodes of apnea by 3% (32). It should be noted that approximately 20% of OSA patients are not obese, so normal weight does not preclude the possibility of OSA. Unfortunately, OSA often goes unrecognized and untreated. For example, it has been estimated that 80% of individuals with moderate or severe OSA are undiagnosed (33,34). Underrecognition is high in both ethnic and minority groups, such as African American and older Chinese American people and elderly individuals, in general. Underrecognition of OSA in women may occur from patients reporting symptoms of fatigue rather than sleepiness.

The role of routine screening for OSA is not established. The U.S. Preventive Searches Task Force in 2017 concluded there was insufficient evidence to recommend routine screening for sleep apnea in primary care settings (35). Individuals whose partner complains of their snoring as well as older age and elevated BMI should all be factored into raising questions about potential OSA.

- *Linkages between SDB and CVD*—SDB appears to increase sympathetic nervous system activity. In contrast, during healthy sleep, parasympathetic activity increases which results in decreased levels of blood pressure and heart rate. Increases in sympathetic activity in disordered breathing may result in acute blood pressure elevations and intermittent hypoxia, which can further stimulate the autonomic nervous system and may augment inflammatory and hypercoagulable states as well as exacerbate insulin resistance and lipolysis (36). Oxygen desaturation resulting from apnea and hypopneas may also compromise oxygenation to the myocardial tissue.

- *SDB and hypertension*—It has been estimated that up to 30% of individuals with essential hypertension and 80% of individuals with resistant hypertension have OSA (37). Over 50% of patients with OSA have hypertension. The Joint National Commission on Prevention, Detection and Evaluation and Treatment of High Blood Pressure (JNC7) identified OSA as a treatable cause of hypertension (38). The mainstay of treatment for OSA, continuous positive airway pressure (CPAP) has been shown to reduce both systolic and diastolic pressure by 1.5–3 mm Hg (39). Combining CPAP with other modalities such as medications, weight loss or increased physical activity may generate greater effects than single modality therapy which underscores the importance of lifestyle measures in the treatment of OSA.

- *SDB and coronary artery disease*—SDB contributes to atherosclerosis by a variety of mechanisms including triggering sympathetic nervous system activity and augmenting the release of pro-inflammatory proteins (40,41). In addition, SDB may contribute to dyslipidemia, insulin resistance and endothelial dysfunction. OSA may also contribute to acute ischemia because of decreased oxygen delivery (secondary to obstructive breathing) and increased oxygen consumption (associated with elevated diastolic pressures and cardiac hypertrophy). More than 75% of patients presenting with acute coronary syndrome have been reported to have SDB (42). SDB is an independent risk factor for CHD.

In the prospective Sleep Heart Health Study Cohort, moderate to severe SDB was associated with a 35% increased risk of CHD. Among men younger than age 70 years, the increased risk was 70%. In the Multi-Ethnic

Study of Atherosclerosis (MESA) study, the diagnosis of OSA was associated with an increase of 1.9 adjusted hazard ratio for cardiovascular events and 2.4 higher mortality rate (43). Several large studies have demonstrated that individuals with OSA with CPAP have significantly reduced rates of fatal and nonfatal CVD compared to untreated patients (27).

- *SDB and cardiac function and heart failure*—Both CSA and OSA are common in heart failure and occur in up to 60% of patients with heart failure. This may represent a bidirectional relationship (30,44). Patients with heart failure experience pulmonary vascular congestion that may cause hyperventilation, while SDB may adversely affect cardiac function by contributing to systemic and pulmonary hypertension. Prospective studies have shown that SDB independently predicts new-onset heart failure (HF). Middle-aged men with severe SDB (predominantly OSA) have an estimated 60% increase in HF compared to without SDB. In patients with HF, SDB also predicts HF exacerbations and progression. The American Heart Association in their published HF Guidelines of 2013 recommend screening patients with HF for SDB and treating those who test positive with a particular focus on minimizing fluid overload. Both weight loss and exercise as well as elastic stockings can represent redistribution of fluid into the thoracic compartment.
- *SDB and cardiac arrhythmias*—Patients with SDB are predisposed to both ventricular and atrial arrhythmias largely as a result of underlying cardiac risk factors and CVD (45–47). Apneas and hypopneas are direct triggers of paroxysms of both atrial and ventricular arrhythmias. In one analysis of temporal patterns of overnight arrhythmias, there was a 17-fold increase of arrhythmias during an episode of apnea compared to a period of normal breathing. CPAP use in patients with OSA reduces atrial fibrillation risk by 44% (48).

9.7 SLEEP AND NORMAL AGING

Both the quality and duration of sleep change as people grow older. As many as 50% of older individuals complain about sleep problems including "disturbed" or "light" sleep (49–51), frequent awakenings, early morning awakenings and undesired daytime sleepiness. These changes make it all the more important for individuals practicing in the area of lifestyle medicine to inquire of patients of all ages, but particularly those over the age of 65 years, about their sleep patterns. The most significant change in sleep in older individuals is repeated and frequent interruption of sleep and long periods of wakefulness. This is possibly a result of age-dependent decreases in the sleep homeostatic processes.

It should be noted that even carefully screened older individuals who do not complain of sleep disturbance may still show these changes as described when compared to younger adults. This suggests that some of the sleep disturbances may be part of the aging process per se and independent of any primary sleep disorders. These are often referred to as "age-related sleep changes." For all of these reasons, issues related to lifestyle practices and sleep are important to consultations during every clinical visit. These issues are particularly important since individuals over the age of 65 years are much more likely than younger individuals to have risk factors for heart disease or already have established CVD. Issues of counseling individuals about sleep and cardiovascular disease, with particular interest on lifestyle factors, are discussed in subsequent sections.

9.8   LIFESTYLE FACTORS AND SLEEP

Given the important value of healthy sleep and the relationship between disturbed sleep and increased risk of CVD, it is important to find strategies to help individuals minimize disruptions in their sleeping patterns. This starts with inquiring of patients about both the quality and duration of their sleep. This is frequently neglected in clinical visits but represents one of the major pillars of lifestyle medicine (52). Lifestyle factors that can significantly impact sleep include the following:

- *Weight*—Individuals who are obese are significantly more susceptible to sleep disturbances than individuals who are in the healthy weight range (53). As already indicated, obesity significantly increases the risk of OSA. In addition, obesity represents an independent risk factor for CVD and is associated with multiple other risk factors. The good news is that weight loss in individuals who are obese can reduce the likelihood of OSA by 50%. The relationship between weight and disordered sleep makes it imperative that individuals who are overweight or obese (over 70% of the adult population in the United States) be counseled about the relationship between weight and sleep and how to ameliorate any problems that are occurring. Of course, this also is particularly important for the aging population. By 2030 the proportion of older adults in the U.S. population will rise to 20%. Individuals over the age of 65 years will effectively double to 72 million individuals. These are individuals who are at particular risk for CVD.
- *Physical activity*—As discussed in multiple chapters in this book (see particularly Chapter 4), physical activity is beneficial for many reasons, including lowering the risk of CVD. Studies have determined that physical activity helps people sleep better (54). It is important to understand, however, that how and when individuals exercise may affect sleep in different ways. The best evidence indicates that regular, moderate exercise can help extend sleep duration and improve sleep quality as well as decrease sleep onset.

  In individuals who already have sleep disorders, exercise may be prescribed somewhat differently. One study showed that moderate activity, including resistance training and stretching exercises, benefits people with insomnia (55). Once again, moderate aerobic sessions improve sleep quality, increase sleep duration and decrease time it takes to fall asleep. Thus, there are multiple benefits from physical activity with regard to both the quality and quantity of sleep. This synergy between one of the other pillars of lifestyle medicine and sleep is significant.
- *Nutrition*—Both diet and nutrition can influence the quality of sleep. Certain foods and drinks can make it easier or harder to get the sleep that every individual needs. We discuss nutrition in multiple chapters in this

book, but it is important to specifically understand that nutrition impacts sleep. The best diet for sleep is similar to those recommended for reduction in CVD. The key in nutrition is to consume a healthy diet with ample fruits and vegetables, whole grains and fiber. Diets that follow these principles such as the Mediterranean diet (56) and the DASH diet (57) have both been shown to have positive impacts on sleep.

Conversely, an unhealthy diet can impact sleep disorders. As already discussed in this chapter, obesity is a key risk factor for OSA, and an unhealthy diet that contributes to excess weight may cause or worsen this problem. It is also important to understand that sleep can affect nutrition. Deficient sleep has been associated in multiple studies with an elevated risk of obesity. Other studies have shown that individuals who do not get enough sleep are more likely to increase their food consumption. There is also a body of information that suggests that people who do not get enough sleep have a tendency to select high-calorie foods. This may be driven by hormonal changes that help control appetite and hunger, which are thrown off by inadequate sleep. The good news is that healthy sleep can help individuals lose weight both by reducing the risk of overeating and creating higher levels of daytime energy allowing for more physical activity.

9.9 SLEEP HYGIENE

Creating an optimum environment for healthy sleep may be summarized under the rubric "sleep hygiene" (58). The concept of sleep hygiene means having both the bedroom environment and daily routines that promote consistent, uninterrupted sleep. This involves maintaining a stable sleep schedule, making the bedroom comfortable and free of disruptions, following a relaxing pre-bed routine and building healthy habits throughout the day that can contribute to ideal sleep hygiene. This is where positive lifestyle habits can play such a critical role. Some specific recommendations to establish good sleep hygiene involve the following:

- *Setting a consistent sleep schedule*—This involves establishing a fixed wakeup time regardless of whether it is a weekday or weekend, prioritizing sleep and making gradual adjustments if sleep has become disordered. It is also important not to overdue napping. Napping can be very important for individuals but should be relatively short and take place limited to the early afternoon.
- *Follow a nightly routine*—This involves such issues as making a consistent routine and budgeting 30 minutes for winding down as well as dimming lights and keeping away from bright lights which can hinder the production of melatonin, a hormone the body creates to help to facilitate sleep. Also, it is useful to unplug electronics that may be very difficult in a world that has nonstop email, texting, and so on.
- *Cultivate healthy daily habits*—These include getting enough daylight exposure, being physically active, not smoking cigarettes, reducing alcohol consumption and cutting down on caffeine in the afternoon and evening. It

may also be useful to not dine late, particularly eating heavy or spicy meals, and restricting in-bed activity or sleep with the only exception being sex.

- *Optimizing the bedroom*—Individuals should also develop an environment in the bedroom that makes sleep inviting. This includes having a comfortable mattress and pillow, setting a cooler comfortable temperature, blocking out light and drowning out noise (59,60).

All of these are essential lifestyle habits, although people frequently neglect them. Since sleep is such an important lifestyle component, these factors can play a critical role not only in overall health and quality of life but also in lowering the risk of CVD.

9.10 SUMMARY/CONCLUSIONS

Healthy sleep is a critically important component to overall quality of life, particularly to reducing the risk of CVD. Lifestyle measures can play a significant role in helping individuals obtain healthy sleep. For this reason, sleep is considered one of the pillars of lifestyle medicine and is particularly important in the area of CVD. Healthy sleep can lower the risk of CVD, while disordered sleep can not only increase the risk of CVD but can also exacerbate existing CVD. Clinicians typically do not place enough emphasis on sleep and CVD. However, it is very important that clinicians inquire of individuals of all ages, particularly individuals over the age of 65 years, about both the quality and duration of their sleep. Lifestyle measures such as weight loss (particularly for overweight or obese individuals), regular physical activity and proper nutrition can all play significant roles in lowering the risk of disordered sleep and the accompanying increase in CVD.

Clinical Applications

- Physicians should inquire about both duration and quality of sleep in every patient encounter.
- Individuals who are overweight or obese are at particular or higher risk for disordered sleep patterns that can significantly increase the risk of CVD.
- Normal sleep patterns change with age with individuals over the age of 65 years being particularly vulnerable to sleep problems. For this reason, it is particularly important to emphasize to this population the importance of healthy sleep and the links between sleep and CVD.
- For all of these reasons, sleep is a pillar of lifestyle medicine.

REFERENCES

1. Consensus Conference Panel, Watson NF, Badr MS, et al. Joint Consensus Statement of the American Academy of Sleep Medicine and Sleep Research Society on the recommended amount of sleep for a healthy adult: Methodology and discussion. Sleep. 2015;38(8):1161–83. Epub 2015/07/22.
2. Institute of Medicine, Committee on Sleep Medicine and Research, Board of Health Sciences Policy. Sleep Disorders and Sleep Deprivation: An Unmet Public Health Problem. Washington, DC: National Academic Press; 2006.

3. Watson NF, Badr MS, Belenky G, et al. Recommended amount of sleep for a healthy adult: A Joint Consensus Statement of the American Academy of Sleep Medicine and Sleep Research Society. Sleep. 2015;38(6):843–4. Epub 2015/06/04.
4. Office of Disease Prevention and Health Promotion. Sleep Health. U.S. Department of Health and Human Services. Washington, DC: Sleep Health, Healthy People; 2020. Accessed February 10, 2022.
5. Moser D, Anderer P, Gruber G, et al. Sleep classification according to AASM and Rechtschaffen & Kales: Effects on sleep scoring parameters. Sleep. 2009;32(2):139–49. Epub 2009/02/26.
6. Rechtschaffen A, Kales A. A Manual of Standardized Terminology, Techniques and Scoring System for Sleep Stages of Human Subjects. Bethesda, MD: National Institutes of Health, National Institute of Neurological Diseases and Blindness, Neurological Information Network; 1968.
7. National Sleep Foundation. 2014 Sleep Health Index. Arlington, VA: National Sleep Foundation; 2014.
8. Chen X, Wang R, Zee P, et al. Racial/ethnic differences in sleep disturbances: The multi-ethnic study of atherosclerosis (MESA). Sleep. 2014;125:162–7.
9. Ryu HS, Lee SA, Lee GH, et al. Subjective apnoea symptoms are associated with daytime sleepiness in patients with moderate and severe obstructive sleep apnoea: A retrospective study. Clin Otolaryngol. 2016;41(4):395–401. Epub 2016/04/19.
10. Younes M, Hanly PJ. Immediate postarousal sleep dynamics: An important determinant of sleep stability in obstructive sleep apnea. J Appl Physiol. 2016;120(7):801–8. Epub 2016/01/01.
11. Ferri R, Rundo F, Zucconi M, et al. An evidence-based analysis of the association between periodic leg movements during sleep and arousals in restless legs syndrome. Sleep. 2015;38(6):919–24. Epub 2015/01/13.
12. Bailey TS, Grunberger G, Bode BW, et al. American Association of Clinical Endocrinologists and American College of Endocrinology 2016 outpatient glucose monitoring consensus statement. Endocr Pract. 2016;22(2):231–61. Epub 2016/02/06.
13. Pulak LM, Jensen L. Sleep in the intensive care unit: A review. J Intens Care Med. 2016;31(1):14–23. Epub 2014/06/12.
14. Elliott R, Rai T, McKinley S. Factors affecting sleep in the critically ill: An observational study. J Crit Care. 2014;29(5):859–63. Epub 2014/06/29.
15. Vgontzas AN, Tsigos C, Bixler EO, et al. Chronic insomnia and activity of the stress system: A preliminary study. J Psychosom Res. 1998;45(1):21–31. Epub 1998/08/28.
16. Vgontzas AN, Bixler EO, Lin HM, et al. Chronic insomnia is associated with nyctohemeral activation of the hypothalamic-pituitary-adrenal axis: Clinical implications. J Clin Endocrinol Metab. 2001;86(8):3787–94. Epub 2001/08/15.
17. Bonnet MH, Berry RB, Arand DL. Metabolism during normal, fragmented, and recovery sleep. J Appl Physiol. 1991;71(3):1112–18. Epub 1991/09/01.
18. Tiemeier H, Pelzer E, Jonck L, et al. Plasma catecholamines and selective slow wave sleep deprivation. Neuropsychobiology. 2002;45(2):81–6. Epub 2002/03/15.
19. Ali T, Choe J, Awab A, et al. Sleep, immunity and inflammation in gastrointestinal disorders. World J Gastroenterol. 2013;19(48):9231–9. Epub 2014/01/11.
20. Hurtado-Alvarado G, Dominguez-Salazar E, Pavon L, et al. Blood-brain barrier disruption induced by chronic sleep loss: Low-grade inflammation may be the link. J Immunol Res. 2016;2016:4576012. Epub 2016/10/16.
21. Irwin M, Thompson J, Miller C, et al. Effects of sleep and sleep deprivation on catecholamine and interleukin-2 levels in humans: clinical implications. J Clin Endocrinol Metab. 1999;84(6):1979–85. Epub 1999/06/18.

22. Ekstedt M, Akerstedt T, Soderstrom M. Microarousals during sleep are associated with increased levels of lipids, cortisol, and blood pressure. Psychosom Med. 2004;66(6):925–31. Epub 2004/11/27.

23. Knutson KL, Van Cauter E, Rathouz PJ, et al. Association between sleep and blood pressure in midlife: The CARDIA sleep study. Arch Intern Med. 2009;169(11):1055–61. Epub 2009/06/10.

24. Phillips B, Mannino DM. Do insomnia complaints cause hypertension or cardiovascular disease? J Clin Sleep Med. 2007;3(5):489–94. Epub 2007/09/07.

25. Rod NH, Vahtera J, Westerlund H, et al. Sleep disturbances and cause-specific mortality: Results from the GAZEL cohort study. Am J Epidemiol. 2011;173(3):300–9. Epub 2011/01/05.

26. Meisinger C, Heier M, Lowel H, et al. Sleep duration and sleep complaints and risk of myocardial infarction in middle-aged men and women from the general population: The MONICA/KORA Augsburg cohort study. Sleep. 2007;30(9):1121–7. Epub 2007/10/04.

27. Javaheri S, Barbe F, Campos-Rodriguez F, et al. Sleep apnea: Types, mechanisms, and clinical cardiovascular consequences. J Am Coll Cardiol. 2017;69(7):841–58. Epub 2017/02/18.

28. McEvoy RD, Antic NA, Heeley E, et al. CPAP for prevention of cardiovascular events in obstructive sleep apnea. N Engl J Med. 2016;375(10):919–31. Epub 2016/08/30.

29. Eckert DJ, White DP, Jordan AS, et al. Defining phenotypic causes of obstructive sleep apnea: Identification of novel therapeutic targets. Am J Respir Crit Care Med. 2013;188(8):996–1004. Epub 2013/06/01.

30. Jordan AS, McSharry DG, Malhotra A. Adult obstructive sleep apnoea. Lancet. 2014;383(9918):736–47. Epub 2013/08/06.

31. Jordan AS, Wellman A, Edwards JK, et al. Respiratory control stability and upper airway collapsibility in men and women with obstructive sleep apnea. J Appl Physiol. 2005;99(5):2020–7. Epub 2005/07/05.

32. Peppard PE, Young T, Barnet JH, et al. Increased prevalence of sleep-disordered breathing in adults. Am J Epidemiol. 2013;177(9):1006–14. Epub 2013/04/17.

33. Redline S, Sotres-Alvarez D, Loredo J, et al. Sleep-disordered breathing in Hispanic/Latino individuals of diverse backgrounds: The Hispanic Community Health Study/Study of Latinos. Am J Respir Crit Care Med. 2014;189(3):335–44. Epub 2014/01/08.

34. Physical Activity Guidelines Advisory Committee. 2018 Physical Activity Guidelines Advisory Committee. 2018 Physical Activity Guidelines Advisory Committee Scientific Report. Washington, DC: U.S. Department of Health and Human Services; 2018.

35. Jonas DE, Amick HR, Feltner C, et al. Screening for obstructive sleep apnea in adults: Evidence report and systematic review for the U.S. Preventive Services Task Force. JAMA. 2017;317(4):415–33. Epub 2017/01/25.

36. Baltzis D, Bakker JP, Patel SR, et al. Obstructive sleep apnea and vascular diseases. Compr Physiol. 2016;6(3):1519–28. Epub 2016/06/28.

37. Pedrosa RP, Drager LF, Gonzaga CC, et al. Obstructive sleep apnea: The most common secondary cause of hypertension associated with resistant hypertension. Hypertension. 2011;58(5):811–17. Epub 2011/10/05.

38. Chobanian AV, Bakris GL, Black HR, et al. Seventh report of the Joint National Committee on Prevention, Detection, Evaluation, and Treatment of High Blood Pressure. Hypertension. 2003;42(6):1206–52. Epub 2003/12/06.

39. Liu L, Cao Q, Guo Z, et al. Continuous positive airway pressure in patients with obstructive sleep apnea and resistant hypertension: A meta-analysis of randomized controlled trials. J Clinical Hypertension. 2016;18(2):153–8. Epub 2015/08/19.

40. Lavie L. Oxidative stress in obstructive sleep apnea and intermittent hypoxia: Revisited-the bad ugly and good: implications to the heart and brain. Sleep Med Rev. 2015;20:27–45. Epub 2014/08/27.

41. Thunstrom E, Glantz H, Fu M, et al. Increased inflammatory activity in nonobese patients with coronary artery disease and obstructive sleep apnea. Sleep. 2015;38(3):463–71. Epub 2014/10/18.

42. Fox H, Purucker HC, Holzhacker I, et al. Prevalence of sleep-disordered breathing and patient characteristics in a coronary artery disease cohort undergoing cardiovascular rehabilitation. J Cardiopulm Rehabil Prev. 2016;36(6):421–9. Epub 2016/10/26.

43. Yeboah J, Redline S, Johnson C, et al. Association between sleep apnea, snoring, incident cardiovascular events and all-cause mortality in an adult population: MESA. Atherosclerosis. 2011;219(2):963–8. Epub 2011/11/15.

44. Pearse SG, Cowie MR. Sleep-disordered breathing in heart failure. Eur J Heart Failure. 2016;18(4):353–61. Epub 2016/02/13.

45. Mehra R, Stone KL, Varosy PD, et al. Nocturnal Arrhythmias across a spectrum of obstructive and central sleep-disordered breathing in older men: Outcomes of sleep disorders in older men (MrOS sleep) study. Arch Intern Med. 2009;169(12):1147–55. Epub 2009/06/24.

46. Hohl M, Linz B, Bohm M, et al. Obstructive sleep apnea and atrial arrhythmogenesis. Curr Cardio Rev. 2014;10(4):362–8. Epub 2014/07/10.

47. Ayas NT, Taylor CM, Laher I. Cardiovascular consequences of obstructive sleep apnea. Curr Opin Cardiol. 2016;31(6):599–605. Epub 2016/10/18.

48. Qureshi WT, Nasir UB, Alqalyoobi S, et al. Meta-analysis of continuous positive airway pressure as a therapy of atrial fibrillation in obstructive sleep apnea. Am J Cardiol. 2015;116(11):1767–73. Epub 2015/10/21.

49. Foley DJ, Monjan AA, Brown SL, et al. Sleep complaints among elderly persons: An epidemiologic study of three communities. Sleep. 1995;18(6):425–32. Epub 1995/07/01.

50. Foley DJ, Monjan A, Simonsick EM, et al. Incidence and remission of insomnia among elderly adults: An epidemiologic study of 6,800 persons over three years. Sleep. 1999;22 Suppl 2:S366–72. Epub 1999/07/08.

51. Vitiello M, Foley DJ, Stratton K, et al. Prevalence of sleep complaints and insomnia in the vitamins and lifestyle (VITAL) study cohort of 77,000 older men and women. Sleep. 2004;27:120.

52. Rippe JM. Manual of Lifestyle Medicine. Boca Raton, FL: CRC Press; 2021.

53. Lauderdale DS, Knutson KL, Rathouz PJ, et al. Cross-sectional and longitudinal associations between objectively measured sleep duration and body mass index: The CARDIA sleep study. Am J Epidemiol. 2009;170(7):805–13. Epub 2009/08/05.

54. Dolezal BA, Neufeld EV, Boland DM, et al. Interrelationship between sleep and exercise: A systematic review. Adv Prev Med. 2017;2017:1364387. Epub 2017/05/02.

55. D'Aurea CVR, Poyares D, Passos GS, et al. Effects of resistance exercise training and stretching on chronic insomnia. Braz J Psychiatry. 2019;41(1):51–7. Epub 2018/10/18.

56. Medline Plus. National Library of Medicine. (review date 7/13/2020) A.D.A.M. Medical Encyclopedia. Mediterranean Diet. Accessed February 2, 2022. Mediterranean diet: MedlinePlus Medical Encyclopedia.

57. Medline Plus. National Library of Medicine. (review date 8/13/2020) A.D.A.M. Medical Encyclopedia. Understanding the DASH Diet. Accessed February 2, 2022. Understanding the DASH diet: MedlinePlus Medical Encyclopedia.

58. National Institute of Health (NIH) (2012, January). NIH News in Health: Breaking Bad Habits. Accessed February 2, 2022. Breaking Bad Habits, NIH News in Health.
59. Harding EC, Franks NP, Wisden W. The temperature dependence of sleep. Front Neurosci. 2019;13:336. Epub 2019/05/21.
60. Hume KI, Brink M, Basner M. Effects of environmental noise on sleep. Noise Health. 2012;14(61):297–302. Epub 2012/12/22.

Part II

Assessment and Treating Cardiovascular Risk Factors

10 Framework for Assessing Risk Factors

KEY POINTS

- There is a substantial and positive link between the modalities of lifestyle medicine and lowering the risk of cardiovascular disease.
- Lifestyle medicine modalities should be combined with standardized risk assessment tools (e.g., Framingham Risk Tables) in order to maximize risk reduction.
- New understandings of the pathophysiology of atherosclerosis, which is the underlying process for coronary heart disease, stroke and peripheral vascular disease, emphasize factors such as cholesterol lowering and reduction of inflammation, all of which are key components of lifestyle medicine.

10.1 INTRODUCTION

A key for the lifestyle medicine approach to cardiovascular disease is to utilize lifestyle medicine modalities and background as components of the framework for assessing risk factors (1). Multiple risk factors increase the risk for cardiovascular disease (CVD). Many of these risk factors have a significant lifestyle component.

Physician visits are an ideal opportunity to stress the importance of lifestyle habits and practices to reduce the risk of CVD. In this chapter, we focus on traditional methods of assessing risk of CVD with an emphasis on how lifestyle medicine concepts and modalities can be applied to provide more in-depth and specific risk assessments.

It is important to underscore, as we have in multiple chapters, that poor lifestyle habits and practices represent significant contributions to the ongoing pandemic of CVD around the world (2). Lifestyle factors play a particularly prominent role in the development and pathogenesis of CVD. Five of the major risk factors for developing CVD, which are incorporated into traditional risk factor assessments, are based on lifestyle practices including the following: choice not to use tobacco products, level of physical activity, control of lipids, diabetes and obesity.

Traditional risk factor assessment tools such as the Framingham Risk Study (3) have deemphasized lifestyle issues such as physical activity, obesity and inflammation, all of which are prominent in the risk of CVD and all of which may be potentially ameliorated through lifestyle practices and habits.

10.2 THE ROLE OF LIFESTYLE MEDICINE IN ASSESSING AND TREATING THE RISK OF CARDIOVASCULAR DISEASE

While considerable progress has been made in determining and treating traditional risk factors for CVD, there are multiple important roles for lifestyle medicine

DOI: 10.1201/b23245-12

modalities. For example, the traditional risk factors for CVD, including cigarette smoking, obesity, poor nutrition, an inactive lifestyle and high blood pressure, all have a significant component of lifestyle medicine modalities in both the underlying risk factor and how it is treated. Other lifestyle medicine modalities such as stress reduction, sleep and positive relationships with others should also play a very important role. All of these issues are discussed in this chapter and in multiple other chapters throughout this book.

10.3   THE PATHOPHYSIOLOGY OF ATHEROSCLEROSIS

Atherosclerosis is the underlying cause of coronary heart disease (CHD), most of the prevalence of strokes and also peripheral vascular disease. The understanding of the pathophysiology of atherosclerosis has significantly advanced in the past 15 years (4). New understandings of atherosclerotic heart disease (ASCVD) have provided crucial links to the role of various lifestyle interventions to reduce the risk not only of CHD but other aspects of CVD. In addition to the traditional risk factors for atherosclerosis, such as dyslipidemia and hypertension, in the past decade a significant role for inflammation as an initiating event in the process of ASCVD has begun to be elucidated (5–8). Multiple other entities such as obesity, diabetes and glucose intolerance and the metabolic syndrome have significant overlap, and it may, indeed, be a component of systemic inflammation that unites all of these processes. The pathophysiology of atherosclerosis is so important that we have devoted an entire chapter to new understandings in this area. (See Chapter 11.)

10.4   THE CONCEPT OF RISK FACTORS

The concept of risk factors is relatively new in the history of medicine. Until the initial findings from the Framingham Study were published in 1960s, the concept of risk factors for CVD did not formally exist (3). Framingham data showed conclusively that factors such as cigarette smoking, diabetes (T2DM), dyslipidemia and high blood pressure independently and significantly increased the risk of CVD.

Subsequently, the concept of CVD risk factors has been expanded to include physical inactivity and obesity. These risk factors are also areas where there is a clear component of lifestyle medicine. In addition, other factors that should be evaluated by lifestyle medicine physicians such as sleep, mental health and relationship with others all contribute to the likelihood of developing CVD and should be considered risk factors to be evaluated and discussed in every clinical encounter.

It is important to understand that Framingham data also demonstrated that risk factors act synergistically and tend to cluster with each other. In fact, over half of all CVD occurs in individuals who have two or more risk factors (9–11). Individuals who have two risk factors quadruple their chance of developing CVD compared to individuals with no risk factors. Individuals with three risk factors increase their risk of developing CHD between 8- and 20-fold compared to individuals with no risk factors.

TABLE 10.1
Framingham Risk Score

Step 1

Age		
Years	LDL Pts	Chol Pts
30–34	–1	[–1]
35–39	0	[0]
40–44	1	[1]
45–49	2	[2]
50–54	3	[3]
55–59	4	[4]
60–64	5	[5]
65–69	6	[6]
70–74	7	[7]

Step 2

LDL-C		
(mg/dl)	(mmol/L)	LDL Pts
< 100	< 2.59	–3
100–129	2.60–3.36	0
130–159	3.37–4.14	0
160–190	4.15–4.92	1
≥ 190	≥ 4.92	2

Cholesterol		
(mg/dl)	(mmol/L)	Chol Pts
< 160	< 4.14	[–3]
160–199	4.15–5.17	[0]
200–239	5.18–6.21	[1]
240–279	6.22–7.24	[2]
≥ 280	≥ 7.25	[3]

Step 3

HDL-C			
(mg/dl)	(mmol/L)	LDL Pts	Chol Pts
< 35	< 0.90	2	[2]
35–44	0.91–1.16	1	[1]
45–49	1.17–1.29	0	[0]
50–59	1.30–1.55	0	[0]
≥ 60	≥ 1.56	–1	[–2]

Step 4

Systolic (mm Hg)	Blood Pressure				
	Diastolic (mm Hg)				
	< 80	80–84	85–89	90–99	≥ 100
< 120	0 [0] pts				
120–129		0 [0] pts			
130–139			1 [1] pt		
140–159				2 [2] pts	
≥ 160					3 [3] pts

Note When systolic and diastolic pressures provide different estimates for point scores, use the higher number

Step 5

Diabetes		
	LDL Pts	Chol Pts
No	0	[0]
Yes	2	[2]

Step 6

Smoker		
	LDL Pts	Chol Pts
No	0	[0]
Yes	2	[2]

Step 7   (sum from steps 1–6)

Adding up the points	
Age	
LDL-C or Chol	
HDL-C	
Blood Pressure	
Diabetes	
Smoker	
Point Total	

Step 8   (determine CHD risk from point total)

CHD Risk			
LDL Pts Total	10-Yr CHD Risk	Chol Pts Total	10-Yr CHD Risk
< –3	1%		
–2	2%		
–1	2%	[< –1]	[2%]
0	3%	[0]	[2%]
1	4%	[1]	[3%]
2	4%	[2]	[4%]
3	6%	[3]	[5%]
4	7%	[4]	[7%]
5	9%	[5]	[8%]
6	11%	[6]	[10%]
7	14%	[7]	[13%]
8	18%	[8]	[16%]
9	22%	[9]	[20%]
10	27%	[10]	[25%]
11	33%	[11]	[31%]
12	40%	[12]	[37%]
13	47%	[13]	[45%]
≥ 14	≥ 56%	[≥ 14]	[≥ 53%]

Step 9   (compare to average person your age)

Comparative Risk			
Age (years)	Average 10-Yr CHD Risk	Average 10-Yr Hard* CHD Risk	Low† 10-Yr CHD Risk
30–34	3%	1%	2%
35–39	5%	4%	3%
40–44	7%	4%	4%
45–49	11%	8%	4%
50–54	14%	10%	6%
55–59	16%	13%	7%
60–64	21%	20%	9%
65–69	25%	22%	11%
70–74	30%	25%	14%

Relative Risk	
	Very low
	Low
	Moderate
	High
	Very high

* Hard CHD events exclude angina pectoris

† Low risk was calculated for a person the same age, optimal blood pressure, LDL-C 100–129 mg/dl or cholesterol 160–199 mg/dl, HDL-C 45 mg/dl for men or 55 mg/dl for women, nonsmoker, no diabetes

Risk estimates were derived from the experience of the Framingham Heart Study, a predominantly Caucasian population in Massachusetts, USA

Source: Wilson P, D'Agostino R, Levy D, et al. Prediction of coronary heart disease using risk factor categories. *Circulation*. 1998;97(18):1837–47.

In addition to lifestyle risk factors identified in the Framingham study, other risk factors have been determined including age, gender, family history of CVD, hemostatic factors, excessive alcohol consumption and hypertriglyceridemia. An enormous literature exists demonstrating that reducing risk factors for CVD can significantly decrease its likelihood. In these areas, lifestyle measures are powerful and effective tools as well as a cost-effective way of lowering risk factors. These measures are low risk, cost effective and many of them simultaneously reduce multiple risk factors.

10.5   EVIDENCE-BASED VERSUS RISK-BASED APPROACHES TO PREVENTION OF CARDIOVASCULAR DISEASE

The traditional method for assessing risk factors for CVD comes from Framingham data and is considered to be "risk based." That is, given certain risk factors, the equations from the Framingham Risk Evaluation estimate a 10-year likelihood for both men and women of developing CVD. The tables for Framingham Risk Scores are found in Tables 10.1 and 10.2. This approach is considered "risk based" since it lumps all individuals who are either of a certain age or have certain risk factors together when making predictions of the likelihood of developing CVD in the next 10 years. Recently, many preventive cardiologists have suggested that a more precise way of assessing risk would be based on evidence-based alternatives with the evidence coming from randomized controlled trials (RCTs) rather than the traditional risk-based approach. This new approach has been called "what works and in whom" (12).

The widespread use of statin medications is the classic example of this new approach to developing risk factor guidelines. The Institute of Medicine has also recommended that any guidelines that are subsequently developed should be based on RCTs rather than on composite risk factors. In the area of statins, preventive cardiologists in the United States, Canada and Europe have suggested five simple and easily understood guidelines for their use for the prevention of CVD. The recommended five components of these guidelines for the use of statin therapy are the following:

- On the basis of high-quality, RCT data, statin therapy should be used as an adjunct to diet, exercise and smoking cessation for secondary prevention in individuals with a previous history of myocardial infarction (MI), stroke or clinically apparent atherosclerosis.
- High-quality RCTs support the use of statin therapy as an adjunct to diet, exercise and smoking cessation as a component of primary prevention for individuals over the age of 50 years with diabetes, elevated LDL cholesterol, low HDL cholesterol or elevated high-sensitivity C-reactive protein (hs-CRP) or multiple risk factors.
- On the basis of high quality RCTs in prescribing statin therapies physicians should seek to maximize the intensity of the regimen and then focus efforts on compliance and long term adherence.
- On the basis of high-quality RCTs the use of nonstatin lipid-lowering agents for monotherapy or in combination with statins should be limited awaiting evidence that such an approach further reduces CVD event rates to specific patient groups.
- Guidelines based on trial evidence should determine what works and on trial entry criteria. These guidelines that ascertain in whom to use statins are simple, practical and consistent with evidence-based principles and should therefore result in broad clinical acceptance.

This approach is fundamentally different than utilizing Framingham Risk Scores and has now been widely accepted in the preventive cardiology community.

A particular benefit of this approach is that it may be more effective in providing appropriate statin therapy for individuals at the low or middle risk of previous risk assessments, such as Framingham Risk, the Reynold's Risk, or the European System of Coronary Risk Evaluation (SCORE). This new approach to guideline development is thought to be more effective in recognizing the individuals after lowering the intermediate risk and reserving aggressive pharmaceutical intervention such as the use of statins for those in "higher"-risk profiles. It should be noted that this new approach still emphasizes lifestyle therapies as key components of all risk reduction approaches.

10.6   RELATIVE RISK VERSUS ABSOLUTE RISK

It is important to differentiate between "relative" and "absolute" risk since this distinction underlies the treatment strategies for risk factor reduction in CVD. *Relative risk* is a comparison between different risk levels (13–15). This compares the likelihood that an individual who possesses a significant risk factor will develop CVD in comparison to an individual without that risk factor. *Absolute risk* represents the likelihood of developing CVD over a specified period of time. Framingham Risk Scores, for example, represent the absolute risk of developing CVD over a 10-year period.

The difference between relative and absolute risk impacts clinical decision-making. For example, a young individual with slightly elevated blood pressure or abnormal lipids would be treated differently than an older individual with these risk factors since while their relative risk may be the same, their absolute risk may be quite different.

Relative risk may also be viewed as an indication of how rapidly an individual may move to absolute risk. For example, a young individual with high relative risk would be at a greater risk for ultimately developing high absolute risk. This should motivate a clinician's advice strategy for lowering risk as a means of slowing the early stages of developing CVD. Individuals with somewhat high relative risk would preferentially be treated with lifestyle measures that would be adopted for a long period of time and carry multiple benefits with relatively little risk or expense. This may ultimately result in a decrease in both relative and absolute risk by employing lifestyle measures.

10.7   PRIMARY VERSUS SECONDARY PREVENTION

It is also important to distinguish between "primary" and "secondary" prevention for risk factor reduction. Primary prevention is based on the goal of preventing or delaying the development of CVD, while secondary prevention focuses on interventions designed to reduce the likelihood of repeat cardiovascular events and/or mortality in individuals who have established CVD.

10.8   PRIMORDIAL PREVENTION AND "IDEAL" CARDIOVASCULAR HEALTH

An important new concept was introduced in 2010 by the American Heart Association (AHA) in their Strategic Plan for the Year 2020 and Beyond (16). This new concept was "primordial" prevention. The AHA articulated the goal in this area that "by 2022 improved cardiovascular health of Americans by 20%, while reducing deaths from cardiovascular disease and stroke by 20%." This statement is based on a recognition from the AHA that "health is a broader more positive construct than just the absence of clinically evident disease."

The AHA has defined primordial prevention as the process to avoid adverse levels of risk factors in the first place rather than try to reduce risk factors when they are already present or treating established disease. New advances in the inflammatory component of atherosclerosis and the potential for determining underlying genetic bases for CVD hold great promise in the area of primordial prevention. This broad risk strategy is completely consistent with the goals and vision of lifestyle medicine that emphasizes techniques that can be adopted throughout the life span to help lower the risk of ever-developing risk factors. This strategy is particularly relevant for children and young adults.

In addition, in their Strategic Plan, the AHA put forth a concept of "ideal" cardiovascular health that was defined as the following: "the simultaneous presence of four favorable health behaviors: absence of smoking within the last year, physical activity at goal, consumption of a heart healthy dietary pattern, and an ideal body mass index." The concept of "ideal" cardiovascular health also included favorable health factors such as untreated cholesterol (<200 mg/dL), untreated blood pressure (<120/80 mm Hg), the absence of T2DM, the absence of clinical cardiovascular disease (including CVD, stroke and heart failure), and so on. Both primordial prevention and ideal cardiovascular health are concepts where lifestyle medicine has the potential to play a critically important and central role.

10.9   IMPLEMENTING RISK FACTOR REDUCTION GUIDELINES

An important trend in the area of risk factor reduction comes from guideline statements from a variety of professional organizations including the AHA Scientific Statement on Implementing Pediatric and Adult Nutrition Guidelines, the Dietary Guidelines for Americans 2020–2025 (17), and the Physical Activity Guidelines for Americans 2018 (18). All three of these guidelines have emphasized the real-world active implementation of recommendations. It is important that lifestyle medicine practitioners pay close attention to these three, widely read and influential documents and continue to counsel patients in the area of how to employ risk factor reduction strategies in their daily lives.

10.10   PREDICTING RISK

The first step prior to utilizing lifestyle measures to lower the risk factors for CVD involves predicting risk. As already indicated, most currently employed evidence-based frameworks for lowering risk factors for CVD involve assessing absolute risk. That is the process used in both the Framingham Risk Tables and multiple guidelines from the AHA. However, as already indicated, most of these guidelines do not cover the full extent of issues related to lifestyle and CHD risk, so it will be important to

TABLE 10–2
Framingham Risk Score

Step 1

Age		
Years	LDL Pts	Chol Pts
30–34	-9	[9]
35–39	4	[4]
40–44	0	[0]
45–49	3	[3]
50–54	6	[6]
55–59	7	[7]
60–64	8	[8]
65–69	8	[8]
70–74	8	[8]

Step 2

LDL-C		
(mg/dl)	(mmol/L)	LDL Pts
< 100	< 2.59	2
100–129	2.60–3.36	0
130–159	3.37–4.14	0
160–190	4.15–4.92	2
≥ 190	≥ 4.92	2

Cholesterol		
(mg/dl)	(mmol/L)	Chol Pts
< 160	< 4.14	[2]
160–199	4.15–5.17	[0]
200–239	5.18–6.21	[1]
240–279	6.22–7.24	[1]
≥ 280	≥ 7.25	[3]

Step 3

HDL-C			
(mg/dl)	(mmol/L)	LDL Pts	Chol Pts
< 35	< 0.90	5	[5]
35–44	0.91–1.16	2	[2]
45–49	1.17–1.29	1	[1]
50–59	1.30–1.55	0	[0]
≥ 60	≥ 1.56	-2	[-3]

Step 4

Blood Pressure					
Systolic (mm Hg)	Diastolic (mm Hg)				
	< 80	80–84	85–89	90–99	≥ 100
< 120	-3 [-3] pts				
120–129		0 [0] pts			
130–139			0 [0] pts		
140–159				2 [2] pts	
≥ 160					3 [3] pts

Note: When systolic and diastolic pressures provide different estimates for point scores, use the higher number

Step 5

Diabetes		
	LDL Pts	Chol Pts
No	0	[0]
Yes	4	[4]

Step 6

Smoker		
	LDL Pts	Chol Pts
No	0	[0]
Yes	2	[2]

Step 7 (sum from steps 1–6)

Adding up the points	
Age	
LDL-C or Chol	
HDL-C	
Blood Pressure	
Diabetes	
Smoker	
Point Total	

Step 8 (determine CHD risk from point total)

CHD Risk			
LDL Pts Total	10-Yr CHD Risk	Chol Pts Total	10-Yr CHD Risk
< -2	1%	[< -2]	[1%]
-1	2%	[-1]	[2%]
0	2%	[0]	[2%]
1	2%	[1]	[2%]
2	3%	[2]	[3%]
3	3%	[3]	[3%]
4	4%	[4]	[4%]
5	5%	[5]	[4%]
6	6%	[6]	[5%]
7	7%	[7]	[6%]
8	8%	[8]	[7%]
9	9%	[9]	[8%]
10	11%	[10]	[10%]
11	13%	[11]	[11%]
12	15%	[12]	[13%]
13	17%	[13]	[15%]
14	20%	[14]	[18%]
15	24%	[15]	[20%]
16	27%	[16]	[24%]
≥ 17	≥ 32%	[≥ 17]	[≥ 27%]

Step 9 (compare to average person your age)

Comparative Risk			
Age (years)	Average 10-Yr CHD Risk	Average 10-Yr Hard* CHD Risk	Low† 10-Yr CHD Risk
30–34	< 1%	< 1%	< 1%
35–39	< 1%	< 1%	1%
40–44	2%	1%	2%
45–49	5%	2%	3%
50–54	8%	3%	5%
55–59	12%	7%	7%
60–64	12%	8%	8%
65–69	13%	8%	8%
70–74	14%	11%	8%

Relative Risk	
	Very low
	Low
	Moderate
	High
	Very high

* Hard CHD events exclude angina pectoris

† Low risk was calculated for a person the same age, optimal blood pressure, LDL-C 100–129 mg/dl or cholesterol 160–199 mg/dl, HDL-C 45 mg/dl for men or 55 mg/dl for women, nonsmoker, no diabetes

Risk estimates were derived from the experience of the Framingham Heart Study, a predominantly Caucasian population in Massachusetts, USA

Source: Wilson P, D'Agostino R, Levy D, et al. Prediction of coronary heart disease using risk factor categories. *Circulation.* 1998;97(18):1837–47.

expand upon them in counseling sessions to fully apply the power of lifestyle medicine techniques to lowering the risk of CHD.

Available guidelines related to risk factors for CVD include those from ATP IV, the American Diabetes Association Guide for Managing Diabetes and the most recent report from the AHA on Prevention, Detection, Evaluation and Treatment of High Blood Pressure as well as the 2018 AHA/ACC Practice Guidelines.

All of these guidelines recommend lowering LDL, managing blood pressure, avoiding cigarette smoking, and so on. These guidelines also follow the new protocol for guideline development that was published by the Guideline Development Committee for the Institute for Medicine (IOM) (19). The IOM report emphasized the need for employing evidence-based medicine in guideline development, which outlines that recommendations should be mainly on evidence obtained from RCTs.

These guidelines can be confusing to clinicians, but they are not a substitute for clinical judgment. It should also be emphasized that all of these guidelines place a high value on lifestyle medicine techniques. Details about these guidelines can be found in a variety of resources that are indicated in the footnotes for this chapter.

10.11   CLASSIFYING INTERVENTIONS FOR MODIFIABLE RISK FACTORS FOR CARDIOVASCULAR DISEASE

The ACC and AHA designated interventions to reduce risk factors in the four categories based on level of evidence that lowering a particular risk factor will result in lowering risk of CHD. The following four classifications are those used by the AHA and ACC:

- *Class 1 interventions*—These are interventions that involve risk factor reduction strategies that have been proven to reduce risk when used.
- *Class 2 interventions*—This classification includes risk factors for interventions that are deemed likely to lower the incidence of CHD.
- *Class 3 interventions*—This classification includes risk factors that have been clearly associated with increased risk of CHD which, if modified, might lower the likelihood of a coronary event.
- *Class 4 interventions*—This classification includes risk factors that have been associated with increased risk of CHD which, if modified, are not likely to decrease the risk of CHD or cannot be modified.

These classifications are listed in Table 10.3.

10.12   LIFESTYLE MEDICINE APPROACH TO RISK FACTOR REDUCTION

Abundant evidence is now available about the power of various lifestyle habits and practices to lower the risk of all forms of CVD and, in particular, CHD. Thus, it is important for evidence-based lifestyle medicine practitioners to utilize the power

TABLE 10.3

Framework for Risk Factor Reduction Interventions

Class 1 Interventions
- Cigarette smoking cessation
- Management of dyslipidemias
- Management of hypertension
- Pharmaceutical measures for cardiac protection

Class 2 Interventions
- Obesity prevention and management
- Diabetes/glucose intolerance management
- Physical inactivity

Class 3 Interventions
- Nutritional counseling
- Psychological risk factors/counseling
- No alcohol consumption

Class 4
- Age
- Male gender
- Low socioeconomic status
- Family history of early-onset CVD

of these various lifestyle measures when counseling patients. The following issues should be discussed in all clinical encounters:

- *Physical activity*—Abundant evidence exists that individuals who obtain the amount of physical activity recommended by the Physical Activity Guidelines for Americans 2018 substantially reduce their risk of heart disease (18). In fact, physically active people cut their risk of heart disease in half.
- *Nutrition*—Lowering fat in the diet substantially lowers the risk of heart disease. Evidence for this can be found in multiple places, perhaps most conveniently in the Dietary Guidelines for Americans 2020–2025 (17).
- *Weight management*—Overweight and obesity substantially increase the risk for multiple chronic diseases, particularly CVD and CHD (20). Individuals should be weighed and their body mass index computed and discussed with them. Ideally, waist circumference would also be measured since accumulation of abdominal fat further increases the risk of heart disease.
- *Smoking cessation*—There are multiple reasons for cessation of smoking (21–23). Multiple pharmaceutical aids are available to help with this process, as is counseling. Using counseling and pharmaceutical therapy in conjunction with each other is the optimal approach.
- *Sleep*—Disordered sleep and sleep apnea have both been shown to increase the risk of CVD by 30%–40% (17). Quality and duration of individuals' sleep should be assessed in every patient.

- *Mental health*—Both anxiety and depression as well as stress increase the risk of heart disease. These should all be assessed in every clinical encounter.
- *Relationships with others*—Positive relationships with others have been associated with decreased risk of heart disease and should be assessed in clinical encounters.
- *Age*—Of course, age is a risk factor for heart disease. Even for individuals over the age of 65 years, lifestyle measures are very important, since these individuals are likely to live to at least the age of 85 years.

All of these issues are discussed in separate chapters in this book.

10.13 COUNSELING, MOTIVATIONAL INTERVIEWING AND BEHAVIORAL CHANGES

Most of the modalities for lifestyle medicine to improve daily lifestyle habits and actions involve changes in behavior. For this reason, it is essential that physicians become skilled in how to counsel patients to remove barriers that may get in the way of making behavioral changes (24). One established technique for accomplishing this is motivational interviewing (25). Motivational interviewing is a technique where the patient's needs, desires and realities are placed at the center of the counseling session. Multiple resources are available for physicians to learn how to do motivational interviewing if they have not already been involved in this.

In addition, health coaching has become a recognized and useful modality for helping people to make behavioral changes. A number of resources are available that may be of value for physicians who want their patients to get additional counseling sessions (26).

10.14 SUMMARY/CONCLUSIONS

To maximize the ability to lower risk factors for CVD, it is essential to establish a framework. A number of frameworks are currently available and widely used such as the Framingham Risk Tables and also the Reynold's Risk Score. However, for lifestyle medicine practitioners, the opportunity to go beyond these currently available risk frameworks is substantial. Lifestyle medicine modalities such as physical activity, proper nutrition, weight management, smoking cessation, sleep, mental health issues and relationships with others are all key components of the overall field of lifestyle medicine. These issues should be discussed with patients in every clinical encounter to maximize the ability to lower risk factors for CVD.

Clinical Applications

- There is a strong association between lifestyle medicine habits and practices and risk of CVD.
- The optimal approach for lifestyle medicine practitioners for lowering risk of CVD involves both the use of currently available risk factor

assessment tools (e.g., Framingham Risk Profile Tables or Reynold's Risk Scores) and multiple components within the field of lifestyle medicine such as counseling for increased physical activity, proper nutrition, weight management, smoking cessation, sleep, mental health and relationships with others.

- The opportunity to incorporate all of these lifestyle medicine modalities in counseling sessions will maximize patients' ability to lower their risk of CVD and emphasize the relationship between lifestyle medicine and CVD risk reduction.

REFERENCES

1. Rippe JM. Lifestyle Medicine. 3rd ed. Boca Raton, FL: CRC Press; 2019.
2. Rippe JM. Lifestyle strategies for risk factor reduction, prevention, and treatment of cardiovascular disease. Am J Lifestyle Med. 2019;13(2):204–12. Epub 2019/02/26.
3. Wilson PW, D'Agostino RB, Levy D, Belanger AM, Silbershatz H, Kannel WB. Prediction of coronary heart disease using risk factor categories. Circulation. 1998;97(18):1837–47. Epub 1998/05/29.
4. Bhatt DL, Steg PG, Ohman EM, et al. International prevalence, recognition, and treatment of cardiovascular risk factors in outpatients with atherothrombosis. JAMA. 2006;295(2):180–9. Epub 2006/01/13.
5. Moulton KS. Angiogenesis in atherosclerosis: Gathering evidence beyond speculation. Curr Opin Lipidol. 2006;17(5):548–55. Epub 2006/09/09.
6. Libby P. Molecular and cellular mechanisms of the thrombotic complications of atherosclerosis. J Lipid Res. 2009;50 Suppl(Suppl):S352–7. Epub 2008/12/20.
7. Libby P. The vascular biology of atherosclerosis. In Mann DL, Zipes DP, Libby P, Bonow RO, eds. Braunwald's Heart Disease: A Textbook of Cardiovascular Medicine. 10th ed. Amsterdam: Elsevier; 2014, pp. 873–90.
8. Libby P, Theroux P. Pathophysiology of coronary artery disease. Circulation. 2005;111(25):3481–8. Epub 2005/06/29.
9. Garcia MJ, McNamara PM, Gordon T, et al. Morbidity and mortality in diabetics in the Framingham population: Sixteen year follow-up study. Diabetes. 1974;23(2):105–11. Epub 1974/02/01.
10. Kannel WB, McGee DL. Diabetes and cardiovascular risk factors: The Framingham study. Circulation. 1979;59(1):8–13. Epub 1979/01/01.
11. Wilson PW, Garrison RJ, Castelli WP, et al. Prevalence of coronary heart disease in the Framingham offspring study: Role of lipoprotein cholesterols. Am J Cardiol. 1980;46(4):649–54. Epub 1980/10/01.
12. Ridker M, Libby P, Buring J. Risk markers for and the primary prevention of cardiovascular disease. In Bonow RO, Mann DL, Zipes DP, Libby P, eds. Braunwald's Heart Disease. 11th ed. Ch 42. Amsterdam: Elsevier; 2015, pp. 891–931.
13. Klag MJ, Ford DE, Mead LA, et al. Serum cholesterol in young men and subsequent cardiovascular disease. N Engl J Med. 1993;328(5):313–8. Epub 1993/02/04.
14. Law MR, Wald NJ, Wu T, et al. Systematic underestimation of association between serum cholesterol concentration and ischaemic heart disease in observational studies: Data from the BUPA study. BMJ. 1994;308(6925):363–6. Epub 1994/02/05.
15. Law MR, Wald NJ, Thompson SG. By how much and how quickly does reduction in serum cholesterol concentration lower risk of ischaemic heart disease? BMJ. 1994;308(6925):367–72. Epub 1994/02/05.

16. Lloyd-Jones DM, Hong Y, Labarthe D, et al. Defining and setting national goals for cardiovascular health promotion and disease reduction: The American Heart Association's strategic Impact Goal through 2020 and beyond. Circulation. 2010;121(4):586–613.

17. U.S. Department of Agriculture and U.S. Department of Health and Human Services. U.S. Department of Agriculture and U.S. Department of Health and Human Services. Dietary Guidelines for Americans, 2020–2025. 9th ed.; December 2020. DietaryGuidelines.gov. www.dietaryguidelines.gov/resources/2020-2025-dietary-guidelines-online-materials.

18. U.S. Department of Health and Human Services. Physical Activity Guidelines for Americans. 2nd ed. Washington, DC; 2018. Physical Activity Guidelines for Americans, 2nd ed. I HealthySD.gov. Accessed February 11, 2022.

19. Ridker PM, Wilson PW. A trial-based approach to statin guidelines. JAMA. 2013;310(11):1123–4. Epub 2013/08/15.

20. Fryar CD, Carroll MD, Ogden CL. Prevalence of Overweight, Obesity, and Severe Obesity among Adults Aged 20 and Over: United States, 1960–1962 through 2015–2016 by Division of Health and Nutrition Examination Surveys. Centers for Disease Control and Prevention Prevalence of Overweight, Obesity, and Severe Obesity among Adults Aged 20 and Over: United States, 1960–1962 through 2015–2016. cdc.gov. Accessed February 11, 2022.

21. Centers for Disease Control and Prevention (US); National Center for Chronic Disease Prevention and Health Promotion (US); Office on Smoking and Health (US). How Tobacco Smoke Causes Disease: The Biology and Behavioral Basis for Smoking-Attributable Disease: A Report of the Surgeon General. Atlanta (GA): Centers for Disease Control and Prevention (US); 2010. www.ncbi.nlm.nih.gov/books/NBK53017/. Accessed February 11, 2022.

22. Centers for Disease Control Prevention. Smoking-attributable mortality, years of potential life lost, and productivity losses—United States, 2000–2004. MMWR Morb Mortal Wkly Rep. 2008;57(45):1226–8. Epub 2008/11/15.

23. Jha P, Ramasundarahettige C, Landsman V, et al. 21st-century hazards of smoking and benefits of cessation in the United States. N Engl J Med. 2013;368(4):341–50. Epub 2013/01/25.

24. Linke SE, Robinson CJ, Pekmezi D. Applying psychological theories to promote healthy lifestyles. Am J Lifestyle Med. 2013;8(1):4–14.

25. Fifield P, Suzuki J, Minski S, et al. Motivational interviewing and lifestyle change. In James Rippe MD, ed. Lifestyle Medicine. 3rd ed. Boca Raton, FL: CRC Press; 2019, Chapter 17, pp. 207–18.

26. Lawson K, Moore M, Clark MM. Health coaching and behavior change. In James Rippe MD, ed. Lifestyle Medicine. 3rd ed. Boca Raton, FL: CRC Press; 2019, Ch. 24, pp. 229–310.

11 Lifestyle Medicine and Atherosclerosis

KEY POINTS

- In the past decade, an increasing role for inflammation has been determined as a key component of the development of atherosclerosis.
- Atherosclerosis is a chronic condition that is highly prevalent throughout the world.
- The standard therapy to lower LDL cholesterol remains the mainstay for treating atherosclerosis, but lowering inflammatory markers have increasingly also played a role.
- Lifestyle medicine modalities contribute to lowering LDL cholesterol and also lowering inflammation.
- Regular physical activity and plant-based diets have been shown to also modulate genetic factors that may impact atherosclerosis.

11.1 INTRODUCTION

In the last 20 years, there has been a substantial revision of how we regard the process of atherosclerosis. As the world has entered into the current stage of epidemiologic transition that people have called the period of "obesity and inactivity," there has been a corresponding rise in atherogenesis, which is stimulated by poor dietary habits (e.g., large numbers of saturated fats and increased calories) and diminished physical activity. These factors have contributed to the rise of atherosclerosis around the world (1).

In addition, the view of arteries has undergone significant changes in the past 20 years. Initially, arteries were viewed as inanimate tubes, but by the mid-19th century, it was clear that there was a link between atherosclerosis and the lining of the arteries. By the early 20th century, experiments done, initially in rabbits, showed that a diet high in fat would result in fatty deposition in the arteries, and cholesterol was initially identified as the culprit. As a more sophisticated view of lipoprotein particles in the 20th century arose, an understanding became available concerning lipoprotein particles, and a more sophisticated view of atherosclerosis emerged (2).

With the ability to significantly lower LDL cholesterol, it was felt that we were on the verge of substantially reducing the risk for atherosclerosis. However, this has clearly not happened. The level of symptomatic atherosclerosis (3) (e.g., myocardial infarction, stroke and hypertension and angina) has decreased, but these manifestations of atherosclerosis are still highly prevalent. Coronary heart disease (CHD) is the leading cause of death in the United States and worldwide (4).

A more sophisticated view of atherosclerosis has emerged in the past decade. This view involves the interaction between the inner lining of the arteries (endothelium), lipids

DOI: 10.1201/b23245-13

within the lumen of the artery and inflammatory cells that invade below the endothelium. Both the lipid component and the inflammatory component are extremely important to the process of atherosclerosis. Both are, thus, highly relevant to practitioners of lifestyle medicine. Lifestyle medicine modalities can be utilized not only to lower lipids within the arteries but also to substantially reduce inflammation, which has increasingly become a hallmark of the modern understanding of atherosclerosis. In addition, evidence now exists that substantial lifestyle medicine changes (e.g., significant reduction in fat in the diet and increased physical activity) can substantially change the role of genetics within the coronary arteries and further reduce the risk of atherosclerosis.

Many unknowns still exist when it comes to atherosclerosis. It is clear, however, that practitioners of lifestyle medicine need to have a basic understanding of this process and how lifestyle medicine modalities can impact it.

11.2   THE EPIDEMIOLOGY OF ATHEROSCLEROSIS

Atherosclerosis is the leading cause of vascular disease worldwide. Clinical manifestations of atherosclerosis include CHD, ischemic stroke and peripheral vascular disease (5). In high-income countries, over the past 50 years a significant decline has occurred in the instance and mortality from both CHD and ischemic stroke (cerebrovascular accident [CVA]). For example, in the United Kingdom, the probability of death from vascular disease in middle-age men (35–69 years old) has decreased from 22% in 1950 to 6% in 2010 (6).

The decline in mortality from atherosclerosis has been largely a result of increased diagnosis and more sophisticated cardiovascular procedures. Lifestyle modalities, however, such as increased physical activity, better control of blood pressure and some improvements in diet have also contributed in significant ways.

Unfortunately, in middle-income countries, the declines in mortality have been much less dramatic. In some countries, there have been increases in atherosclerosis (e.g., Eastern Europe and Asia).

Lifestyle modalities have been clearly identified in atherosclerosis, including inactivity, smoking, obesity, high blood pressure, dyslipidemia and type 2 diabetes mellitus (T2DM). These risk factors that largely result from lifestyle habits and practices offer the most compelling opportunities for reducing the worldwide epidemic of atherosclerosis.

The need to reduce smoking and control the accelerating obesity epidemic are particularly important. These factors, along with physical activity, control of blood pressure and improvements in diet are all key components of the initiative from the World Health Organization (WHO) to combat noncommunicable diseases, in general, and cardiovascular (CVD), in particular (7). Thus, lifestyle medicine practitioners should recognize the importance of these modalities in treating the leading killer of adults worldwide.

11.3   STRUCTURE OF THE NORMAL ARTERY

Normal arteries have what is called a "truliminer" structure. The innermost layer is called the tunica intima. Within it reside the cells that line the arteries that are called endothelial cells (ECs) (8). The ECs are remarkable structures that play a critical role in the function of arteries. Problems that arise with these cells represent a critical first step in the pathogenesis of arterial diseases. For example, ECs provide one of the only surfaces that can maintain blood in a liquid state during protracted contact. This is derived in part from heparin sulfate glycosaminoglycan molecules on the surface of ECs. In addition, ECs produce other substances such as nitric oxide that are responsible for the dilation and contraction of arteries. When these cells are disrupted, the ability of arteries to dilate and constrict is significantly hampered.

The second major cell type in a normal arterial wall is smooth muscle cells (SMCs) (9). These cells are also responsible for contracting and relaxing to control blood flow. Once again, atherosclerotic changes can inhibit these cells' ability to both expand and contract to meet physiologic needs. The SMCs are largely contained in the second layer of the normal artery, which is called the tunica media.

The final layer of the normal artery is called the adventitia that contains largely collagen fibrils and blood vessels that supply the artery.

11.4 INITIATION OF ATHEROSCLEROSIS

The first step in the initiation of atherosclerosis is thought to be the accumulation of lipoprotein particles. These particles initially appear in the lumen of the artery and then begin to migrate to the intima and aggregate with each other. These lipoprotein molecules then may be oxidized in a process that is thought to be part of the early process of atherosclerosis.

The next step in atherosclerosis involves recruitment of leukocytes (10–12). Normally the endothelium resists interactions and adhesions of leukocytes, but in the presence of elevated blood lipids, these white blood cells adhere to the endothelium and penetrate through the ECs, begin to accumulate lipids and become what are called foam cells. These cells also generate a variety of adhesion modules. This class of leukocytes start out as monocytes, but as they enter the interior wall, they become macrophages utilizing adhesion molecules to start to accumulate cholesterol.

The monocytes consume lipids and become a foam cell or lipid-laden macrophage (13). Once this process occurs, these macrophages can replicate and proliferate to establish lesions (14). These lesions may ultimately progress to more complicated features such as fibrosis and thrombosis and quantification. Initially, however, they manifest as fatty streaks. In the process of lipid lowering, this process may reverse itself. In this stage, lifestyle measures as well as perhaps pharmaceutical treatment to lower lipids may be particularly beneficial.

11.5 IMMUNITY AND INFLAMMATION

Over the past 10 years, an important role for inflammation and immunity has emerged in the area of atherogenesis. The macrophage foam cells recruited in the artery function not only as a reservoir for excess lipids, but as the atherosclerotic lesion develops, they also furnish many pro-inflammatory mediators. These inflammatory mediators can promote inflammation in the plaque and thereby contribute to its progression. This process is termed *innate immunity* (15).

In addition to *innate immunity*, an important role for antigen-specific or "adaptive" immunity emerges as plaques progress (16). In addition to the mononuclear phagocytes, cells in the atherosclerotic lesions present antigens to T cells that represent an important component of the leukocytes in atherosclerotic lesions. These activated T cells then secrete large quantities of cytokines that continue to enhance atherogenesis. Cytokines can also lead to plaque destabilization and increase thrombogenicity. The death of a variety of cell types within the atherosclerotic lesion may contribute to its progression and complications. Humeral immunity, including the role of B cells, remains under active investigation.

Eventually SMCs become involved in the atherosclerotic process, too. Once a plaque experiences disruption from thrombosis (see subsequent section), SMC activities may substantially increase. In addition to replicating, the SMCs may experience death and may further complicate the atherosclerotic plaque. Thus, SMCs experience not only replication but also cell death. In addition, the atherosclerotic plaques can develop their own microcirculation as they grow. These micro vessels can potentially play an important role in the disruption of plaque since they provide a mechanism for leukocytes to travel. In addition, these micro vessels are very fragile and prone to rupture.

11.6   GENETICS OF ATHEROSCLEROSIS

Genetic factors have been demonstrated to play a significant role in the risk of CHD. Genome-wide association studies (GWASs) have shown up to 60 genes with minor abnormalities that are associated with increased risk of CHD (17). While this may seem incredibly complicated, it begins to explain the estimated 28% inheritability of CHD. While these studies have not yet provided information with direct clinical significance, it is an area of intense investigation that ultimately may lead to genetic risk scores that can help determine which individuals are at increased risk for atherosclerosis.

11.7   THE ROLE OF LIFESTYLE MODALITIES IN ATHEROSCLEROSIS

There is no question that a variety of lifestyle medicine modalities significantly impact various aspects of atherosclerosis. Specifically, lower-fat diets have been demonstrated to lower lipids in the bloodstream and have been demonstrated to significantly lower the risk of CHD. Physical activity has also been demonstrated to decrease the risk of CHD, and this may also be true in genetic alterations. In one study in which participants dramatically lowered the fat in the diet (from 60% to 10%) and increased physical activity, a number of new genes were discovered in peripheral blood, and the number of previously existing genes were found to be suppressed. This altered genetic profile specifically related to the development of leukocytes, which are a key component of inflammation.

In contrast, there is now some evidence that red meat that is consumed may alter microbiota in the gut in ways that increase inflammation. Several small studies have shown that plant-based eating, regular physical activity and stress reduction lower angiographically demonstrated lesions in coronary arteries. These findings undoubtedly result from decreased levels of lipids in the blood and decreased inflam-mation in atherosclerotic plaques, which allow them to stabilize. Clearly, obesity and diabetes share a component of inflammation. Lifestyle treatments of both obesity and T2DM carry significant implications for the development of atherosclerosis. Thus, lifestyle modalities not only impact established risk factors such as dyslipidemia, obesity and diabetes, but they may also interact with underlying genetic changes that can result in decreased inflammatory markers.

11.8   COMPLICATIONS OF ATHEROSCLEROSIS

The process of atherosclerosis typically lasts for many years during which time the individual with atherosclerosis may not experience any symptoms (18). When the burden of atherosclerosis achieves the capacity of the artery to remodel itself, it begins to encroach on arterial lumens (18,19). Eventually, the stenosis may progress to a degree that blood flow is inhibited to the artery. This is particularly true when the stenosis is greater than 60%. This type of atherosclerotic disease commonly pro-duces chronic stable angina or, if found in the legs, intermittent claudication, particu-larly during episodes of increased demand.

In contrast, in many instances of myocardial infarction (MI), there is no previ-ous history of stable angina. Acute coronary syndromes may result from thrombi due to disruption of plaque (19,20). The larger stenoses, however, are more likely to cause MI. Lesser stenoses, however, are also capable of causing MI if the plaque is disrupted.

In about two-thirds of acute MIs, plaque rupture occurs leading to thrombosis. This typically involves rupture of the plaque's fibrous cap that usually results from imbalance between forces affecting the cap and the mechanical strength of the cap. This may be due to cytokines produced by leukocytes or mediators released by plate-lets within the fibrous cap. The macrophages in the atherosclerotic plaque may also produce chemicals that can break down the collagen within the fibrous cap, repre-senting another link of inflammatory response to thrombotic complications of the atherosclerotic plaque.

Plaques that rupture may also have a prominent accumulation of macrophages and a large lipid pool. Lipid-lowering therapy may result in both the reduction of lipids and decrease of inflammation that lowers the risk of plaque rupture (21,22). In addition to the potential for plaque rupture, there may be superficial erosion of plaque. The type of plaque that this occurs in is very different from those that rup-ture. These plaques also contain multiple white blood cells and acute inflamma-tory cells. These may result in endothelial alterations that predispose to superficial erosion.

11.9   ENDOTHELIAL DYSFUNCTION

When the endothelium of the artery is disrupted, atherosclerotic plaque is promul-gated. It is the key lesion behind CHD. As already indicated, both acute and chronic inflammatory reactions occur within the arterial wall, furthering endothelial cell dys-function. Both lipids and inflammation are involved in endothelial cell dysfunction.

In addition, endothelial gene expression can be changed at both genetic and epigenetic levels. For example, in one recent study, DNA transfer activity occurred when alterations flow within the vessels occurred because of atherosclerosis. Recent studies have shown that an inflammatory marker C-reactive protein (hs-CRP) is a key marker in development of atherosclerotic vascular disease (ACVD). This may be a function of inflammatory reaction activation of endothelial cells. In the JUPITER Trial, individuals with high levels of hs-CRP had a higher risk of CHD than did individuals with elevated LDL (23). It should also be noted that endothelial cells generate nitric oxide (NO), which is responsible for both dilation and constriction of coronary arteries. Thus, when endothelial cells are disrupted and NO synthesis is curtailed, arteries are less able to both dilate and constrict in response to increased or decreased loads.

11.10   INFECTIONS, MICROBIOME AND ATHEROSCLEROSIS

There is ongoing interest in the possibility that interactions with infections may cause atherosclerosis (24). Much of the interest is based on the fact that infections often cause an inflammatory response, and there is clear evidence that inflammation within the walls of arteries contributes to atherosclerosis. In addition, there is a high level of atherosclerosis in developed countries where there is evidence of previous infections. There is also reasonable evidence that infections may exacerbate additional risk factors such as hypercholesterolemia.

As already indicated, there has been an increased interest in the intestinal microbiome and the potential ability of bacteria in the biome to create signals that could alter systemic risk factors and contribute to inflammation in adipose tissue or contribute to insulin resistance (25). In addition, metabolites produced by gut microflora may create metabolites that may augment atherosclerosis.

Finally, acute infections may lead to hemodynamic alterations that could stimulate coronary events. For example, increased metabolic demands could increase tachycardia and other hemodynamic changes that lead to ischemia in an otherwise asymptomatic, stable individual.

11.11   THERAPIES TO REDUCE INFLAMMATION

The evidence implicating inflammation as a component of atherosclerosis has led to research in various potential therapies for lowering inflammation directly. In one ongoing trial, antibiotics have been studied in humans to reduce IL-1B as an attempt to reduce measures of inflammation (hs-CRP, AL-6 and fibrinogen) without influencing lipids. Another trial of 7,000 individuals with coronary artery disease and metabolic syndrome compared low-dose methotrexate to usual care to explore whether reducing inflammation in this manner would lower the risk of CHD. These therapies are under investigation and are not ready for clinical use. The mainstay for reducing risk of atherosclerosis remains in controlling lipids. A target that has been established for many years and shown in many studies to lower the risk of CHD is lowering LDL cholesterol. In addition, there has been recent interest in lowering triglycerides, since triglyceride-rich lesions in coronary arteries contribute to atherosclerosis.

11.12 SUMMARY/CONCLUSIONS

The field of atherosclerosis is an important one for individuals practicing in the area of lifestyle medicine. In the past decade, discovery of the key role that inflammation plays in the development of atherosclerotic plaque has underscored why therapies such as weight loss, physical activity and lower-fat diets may all contribute to reducing inflammation and thereby contribute to reducing the risk of atherosclerosis. These therapies, in addition to the established therapies for lowering LDL cholesterol, are all areas where practitioners of lifestyle medicine can play an important role. Thus, atherosclerosis is a key area where lifestyle medicine has modalities and treatment that can yield multiple benefits for reducing risk of CHD.

Clinical Applications

- Many traditional lifestyle medicine modalities can reduce the risk of atherosclerosis by reducing the level of LDL cholesterol and inflammation, both of which contribute to the development of atherosclerosis.
- Such modalities as plant-based diets and regular physical activity have also been demonstrated to contribute to changes in the genome that impact the likelihood of developing atherosclerosis.
- Since atherosclerosis is the underlying process that contributes to multiple complications such as stable angina, unstable angina, MI and stroke, the role for lifestyle medicine plays a very important and increasing role in the area of cardiovascular disease prevention.

REFERENCES

1. Herrington W, Lacey B, Sherliker P, et al. Epidemiology of atherosclerosis and the potential to reduce the global burden of atherothrombotic disease. Circ Res. 2016;118(4):535–46. Epub 2016/02/20.
2. Libby P, Bornfeldt KE, Tall AR. Atherosclerosis: Successes, surprises, and future challenges. Circ Res. 2016;118(4):531–4. Epub 2016/02/20.
3. Shapiro MD, Fazio S. From lipids to inflammation: New approaches to reducing atherosclerotic risk. Circ Res. 2016;118(4):732–49. Epub 2016/02/20.
4. Mozaffarian D, Benjamin EJ, Go AS, et al. Heart disease and stroke statistics—2015 update: A report from the American Heart Association. Circulation. 2015;131(4):e29–322. Epub 2014/12/19.
5. Moran AE, Forouzanfar MH, Roth GA, Mensah GA, Ezzati M, Murray CJ, et al. Temporal trends in ischemic heart disease mortality in 21 world regions, 1980 to 2010: The global burden of disease 2010 study. Circulation. 2014;129(14):1483–92. Epub 2014/02/28.
6. Bennett DA, Krishnamurthi RV, Barker-Collo S, et al. The global burden of ischemic stroke: Findings of the GBD 2010 study. Glob Heart. 2014;9(1):107–12. Epub 2014/11/30.
7. World Health Organization. Noncomunicable Disease. www.who.int/teams/surveillance-of-noncommunicable-diseases/about/ncds#:~:text=The%20%E2%80%98Internal%20horizontal%20network%20for%20collective%20action%20to,screening%2C%20early%20diagnosis%2C%20and%20appropriate%20treatment%20of%20NCDs.?msclkid=ce82f946aace11ecb469b1b4e0121ab8. Accessed March 23, 2022.

8. Gimbrone MA, Jr., Garcia-Cardena G. Endothelial cell dysfunction and the pathobiology of atherosclerosis. Circ Res. 2016;118(4):620–36. Epub 2016/02/20.

9. Bennett MR, Sinha S, Owens GK. Vascular smooth muscle cells in atherosclerosis. Circ Res. 2016;118(4):692–702. Epub 2016/02/20.

10. Muller WA. How endothelial cells regulate transmigration of leukocytes in the inflammatory response. Am J Pathol. 2014;184(4):886–96. https://doi.org/10.1016/j.ajpath.2013.12.033

11. Gerhardt T, Ley K. Monocyte trafficking across the vessel wall. Cardiovasc Res. 2015;107(3):321–30. Epub 2015/05/21.

12. Li J, Ley K. Lymphocyte migration into atherosclerotic plaque. Arterioscler Thromb Vasc Biol. 2015;35(1):40–9. Epub 2014/10/11.

13. Moore KJ, Sheedy FJ, Fisher EA. Macrophages in atherosclerosis: A dynamic balance. Nat Rev Immunol. 2013;13(10):709–21. Epub 2013/09/03.

14. Robbins CS, Hilgendorf I, Weber GF, et al. Local proliferation dominates lesional macrophage accumulation in atherosclerosis. Nat Med. 2013;19(9):1166–72. Epub 2013/08/13.

15. Libby P, Lichtman AH, Hansson GK. Immune effector mechanisms implicated in atherosclerosis: From mice to humans. Immunity. 2013;38(6):1092–104. Epub 2013/07/03.

16. Ketelhuth DF, Hansson GK. Adaptive response of T and B cells in atherosclerosis. Circ Res. 2016;118(4):668–78. Epub 2016/02/20.

17. McPherson R, Tybjaerg-Hansen A. Genetics of coronary artery disease. Circ Res. 2016;118(4):564–78. Epub 2016/02/20.

18. Libby P. Mechanisms of acute coronary syndromes and their implications for therapy. N Engl J Med. 2013;368(21):2004–13. Epub 2013/05/24.

19. Bentzon JF, Otsuka F, Virmani R, et al. Mechanisms of plaque formation and rupture. Circ Res. 2014;114(12):1852–66. Epub 2014/06/07.

20. Luscher TF. Substrates of acute coronary syndromes: New insights into plaque rupture and erosion. Eur Heart J. 2015;36(22):1347–9. Epub 2015/06/09.

21. Yla-Herttuala S, Bentzon JF, Daemen M, et al. Stabilization of atherosclerotic plaques: An update. Eur Heart J. 2013;34(42):3251–8. Epub 2013/08/24.

22. Libby P. How does lipid lowering prevent coronary events? New insights from human imaging trials. Eur Heart J. 2015;36(8):472–4. Epub 2015/01/13.

23. Ridker PM. The JUPITER trial: Results, controversies, and implications for prevention. Circ Cardiovasc Qual Outcomes. 2009;2(3):279–85. Epub 2009/12/25.

24. Campbell LA, Rosenfeld ME. Persistent *C. pneumoniae* infection in atherosclerotic lesions: Rethinking the clinical trials. Front Cell Infect Microbiol. 2014;4:34. Epub 2014/04/09.

25. Piya MK, Harte AL, McTernan PG. Metabolic endotoxaemia: Is it more than just a gut feeling? Curr Opin Lipidol. 2013;24(1):78–85. Epub 2013/01/10.

12 Lifestyle Strategies for Managing Dyslipidemia

KEY POINTS

- Dyslipidemia including elevations of total cholesterol, LDL, triglycerides and reduced level of HDL are all significant risk factors in coronary heart disease.
- Lifestyle management represents a foundational element of the treatment of dyslipidemia including proper diet, regular physical activity, maintenance of a healthy weight, tobacco avoidance and moderate consumption of alcohol.
- Pharmacologic therapy of dyslipidemia focuses primarily on the utilization of HMG-CoA reductase inhibitors (statins). Alternate medicines may also be utilized depending on patient comorbidities.

12.1 INTRODUCTION

A compelling body of information exists that various forms of dyslipidemia are important risk factors for increasing the likelihood of all forms of atherosclerotic cardiovascular disease (ASCVD). A high prevalence of dyslipidemia exists in the United States. In particular, elevated total cholesterol and low-density lipoprotein cholesterol (LDL-C) as well as high-density lipoprotein cholesterol (HDL-C). The overall prevalence of dyslipidemia in the United States is 53% with LDL-C elevations in 27% and low HDL-C in 23% of American adults (1). In addition, 30% of individuals have an elevated level of triglycerides. However, many of these individuals also have low HDL or high LDL, so this prevalence of elevated triglycerides should not be counted separately.

Lifestyle measures contribute in significant ways to the treatment of dyslipidemias. This fact is recognized by the major guidelines published by the American Heart Association (AHA) and the American College of Cardiology (ACC) including the 2018 AHA/ACC Guidelines for the Management of Blood Cholesterol (2). Such factors as proper nutrition, weight management, regular physical activity and cessation of cigarette smoking are all important lifestyle factors that interact with the management of dyslipidemias. In fact, in the 2018 AHA/ACC Guideline on the Management of Blood Cholesterol, the number one take home message emphasizes a heart healthy lifestyle. Here is what the AHA/ACC number one take home message is:

> In all individuals should emphasize a heart healthy lifestyle across the life course. A healthy lifestyle reduces atherosclerotic cardiovascular disease (ASCVD) risk at all ages. In younger individuals, healthy lifestyles can reduce the development of risk factors and is a foundation of ASCVD risk factor reduction. In young adults 20–39 years

DOI: 10.1201/b23245-14

of age an assessment of lifetime risks facilitates the clinician-patient risk discussion and emphasizes intensive lifestyle efforts. In all age groups lifestyle therapy is the primary intervention for metabolic syndrome.

In addition, the recently released 2021 ACC Expert Consensus Decision Pathway on the Management of ASCVD Risk Reduction in Patients with Persistent Hypertriglyceridemia places strong emphasis on multiple components of lifestyle medicine (3). With these documents as background, it is incumbent upon all physicians, but particularly those interested in lifestyle medicine, to address lifestyle factors in the management of dyslipidemias.

12.2   BACKGROUND/DEFINITION

Dyslipidemia is defined as elevated fasting blood levels of total cholesterol (TC), LDL cholesterol, triglycerides (TG) and/or a reduced level of HDL alone or in combination (4,5). Although lipids contribute to many vital functions in the body, abnormal blood levels of lipids and their lipoprotein carriers contribute significantly to the pathophysiology of ASCVD and the development and progression of coronary heart disease (CHD). There is a strong genetic, environmental and lifestyle contribution to dyslipidemia. LDL cholesterol is the best established risk factor for ASCVD.

12.3   LDL CHOLESTEROL

Elevated LDL cholesterol has been clearly linked to both incident myocardial infarction (MI) and cardiovascular death. High LDL cholesterol levels consistently predict cardiovascular events. Longitudinal observational studies have demonstrated a positive association with TC and cardiovascular disease. (Above 180 mg/dL, a 2% increase in CHD risk occurs for every 1% increase in the presence of other major risk factors [6,7].) Observational studies have also suggested that a concentration of apolipoprotein B100 (apoB-100) is even stronger in predicting CHD than LDL-C (8,9).

Randomized controlled clinical trials of the cholesterol-lowering drug HMG-CoA reductase inhibitors (statins) have been uniformly successful in reducing CHD risk (10–13). A meta-analysis that includes the results of large-scale, placebo-controlled, statin trials involving greater than 30,000 participants over an average of 5.4 years indicated that statins resulted in a mean reduction of 30% in initial or recurrent CHD events (13).

Evidence also suggests that what may be regarded as "normal" cholesterol levels in Western society typically exceed levels that good health requires. Elevations in LDL cholesterol (greater than 200 mg/dL) are the most prevalent dyslipidemia found, occurring in 27% of adults. Importantly, cholesterol levels measured early in life are strongly associated with long-term cardiovascular risk, including risk of elevated CVD and elevated cholesterol.

All patients with elevated LDL cholesterol should be counseled to participate in aggressive diet and exercise programs before the initiation of pharmacologic therapy. Even though statins have been clearly demonstrated to lower LDL cholesterol, these lifestyle measures remain the initial therapy and play a synergistic role with statins.

While statin therapy represents the cornerstone for pharmacologic reduction of LDL-C, considerable interest has emerged in the monoclonal antibodies that inhibit PCSK9 binding, and consequently prolong the effect of half-life surface LDL markers (14). These agents substantially reduce LDL-C monotherapy and act as adjuncts to statin therapy. They may be particularly useful for those who have statin intolerance. These agents are currently under active research.

12.4 HIGH-DENSITY LIPOPROTEIN

Numerous studies have demonstrated an inverse relationship between HDL cholesterol and vascular risk (15). Data from observational studies suggest that for every incremental increase in HDL cholesterol of 1 mg/dL, there is a 2%–3% decrease in total CVD. For this reason, measurement of HDL is a component of all risk algorithms, and the ratio of total to HDL cholesterol is a potent lipid-based predictor of cardiovascular risk.

HDL functions in the body to remove cholesterol in the cell membrane and transport it to the liver in the bile as bile acids (16). Unfortunately, pharmacologic attempts to raise HDL have failed to improve cardiovascular outcomes in clinical trials to date.

It is important to note that regular physical activity and fitness are both associated with increases in HDL, further underscoring the importance of lifestyle factors in reduction of risk for CVD.

12.5 TRIGLYCERIDES

Elevated triglycerides also represent a risk for ASCVD (3). A number of studies have shown that despite use of statin therapy, ASCVD rates remain high in patients with elevated triglycerides.

TG levels in the blood are elevated for about an hour following meals, and in the fasting state they are primarily carried by very low-density lipoprotein (VLDL). Triglycerides tend to vary inversely with HDL. For this reason, initially triglycerides were thought to be less of a risk factor by themselves because of this inverse association with HDL. Recent data have, in fact, acknowledged that association.

12.6 ROLE OF LIFESTYLE IN THE MANAGEMENT OF DYSLIPIDEMIAS

- *Impact of diet*—The 2018 AHA/ACC Guidelines recommend that fibers bind and prevent reabsorption of bile in the small intestine, thereby upregulating hepatic LDL receptors, enhancing LDL removal and reducing LDL-C levels. It should also be noted that dietary fiber slows gastric emptying and glucose absorption, while decreasing insulin response and thereby promoting satiety. Both THE 2017 (17) and 2018 AHA/ACC Guidelines (2) indicate that more research is necessary on the influence of fiber on lipids and CHD risk. Plant sterols and stanols are plentiful in vegetables, seeds and nuts and may also contribute to reduced levels of LDL-C.

Plant-derived antioxidants such as vitamin E, beta-carotene and vitamin C may reduce the development and progression of CHD by lowering oxidative stress and reducing LDL oxidation and endothelial dysfunction (18,19). It should be noted, however, that large-scale, randomized controlled trials have failed to demonstrate protective effects in CVD mortality by supplementation from antioxidant vitamins such as vitamin E, vitamin C or beta-carotene. There has been interest in recent years about flavonoids such as those found in fruits, vegetables, tea, red wine and cocoa bean products. These phytochemicals have been shown in some in vitro studies to inhibit LDL oxidation. This is an area of research, and current evidence does not clearly support their use in the clinical setting.

Moderate alcohol intake (one to two drinks/day) has been associated with approximately 30% lower risk of mortality from CHD when compared to no alcohol or heavy alcohol consumption (20). This risk reduction may be due to antithrombotic effect or increase in HDL levels. It should be noted, however, that alcohol may produce a concomitant increase in TG and VLDL production and thereby raises non-HDL-C levels. Excessive use of alcohol also raises high blood pressure and can contribute to major health problems in addition to increasing the risk of accidents and violent death. (See Chapter 13 for further discussion.)

- *Weight management*—Dyslipidemia as well as all components of the metabolic syndrome and increased risk of type 2 diabetes mellitus (T2DM) and CHD are all associated with excess body weight (21). Thus, weight reduction is a critical component in the management of dyslipidemia. (See also Chapter 6.)

Furthermore, guidelines from the AHA/ACC and The Obesity Society (TOS) point to numerous health benefits of weight reduction in individuals who are obese (22). A 10% weight loss may result in a significant decrease in TC of over 30 mg/dL (minus 13%), LDL-C of 15.1 mg/dL (minus 11.3%), VLDL-C of 15.5 mg/dL (minus 36.5%), and TG of 58.4 mg/dL (minus 32.2%). HDL-C initially may decline during the active weight loss phase (23) but then increase 5.5 mg/dL (plus 12.6%) after weight stabilization.

Reduced fat and low-carbohydrate diets (e.g., South Beach or Atkins diet) have been compared for weight loss and cardiovascular risk factors. Both were initially successful for weight loss up to 1 year. However, reduction in TC and LDL-C was more favorable in low-fat diets compared to low-carbohydrate diets. Surprisingly, changes in LDL-C (plus 4.6 mg/dL) and TG (minus 22.1 mg/dL) were significantly more favorable in the low-carbohydrate diets. In one meta-analysis of 23 trials in short-term studies, low-carbohydrate diets resulted in further reduction of total cholesterol (2.7 mg/dL) and LDL-C (3.7 mg/dL), a greater increase of HDL-C (3.3 mg/dL), and a greater decrease in triglycerides (14 mg/dL). These findings were not examined for long-term effects (24).

Low-carbohydrate and low-fat diets have also been compared to a restricted calorie Mediterranean-type diet. Weight loss was comparable in the three diets, as was the mean increase in HDL-C. However, TG reduction (23.7 mg/dL) was significantly more favorable in the low-carbohydrate diet. There was no significant change in LDL-C in any group.

A combination of lifestyle measures such as calorie reduction and regular exercise has consistently been shown to be the most effective approach for achieving and maintaining long-term weight reduction. Thus, lifestyle measures remain a centerpiece for weight reduction for multiple reasons including positive impact on dyslipidemia.

- *Physical activity*—Increased physical activity has been demonstrated to be a powerful lifestyle practice to reduce the risk of cardiovascular disease. Moreover, studies have consistently shown that aerobic exercise modestly increases HDL-C of 2–3 mg/dL (25–28). It should be noted that there is a great deal of variability in the HDL elevating effects which may be a result of weight loss. Both the 2013 AHA/ACC and 2018 AHA Guidelines for treating dyslipidemia have advised that increased physical activity is helpful in reducing LDL-C and non-HDL-C, and they advocate that adults should participate in physical activity three to four times per week, 40 minutes per session, of moderate to vigorous activity (29).
- *Cigarette smoking*—Cigarette smoking has been associated with reduced ApoA1 and HDL-C levels of about 4–6 mg/dL or 11%–14% lower than non-smokers (30–32). It is important to note that smoking cessation appears to result in rapid improvement in HDL-C (average of 6–8 mg/dL increase). It should also be noted that smokers have been typically found to have slightly higher LDL-C level than nonsmokers. There are multiple reasons, of course, to stop cigarette smoking, but improvements in dyslipidemia should be considered as a component of this.

12.7 SUMMARY/CONCLUSIONS

Multiple lifestyle components are major contributors to treating dyslipidemia and lowering the risk of CHD. These include improvements in nutrition and increases in physical activity. Multiple eating patterns have been associated with reduced risk of dyslipidemia and CVD, including vegetarian diets, Mediterranean-style diets (33), Dietary Approaches to Stop Hypertension (DASH) diet (34) and multiple diets recommended by the AHA (35) and the Healthy U.S.-Style Dietary Pattern for Adults recommended by the Dietary Guidelines for Americans 2020–2025 (36). Thus, proper nutrition is a central lifestyle-related component of management of dyslipidemia.

As already indicated in this chapter, diets that increase fruits and vegetables, whole grains, legumes and a moderate intake of fish and low-fat dairy products has been routinely recommended for multiple reasons to reduce the risk of CHD. These diets are also foundational for the treatment of dyslipidemia. In addition, low intake of saturated and trans-fat, dietary cholesterol, reduction in red meat, concentrated fats and whole-fat milk have all been shown to increase cholesterol. A combination of proper dietary plan and regular aerobic exercise has been shown to lower TC by 7%, LDL-C by 18%, and TG by 4% and 18%, and increase HDL-C 2%–18%.

Additionally, weight management is important for management of dyslipidemia. Thus, lifestyle factors play a critically important role in managing dyslipidemia, thereby lowering the risk of CHD.

Clinical Applications

- The following clinical applications have been shown to be effective in helping to manage dyslipidemia. These are outlined in Table 12.1.

TABLE 12.1
Clinical Applications

Dietary component or TLC change	TC	LDL-C	HDL-C	TG (and Non-HDL-C)
Decrease SFAs, trans fats, and cholesterol	↓↓	↓↓	↓	↓
Increase omega 6-PUFAs	↓	↓	→ ↓	→
Increase omega 3-PUFAs	→	→ ↑	↑ →	↓↓
Increase MUFAs	→ ↓	→ ↓	↑ →	↓
Increase soluble fiber	↓	↓	→	→
Moderate alcohol	→	→	↑↑	↑↑
Phytosterols	↓	↓	→	→
Soy proteins	↓	↓	→	↓
Vitamin E (recycled by vitamin C)	–	↓ OxLDL	–	–
Negative energy balance (weight loss)	↓	↓	↑	↓↓
Aerobic exercise	↓ →	↓ →	↑	→
Smoking cessation	→	→	↑	↓

- ↑ = Increase, ↓ = decrease, → = no change.

Source: Adapted from Bronas UG, et al. Clinical strategies for managing dyslipidemias. In: Rippe JM. *Lifestyle Medicine*. 3rd ed. CRC Press; 2019. Used with permission of the editor.

REFERENCES

1. Mercado C, DeSimone AK, Odom E, et al. Prevalence of cholesterol treatment eligibility and medication use among adults—United States, 2005–2012. MMWR Morbid Mortal Wkly Rep. 2015;64(47):1305–11.
2. Grundy SM, Stone NJ, Bailey AL, et al. 2018 AHA/ACC/AACVPR/AAPA/ABC/ACPM/ADA/AGS/APhA/ASPC/NLA/PCNA Guideline on the management of blood cholesterol: A report of the American College of Cardiology/American Heart Association Task Force on clinical practice guidelines. Circulation. 2019;139(25):e1082–143. Epub 2018/12/28.

3. Virani SS, Morris PB, Agarwala A, et al. 2021 ACC expert consensus decision pathway on the management of ASCVD risk reduction in patients with persistent hypertriglyceridemia: A report of the American College of Cardiology Solution Set Oversight Committee. J Am Coll Cardiol. 2021;78(9):960–93. Epub 2021/08/02.

4. Rippe JM. Lifestyle strategies for risk factor reduction, prevention, and treatment of cardiovascular disease. Am J Lifestyle Med. 2019;13(2):204–12. Epub 2019/02/26.

5. Bassuk SS, Manson JE. Lifestyle and risk of cardiovascular disease and type 2 diabetes in women: A review of the epidemiologic evidence. Am J Lifestyle Med. 2008;2(3):191–213.

6. Keys A Coronary heart disease-the global picture. Atherosclerosis. 1975;22:149–52.

7. Kannel WB, McGee D, Gordon T. A general cardiovascular risk profile: The Framingham Study. Am J Cardiol. 1976;38:46–51.

8. Mudd, JO, Borlaug, BA, Johnson, PV, et al. Beyond low-density lipoprotein cholesterol. J Am Coll Cardiol. 2007;50:1735–41.

9. Batter PJ, Ballantyne CM, Carhona R, et al. APO B versus cholesterol in estimating cardiovascular risk and in guiding therapy: Report of the thirty-one person/thirty-country panel. J Intern Med. 2006;259:247–58.

10. Committee on Diet and Health, Food and Nutrition Board, Commission on Life Science, National Research Council. Fats and other lipids. In Diet and Health Implications for Reducing Chronic Disease Risk. Washington, DC: National Academy Press; 1989, pp. 154–288.

11. Bergland, L, Anuurad, E. Role of apoprotein (a) in cardiovascular disease: Current and future prospective. Circulation. 2008;52:132–4.

12. Thomopoulos C, Skalis G, Michalopoulou H, Tsioufis C, Makris T. Effect of low-density lipoprotein cholesterol lowering by ezetimibe/simvastatin on outcome incidence: Overview, meta-analyses, and meta-regression analyses of randomized trials: Effect of LDL-C lowering on outcomes. Clin Cardiol. 2015;38(12):763–9.

13. LaRosa, JC, He J, Vuppututi S. Effects of statins on risk of coronary heart disease: A meta-analysis of randomized trials. JAMA. 1999;282:23430–46.

14. Ridker PM, Revkin J, Amarenco P, et al. Cardiovascular efficacy and safety of bococizumab in high-risk patients. N Engl J Med. 2017;376(16):1527–39.

15. Gordon DJ. Probstfield, Garrison, RJ, et al. High-density lipoprotein cholesterol and cardiovascular disease: Four prospective American studies. Circulation. 1989;79:8–19.

16. Baymes JW, Dominiczac MH. Lipids and lipoproteins. In Medical Biochemistry. 2nd ed. Philadelphia: Elsevier Mosby; 2005, pp. 225–43.

17. Lloyd-Jones DM, Morris PB, Ballantyne CM, et al. 2017 Focused update of the 2016 ACC expert consensus decision pathway on the role of non-statin therapies for LDL-cholesterol lowering in the management of atherosclerotic cardiovascular disease risk: A report of the American College of Cardiology Task Force on Expert Consensus Decision Pathways. J Am Coll Cardiol. 2017;70(14):1785.

18. Bettridge DJ, Morrell JM. Clinician's Guide to Lipids and Coronary Heart Disease. 2nd ed. London: Arnold; 2003, pp. 101–235.

19. Fletcher B, Berra K, Braun L, et al. Managing abnormal blood lipids: A collaborated approach. Circulation. 2005;112:3184–209.

20. Law M, Wald N. The relative risk of CHD death according to alcohol consumption in the five largest cohort studies. Br Med J. 1999;318:1471–80.

21. National Institute of Health. Clinical Guidelines on the Identification, Evaluation and Treatment of Overweight and Obesity in Adults. The Evidence Report. Bethesda, MD: NIH Publication, No. 98–408; 1998.

22. Jensen MD, Ryan DH, Apovian CM, et al. 2013 AHA/ACC/TOS guideline for the management of overweight and obesity in adults: A report of the American College of Cardiology/American Heart Association Task Force on Practice Guidelines and the Obesity Society. Circulation. 2014;129(25_suppl_2 Suppl 1):S102–38.

23. Danttilo AM, Kris-Etherton PM. Effects o weight reduction on blood lipids and lipoproteins: A meta-analysis. Am J Clin Nutr. 1992;56:320–8.

24. Hu T, Mills KT, Yao L, et al. Effects of low-carbohydrate diets versus low-fat diets on metabolic risk factors: A meta-analysis of randomized controlled clinical trials. Am J Epidemiol. 2012;176(7):S44–54.

25. Kodama S, Tanaka S, Saito K, et al. Effects of aerobic exercise training on serum levels of high-density lipoprotein cholesterol: A meta-analysis. Arch Intern Med. 2007;167:999–1008.

26. Durstine SL, Grandjean PW, Cox CA, et al. Lipids, lipoproteins, and exercise. J Cardiopulm Rehabil. 2002;22:389–98.

27. Leon AS, Sanchez OA. Response of blood lipids to exercise training alone or combined with dietary intervention. Med Sci Sports Exerc. 2001;33(Supple):S502–15.

28. Leon AS, Rice R, Mandel S, et al. Blood lipid response to 20 weeks of supervised exercise in a large biracial population: The HERITAGE Family Study. Metabolism. 2001;49:S13–20.

29. Eckel RH, Jakicic JM, Ard JD, et al. 2013 AHA/ACC Guideline on lifestyle management to reduce cardiovascular risk: A report of the American College of Cardiology/American Heart Association Task Force on Practice Guidelines. Circulation. 2014;129(25_suppl_2 Suppl 1):S76–99.

30. Kannell, WB. Update on the role of cigarette smoking in coronary artery disease. Am Heart J. 1981;101:319–28.

31. Goldbourt J, Medalie JH. Characteristics of smokers, nonsmokers, and ex-smokers among 10,000 adult males in Israel II: Physiologic biochemical, and genetic characteristics. Am J Epidemiol. 1997;105:75–84.

32. Craig W, Palomaki G, Haddow J. Cigarette smoking and serum lipids and lipoprotein concentrations: Analysis of published data. BMJ. 1989;784–8.

33. Estruch R, Ros E, Salas-Salvado J, et al. Primary prevention of cardiovascular disease with a Mediterranean diet. N Engl J Med. 2013;368(14):1279–90. Epub 2013/02/26.

34. Appel LJ, Moore TJ, Obarzanek E, et al. A clinical trial of the effects of dietary patterns on blood pressure. DASH Collaborative Research Group. N Engl J Med. 1997;336(16):1117–24. Epub 1997/04/17.

35. Lichtenstein AH, Appel LJ, Vadiveloo M, et al. 2021 dietary guidance to improve cardiovascular health: A scientific statement from the American Heart Association. Circulation. 2021;144(23):e472–87. Epub 2021/11/03.

36. U.S. Department of Agriculture and U.S. Department of Health and Human Services. U.S. Department of Agriculture and U.S. Department of Health and Human Services. Dietary Guidelines for Americans, 2020–2025. 9th ed.; December 2020. DietaryGuidelines.gov. www.dietaryguidelines.gov/resources/2020-2025-dietary-guidelines-online-materials. Accessed April 27, 2022.

13 Lifestyle Management and Prevention of Hypertension

KEY POINTS

- Hypertension is extremely common in the United States and throughout the world. (Approximately 80 million individuals have high blood pressure in the United States and over a billion individuals worldwide.)
- There is a strong age-related increase in blood pressure. Even individuals who have normal blood pressure at the age of 60 years have a 90% chance of developing hypertension during their life.
- Multiple lifestyle therapies decrease the risk of developing hypertension and can assist in its therapy, including regular physical activity, proper nutrition (particularly sodium reduction) and weight management (if necessary) as well as smoking cessation.
- For all of these reasons, lifestyle therapies for high blood pressure are extremely important and should be discussed in every clinical encounter. Lifestyle therapies are also key first-line components of all of the major blood pressure control recommendations from the American Heart Association and the American College of Cardiology.

13.1 INTRODUCTION

Hypertension is extremely common both in the United States and around the world (1). High blood pressure (hypertension) affects over 80 million people in the United States and over one billion people worldwide. High blood pressure is the most common, identifiable and reversible risk factor for myocardial infarction (MI), stroke, heart failure, arterial fibrillation, aortic dissection, peripheral vascular disease and cognitive decline.

There is no longer any serious question that lifestyle measures have an enormous potential impact on lowering the burden of high blood pressure (2). Persuasive studies in the area of increased physical activity, weight reduction and proper nutrition as well as cigarette smoking cessation have all clearly demonstrated benefits in terms of lowering the prevalence and assisting in the treatment of high blood pressure.

Unfortunately, the burden of hypertension around the world has been increasing for the past 20 years. This is largely due to increasing obesity as well as the aging population worldwide. It is now projected that high blood pressure may affect as many as 1.5 billion people by 2025 (3). The prevalence of hypertension is increasing rapidly in developing countries (80% of the world) as well as developed countries.

DOI: 10.1201/b23245-15

Hypertension is a particularly significant risk factor for stroke. It is associated with two-thirds of all cerebrovascular accidents (strokes) as well as half of all coronary heart disease (CHD) worldwide (3).

The enormous benefit of lifestyle measures with regard to high blood pressure comes not only from their effectiveness but also because these modalities can be used in conjunction with pharmaceutical therapies if needed. Moreover, lifestyle modalities simultaneously impact multiple risk factors for cardiovascular disease (CVD) and CHD.

Because the vast majority of hypertension is asymptomatic, the diagnosis may be delayed. Moreover, since hypertension is a lifelong condition requiring continued assessment and therapy from physicians, this further contributes to the population-wide difficulty in controlling this condition. It is estimated that blood pressure remains elevated at 140/90 mm Hg or higher in half of affected individuals in the United States and other developed countries.

13.2 HYPERTENSION, LIFESTYLE FACTORS AND CARDIOVASCULAR DISEASE

Major advances have occurred in the understanding of high blood pressure, yet it remains poorly controlled. Despite strong evidence that lifestyle factors play a very important role in lowering the risk of hypertension and assisting in its treatment, pharmaceutical therapy remains a mainstay in many individuals. This is unfortunate, since national evidence-based guidelines have routinely recommended lifestyle measures as the first-line therapy or in conjunction with pharmaceutical therapy. For example, in the 2014 Evidence Based Guidelines for the Management of High Blood Pressure in Adults (JNC VII) (4,5), lifestyle management recommendations included the following:

- Engaging in regular aerobic activity three to four sessions per week lasting an average of 40 minutes per session of moderate to vigorous intensity physical activity. (Consistent with the Physical Activity Guidelines for Americans 2018 recommendations of 150 minutes of moderate-intensity physical activity per week [6].)
- Consuming no more than 2,300 milligrams of sodium per day.
- Consuming a diet high in fruits and vegetables, whole grains and including low-fat dairy, poultry, fish, legumes and nontropical nuts, while eliminating sweets, sugar-sweetened beverages and red meat.

In 2017, the American College of Cardiology (ACC) and American Heart Association (AHA) issued "Guideline for the Prevention, Detection, Evaluation and Management of High Blood Pressure in Adults" and established thresholds that were lower than previous classifications (see subsequent sections) (7). These guidelines also advocated lifestyle measures to prevent and treat hypertension consisting of

- Weight loss to ideal body weight;
- DASH dietary patterns;
- Reduced sodium intake to less than 1,500 milligrams per day;

- Enhanced intake of dietary potassium;
- Physical activity consisting of 120–150 minutes per week of aerobic exercise and three sessions per week of resistance training; and
- Moderation of alcohol intake.

13.3 PREVALENCE

The prevalence of high blood pressure increases with age and is particularly prevalent after the age of 50 years. Before menopause, women have a somewhat lower prevalence of hypertension than men, but after menopause, the prevalence of hypertension increases rapidly in women and surpasses men (8). By the age of 80 years, both men and women will have an almost 90% likelihood of high blood pressure. This is true for both men and women even if their blood pressure is normal at age 60 years.

13.4 DEFINITION OF HYPERTENSION

There have been various definitions of high blood pressure. Traditionally, high blood pressure has been defined as a usual office blood pressure of 140/90 mm Hg or higher. However, data that have accumulated over the past 20 years have suggested that the risk of CVD based on high blood pressure occurs at much lower levels. Thus, the definition of high blood pressure has shifted significantly over this period of time. In the 2017 ACC/AHA "Guideline for the Prevention, Detection, Evaluation and Management of High Blood Pressure in Adults," classifications were established as outlined on Table 13.1.

As summarized in Table 13.1, normal blood pressure is now classified as systolic <120 mm Hg and diastolic <80 mm Hg. Lifestyle measurements are advocated

TABLE 13.1

Categories of Blood Pressure in Adults

BP classification	SBP	DBP	Lifestyle habits	Drug treatment
Normal BP	<120 mm Hg	<80 mm Hg	Promote	None
Elevated BP	120–129 mm Hg	<80 mm Hg	Yes	None
Stage 1 hypertension	130–139 mm Hg	80–89 mm Hg	Yes	May be indicated*
Stage 2 hypertension	≥140 mm Hg	≥90 mm Hg	Yes	indicated+

Note: BP, blood pressure; SBP, systolic blood pressure; DBP, diastolic blood pressure.

Source: Adapted from Whelton PK, Carey RM, Aronow WS, et al. 2017 ACC/AHA/AAPA/ABC/ACPM/ AGS/APhA/ASH/ASPC/NMA/PCNA guideline for the prevention, detection, evaluation, and management of high blood pressure in adults: Executive summary: A Report of the American College of Cardiology/American Heart Association Task Force on Clinical Practice Guidelines. Hypertension 2017.

* Initiate pharmacologic treatment if clinical ASCVD or estimated 10-year CVD risk >10%.

\+ Consideration of two medications from two different classes.

to maintain blood pressure in this category. In the next category of blood pressure (120–129 mm Hg systolic and <80 mm Hg diastolic), improved lifestyle habits are also advocated, and pharmaceutical therapy is not indicated. Stage 1 and Stage 2 hypertension, as indicated in this table, also advocate improved lifestyle habits and note that pharmaceutical therapy may also be indicated.

The reason for the lower levels of blood pressure classification is that it is now clear that increased risk of CVD occurs at levels starting at 115 mm Hg systolic and 75 mm Hg diastolic. For every 10 mm Hg increase above 75 mm Hg diastolic or 20 mm Hg increase above 125 systolic, the risk of CVD doubles (4).

The issue of lower blood pressure treatment targets was investigated in a major study entitled "The Systolic Blood Pressure Intervention Trial (SPRINT)," which was a study of over 9,000 adults at the mean age of 67.9 years at baseline with systolic blood pressure of 130–180 mm Hg (9). This study showed that blood pressure targets of SBP less than 120 mm Hg compared to standards of SBP greater than 140 mm Hg resulted in a 30% decreased risk of heart attack, acute coronary syndromes, stroke, heart failure and death compared to a standard of SBP of 140 mm Hg. It should be noted that achieving these lower levels of blood pressure often requires the use of three pharmaceutical agents, something that may be impractical in the normal clinical setting. This represents another reason why lifestyle measures can play a very important role in lowering blood pressure due to their synergistic effects with pharmaceutical therapies.

13.5 MEASUREMENT OF BLOOD PRESSURE

The 2017 ACC/AHA "Guideline for the Prevention, Detection, Evaluation and Management of High Blood Pressure in Adults" emphasizes that proper technique for blood pressure measurement must be followed and that differences may arise between blood pressure monitoring conducted in different settings. These guidelines outline six clearly defined steps on blood pressure measurement, which include proper patient preparation, proper technique, proper measurements, proper documentation, averaging of readings and providing readings to patients (7). In addition, these six steps highlight the importance of 5 minutes of rest before measurement and the use of correct cuff size applied to the skin, arm placement, bilateral arm measurements and the use of the average of more than two readings obtained on two different occasions. In addition, blood pressure should be measured after 5 minutes of repeated rest and with the patient seated in a chair with their back supported and the arm bare and at the heart level. Tobacco and caffeine should be avoided for at least 30 minutes. Blood pressure should also be measured in both arms and after 5 minutes of standing. Common errors for office-based readings occur because of measurement errors and too small a number of readings. In addition, "white coat" reaction and a large number of other factors may influence blood pressure outside of the medical office.

13.6 BLOOD PRESSURE VARIABILITY AND ITS DETERMINANTS

A number of behaviors can contribute to variability of blood pressure. For example, nicotine in cigarette smoke transiently raises blood pressure by 10–20 mm Hg. Individuals with moderate alcohol consumption (one to two drinks/day) generally have less hypertension than individuals who do not consume alcohol, but the development of hypertension increases in heavy drinkers (three or more drinks/day). Caffeine consumption will typically cause a small and transient rise in blood pressure. This is particularly true when caffeine is consumed in diet sodas, presumably because the antioxidant polyphenols in coffee, which are not present in diet soda, moderate increases in blood pressure. Other dietary habits, which are discussed later in this chapter, that may increase blood pressure include weight gain or elevated body mass index (BMI). There is also considerable evidence that developing hypertension increases with dietary sodium intake and decreases with dietary potassium intake (10). These issues are discussed in subsequent sections of this chapter.

13.7   CAUSES OF HYPERTENSION

Over 90% of all hypertension is of unknown etiology and is called "essential" hypertension. There are, however, three different subtypes of primary hypertension:

- *Systolic hypertension in teenagers and young adults*—The underlying etiology of this type of hypertension in young adults (typically 17–25 years of age) is increased cardiac output and stiff peripheral vascular disease, particularly in the aorta. This may be found in up to 25% of young men but only 2% of young women (11).
- *Diastolic hypertension in middle age (typically 30–50 years old)*—This is typically reflected by the pattern of elevated diastolic pressure and normal systolic pressure. This is the most common pattern in middle age and represents the classic "essential" hypertension. It is more common in men than women and is associated with middle-age weight gain.
- *Isolated systolic hypertension in older adults*—After 55 years of age, isolated systolic hypertension (ISH: SBP >140 mm Hg and DBP <90 mm Hg) is the predominant form of hypertension. This is largely due to an aging phenomenon and reflects stiffening of the aorta that results in widening of the pulse pressure.

13.8   PHYSICAL ACTIVITY AND HYPERTENSION

Several studies have reported an inverse relationship between leisure time physical activity and physical fitness (relative risk 1.5–1.9 in development and severity of hypertension even after adjusting for other risk factors) (12–24). Kokkinos et al reported a 5–9 mm Hg systolic and 4–5 mm Hg diastolic lower mean 24-hour ambulatory blood pressure in individuals with high or moderate physical fitness compared to individuals with low fitness levels (25). A review by Liu et al found a dose-response-related physical activity and hypertension prevention with a relative risk reduction of 6% for every 10 Met hours per week of leisure time physical activity (26).

There are over 70 randomized control trials and 15 meta-analyses that have shown the positive effects of exercise training on blood pressure (27–43). These studies have generally shown that an aerobic exercise training program of 30–60 minutes per session three times a week for 12–16 weeks lowers elevated blood pressure levels (44,45).

The amount of lowering has been reported in normotensive individuals at 2.61–4.7 mm Hg SBP and 1.8–3.1 mm Hg DBP and in individuals with diagnosed hypertension at 6–10 mm Hg SBP and 2.4–7.6 mm Hg DBP with diagnosed hypertension in response to aerobic exercise training progress. Similar reductions were found in 24-hour measurements of SBP of 6–10 mm Hg and DBP of 5–8 mm Hg in hypertensive patients and 3.0–3.3 mm Hg SBP and 3.3–3.5 mm Hg DBP in normotensive individuals (43). These data suggest that 40%–70% of maximal aerobic exercise training of 30–60 minutes 3–5 days per week is effective for both prevention and management of hypertension.

In addition, there are acute benefits of lowering blood pressure following aerobic exercise (reduction in systolic 5–15 mm Hg and diastolic 4–6 mm Hg) (46–48). This may last up to 24 hours. There are multiple possible mechanisms for acute blood pressure reduction including decreases in sympathetic adrenergic stimulation, resetting of arterial cardiopulmonary baroreceptors operating and neural adaptations.

Resistance strength exercise training has been reported in a few studies to result in lowering of blood pressure of approximately 6–7 mm Hg (49). However, not all studies have shown this response. For this reason, it is recommended that resistance training be used as an adjunct to aerobic training for blood pressure control and not as a substrate.

There are multiple postulated mechanisms for exercise-induced reduction of blood pressure including reduction in peripheral vascular resistance, improved vascular endothelial function and improved baroreceptor activity as well as reduced circulating catecholamines. Resistance training may increase skeletal muscle precapillary and capillary vessel numbers. There may also be a genetic impact of exercise-induced reduction in blood pressure, but this is an area of active research. The genetic component may be a function of improving nitrous oxide endothelial activity.

13.9 NUTRITION AND HYPERTENSION

Multiple prestigious medical and nutrition organizations have concluded that healthier diets are an important component in the prevention and management of hypertension. These include recommendations from the AHA (5,50), the ACC and the Dietary Guidelines for American 2020–2025 (DGA 2020–2025) (51). Multiple studies have shown that healthier diets are associated with a decreased likelihood of developing hypertension. The positive effects of healthier diets appear to be through a combination of decreased sodium intake and increased intake of potassium, calcium and magnesium as well as a moderation in alcohol consumption. These dietary recommendations have been supported by numerous randomized controlled trials. Thus, effective dietary interventions for blood pressure control and reduction are similar to those for reduction of risk of CVD, in general. These include a diet that is rich in fruit and vegetables, whole grains, legumes, seeds, nuts, fish and dairy and low in meat, sweets and alcohol. Examples of such diets include the Mediterranean diet and the DASH diet (52). An example of the DASH diet is found in Table 13.2.

The DASH diet, in particular, has been shown in controlled randomized studies to be effective in reducing blood pressure between 5.5 and 11.4 mm Hg in hypertensive patients and 3.5 mm Hg systolic and 2.2 mm Hg diastolic in prehypertensive patients (51). Of note, the DASH diet appears to be more effective in lowering blood pressure in Black study participants compared with White participants.

TABLE 13.2

Dietary Approaches to Stop Hypertension (DASH) Dietary Plan

Nutrient	Percentage of total caloric intake
Total fat (% of total Kcal)	25%–35%
Saturated fat	<7%
Trans fats	<1%
Monounsaturated fats	15%
Polyunsaturated fats	10% or less
(with an omega-6 to 3 ratio of 3 to 4 to 1)	
Cholesterol (% of total Kcal)	≤200 mg/d
Protein (% of total Kcal)	About 18%
Carbohydrates (% of total Kcal)	50%–60%
Dietary fiber (g/day)	31 g/day
Potassium (mg/day)	4,700 mg/day
Calcium (mg/day)	500 mg/day
Sodium (mg/day)	1,500–2,400 mg/day

Number of servings per day based on 2,000 Kcal diet

	Daily servings*	Servings per NIH DASH recommendations+
Fruits	7–8	4–5
Vegetables	4–5	4–5
Grains	4–5	6–8
Low-fat dairy products	2–3	2–3
Meats, poultry, fish	≤2	6 or less
Nuts, seeds, dry beans	4–5	4–5 per week
Fats, oils	2–3	2–3
Sweets	≤5 per week	5 or less per week

Total effect of blood pressure reduction using the DASH diet is approximately 11/6 mm Hg.

* Kingwell BA. Nitric oxide-mediated metabolic regulation during exercise: Effects of training in health and cardiovascular disease. *FASEB J.* 2000;14:1685–1696.

+ National Heart, Lung, and Blood Institute. *DASH Eating Plan* Website. www.nhlbi.nih.gov/health-topics/dash-eating-plan.

Other dietary studies have shown similar reductions in blood pressure of 6–10 mm Hg in normotensive patients versus 12–16 mm Hg reductions in individuals with hypertension following a diet high in fruits and vegetables and plant based (53). Current recommendations from the AHA and the DGA 2020–2025 recognize the DASH dietary pattern, the USDA Healthy Food Pattern and the AHA diet as effective nutritional strategies for lowering the risk of hypertension or helping in its control. The following components of these diets are important and similar:

- *Sodium restriction*—Multiple studies have shown an independent association between sodium intake and blood pressure levels (54,55). The largest dose-response from sodium restriction comes from a modification of the DASH diet to include low sodium (56). In general, sodium restriction reduces elevated SBP by 4.7–7 mm Hg and elevated DBP between 2.5 and 2.7 mm Hg and also reduces the risk of progression from prehypertension to hypertension by about 20%. Unfortunately, the current American diet is high in sodium (average approximately 3,400 milligrams per day). Various recommendations from the JNC VII and JNC VIII reports as well as the AHA Guidelines for Lifestyle Management all support sodium restriction. JNC VIII recommends no more than 2,400 milligrams per day, whereas the 2017 ACC/AHA "Guideline for the Prevention, Detection, Evaluation and Management of High Blood Pressure in Adults" (5) and the previous JNC VII (4) recommend reducing sodium chloride to 2,300 milligrams per day.

- *Effects of raising dietary potassium intake*—Potassium and sodium balance are both critical to fluid homeostasis (57,58). In general, increased sodium levels are responsible for fluid retention, whereas increased potassium levels lead to an increase in sodium excretion. The clinical trials supporting increased potassium to help control blood pressure intake have been somewhat mixed, generally resulting in a 2–4 mm Hg systolic and 1.5–2.5 mm Hg diastolic reduction in patients with hypertension. Decreases in sodium and increases in potassium may be achieved by following the DASH diet or the USDA Healthy Eating Patterns.
- *Alcohol consumption*—Light alcohol consumption has no effect on blood pressure (59–62). However, higher alcohol consumption increases blood pressure levels. Thus, individuals consuming one to two alcoholic beverages a day may have no effect on blood pressure. However, diets that contain three or more alcoholic beverages a day have resulted in an increase in blood pressure of 2 mm Hg systolic and 1 mm Hg diastolic. These consumption levels are similar recommendations that are found in the area of CVD risk, in general.
- *Effect of omega-3 polyunsaturated fatty acids*—Fatty fish and oil are rich in long-chain omega-3 polyunsaturated fatty acids and may play a role in blood pressure regulation via the production of eicosanoids and prostaglandins (63–65). Small studies of supplements suggest that they are associated with a reduction of 2.3–4.0 mm Hg systolic and 2.2–2.5 mm Hg diastolic pressure. Recommendations for consuming two or more fatty fish meals per week for cardioprotective effects are also appropriate for obtaining omega-3 polyunsaturated fats.

13.10 WEIGHT MANAGEMENT

The association between obesity and hypertension is well established in multiple trials (66). Furthermore, the reduction in body weight of 5–10 kg in overweight individuals is a highly effective way of reducing blood pressure, with reductions of 6–12 mm Hg systolic and 5–8 mm Hg diastolic (67–70). The combination of caloric reduction as well as increased physical activity are both important components of weight loss and weight management. A combination of exercise, weight reduction and decreased caloric consumption results in greater blood pressure reduction than individual strategies alone.

For all of these reasons, the AHA recommends that overweight adults with hypertension should be counseled to begin lifestyle changes in the areas of caloric reduction and physical activity to achieve a sustained weight loss of 3%–5% to achieve clinically meaningful health benefits. Intervention trials that include components of these lifestyle medicine modalities, such as the PREMIER (71) and ENCORE (72) studies, have both recorded significant reductions in blood pressure of 11–16 mm Hg SBP and 6–10 mm Hg DBP. Both physical activity and weight loss are independently important lifestyle measures for reduction in the risk of CVD, in general, and are handled in more detail in separate chapters in this book.

13.11   CIGARETTE SMOKING

There is a strong relationship between cigarette smoking and increased blood pressure. Cigarette smoking evokes an increased blood pressure response that slowly dissipates over the next hour or two following each cigarette. Since there are overwhelmingly deleterious effects of smoking on CVD risk, counsel that cigarette smoking cessation is important not only for blood pressure control but for multiple other risks of CVD.

13.12   COMPLEMENTARY THERAPIES

Multiple complementary therapies have been suggested to play a role in the management of high blood pressure through lifestyle modification (73). Most of these therapies (e.g., stress reduction, various types of music, deep breathing exercises, mind-body therapy, yoga, etc.) have had some significant but small effects on blood pressure management. These modalities are important for the risk of CVD, in general, and are treated in more detail in Chapter 10.

13.13   PHARMACOLOGIC MANAGEMENT OF HYPERTENSION

Current practice guidelines outlined in recent AHA documents all recommend first-line therapies of lifestyle medicine (1). In instances where blood pressure is greater than 140/90, however, additional pharmaceutical therapy may be necessary. Current guidelines suggest initial treatment of hypertension with one or more of three classes of first-line blood pressure–lowering medicines:

1. Calcium channel blockers (CCB),
2. Renin-angiotensin system (RAS) inhibitors including angiotensin-converting enzymes inhibitors (ACEIs); and
3. Angiotensin receptor blockers (ARBs) or thiazide-type diuretics.

These drugs also have been shown to reduce risk of fatal or nonfatal CVD events.

Even though beta blockers are first-line drugs for angina and HF, there is some debate about whether or not they should be included as first line drugs for uncomplicated hypertension because of their inferior stroke protection and increased risk for incident diabetes.

Recommendations of drugs within each of these three classifications is beyond the scope of the current chapter. However, detailed information about all of these classes of medications may be found in appropriate cardiovascular textbooks.

13.14 SUMMARY/CONCLUSIONS

As documented in this chapter, multiple lifestyle interventions are highly effective and important for lowering the risk of developing hypertension and important components of its therapy. Lifestyle modalities are synergistic with pharmaceutical therapy and carry virtually no adverse side effects. Moreover, these modalities are important for reducing other risk factors for CVD.

Hypertension remains the most prevalent and easily recognizable risk factor for CVD. It is the leading cause of outpatient visits for virtually every physician practice in the United States. For all of these reasons, lifestyle therapies are an important component of counseling for blood pressure control for every physician who wishes to practice evidence-based medicine. Table 13.3 summarizes some of the appropriate lifestyle modifications for reduction of risk for management of hypertension.

TABLE 13.3
Clinical Applications/Lifestyle Modifications for Management of Hypertension

Modification	Recommendation	Blood pressure reduction
Weight reduction	Maintain a BMI between 18.5 and 24.9	5–20 mm Hg per 10 kg weight loss
Healthy diet	Consume a diet rich in fruits, vegetables and whole grains; moderation in fat-free or low-fat dairy products Reduced saturated fat and cholesterol such as the DASH dietary pattern	8–14 mm Hg
Exercise	Regular aerobic exercise 120–150 min/week; Or 60–90 min/day for weight reduction and maintenance; Dynamic resistance exercise 90–150 min/week; Isometric resistance exercise three sessions/week	4–9 mm Hg
Reduced sodium/ salt intake	Lower salt intake as much as possible (1.5 g/day of sodium or 3.8 g/day of sodium chloride) or at least 1,000 mg reduction in current intake	2–8 mm Hg
Limit alcohol consumption	No more than two drinks/day for men; No more than one drink/day for women	2–4 mm Hg
Increase potassium	Increase intake to 3,500–5,000 mg/day (level of DASH diet); Content from fruits, vegetables, and low-fat dairy products	2–5 mm Hg

Sources: Adapted from Chobanian AV, Bakris GL, Black HR, et al. The seventh report of the Joint National Committee on Prevention, Detection, Evaluation, and Treatment of High Blood Pressure: The JNC 7 report. *JAMA*, 2003;289:2560–2572.

Whelton PK, Carey RM, Aronow WS, et al. 2017 ACC/AHA/AAPA/ABC/ACPM/AGS/APhA/ASH/ASPC/NMA/PCNA guideline for the prevention, detection, evaluation, and management of high blood pressure in adults: Executive summary: A Report of the American College of Cardiology/American Heart Association Task Force on Clinical Practice Guidelines. *Hypertension* 2017.

Appel LJ, Brands MW, Daniels SR, et al. Dietary approaches to prevent and treat hypertension: A scientific statement from the American Heart Association. Hypertension. 2006;47:296–308.

Clinical Applications

- High blood pressure is a significant and very common risk factor for CVD.
- Recent guidelines for blood pressure control have emphasized that even small increases in blood pressure above 115 mm Hg systolic and 75 mm Hg diastolic significantly increase the risk of CVD.
- Multiple lifestyle interventions including regular physical activity, nutritional interventions (particularly salt reduction) and weight management (if needed) and smoking cessation all can profoundly affect the likelihood of developing high blood pressure and assist in its treatment.

REFERENCES

1. Blacher J, Levy BI, Mourad JJ, et al. From epidemiological transition to modern cardiovascular epidemiology: Hypertension in the 21st century. Lancet. 2016;388(10043):530–2. Epub 2016/02/10.
2. Rippe JM. Lifestyle medicine and cardiovascular disease. In Rippe JM, ed. Manual of Lifestyle Medicine. Boca Raton, FL: CRC Press; 2021, p. 61.
3. Poulter NR, Prabhakaran D, Caulfield M. Hypertension. Lancet. 2015;386(9995):801–12. Epub 2015/04/03.
4. Chobanian AV, Bakris GL, Black HR, et al. The seventh report of the Joint National Committee on Prevention, Detection, Evaluation, and Treatment of High Blood Pressure: The JNC 7 report. JAMA. 2003;289(19):2560–72. Epub 2003/05/16.
5. Eckel RH, Jakicic JM, Ard JD, et al. 2013 AHA/ACC guideline on lifestyle management to reduce cardiovascular risk. Circulation. 2014;129(25_suppl_2):S76–99.
6. Physical Activity Guidelines Advisory Committee. 2018 Physical Activity Guidelines Advisory Committee. 2018 Physical Activity Guidelines Advisory Committee Scientific Report. Washington, DC: U.S. Department of Health and Human Services; 2018.
7. Whelton PK, Carey RM, Aronow WS, Casey DE, Jr., Collins KJ, Dennison Himmelfarb C, et al. 2017 ACC/AHA/AAPA/ABC/ACPM/AGS/APhA/ASH/ASPC/NMA/PCNA Guideline for the prevention, detection, evaluation, and management of high blood pressure in adults: Executive summary: A report of the American College of Cardiology/American Heart Association Task Force on Clinical Practice Guidelines. Hypertension. 2018;71(6):1269–324. Epub 2017/11/15.
8. Yoon SS, Carroll MD, Fryar CD. Hypertension prevalence and control among adults: United States, 2011–2014. NCHS Data Brief. 2015(220):1–8. Epub 2015/12/04.
9. Sprint Research Group, Wright JT, Jr., Williamson JD, et al. A randomized trial of intensive versus standard blood-pressure control. N Engl J Med. 2015;373(22):2103–16. Epub 2015/11/10.
10. Buendia JR, Bradlee ML, Daniels SR, et al. Longitudinal effects of dietary sodium and potassium on blood pressure in adolescent girls. JAMA Pediatrics. 2015;169(6):560–8. Epub 2015/04/29.
11. Lurbe E, Agabiti-Rosei E, Cruickshank JK, et al. 2016 European Society of Hypertension guidelines for the management of high blood pressure in children and adolescents. J Hypertens. 2016;34(10):1887–920. Epub 2016/07/29.
12. Kokkinos PF, Giannelou A, Manolis A, et al. Physical activity in the prevention and management of high blood pressure. Hellenic J Cardiol. 2009;50(1):52–9. Epub 2009/02/07.
13. Thijs L, Den Hond E, Nawrot T, et al. Prevalence, pathophysiology and treatment of isolated systolic hypertension in the elderly. Expert Rev Cardiovasc Ther. 2004;2(5):761–9. Epub 2004/09/08.

14. Paffenbarger RS, Jr., Wing AL, Hyde RT, et al. Physical activity and incidence of hypertension in college alumni. Am J Epidemiol. 1983;117(3):245–57. Epub 1983/03/01.
15. Haapanen N, Miilunpalo S, Vuori I, et al. Association of leisure time physical activity with the risk of coronary heart disease, hypertension and diabetes in middle-aged men and women. Int J Epidemiol. 1997;26(4):739–47. Epub 1997/08/01.
16. Reaven PD, Barrett-Connor E, Edelstein S. Relation between leisure-time physical activity and blood pressure in older women. Circulation. 1991;83(2):559–65. Epub 1991/02/01.
17. Staessen JA, Fagard R, Amery A. Life style as a determinant of blood pressure in the general population. Am J Hypertens. 1994;7(8):685–94. Epub 1994/08/01.
18. Gibbons LW, Blair SN, Cooper KH, et al. Association between coronary heart disease risk factors and physical fitness in healthy adult women. Circulation. 1983;67(5):977–83. Epub 1983/05/01.
19. Blair SN, Goodyear NN, Gibbons LW, et al. Physical fitness and incidence of hypertension in healthy normotensive men and women. JAMA. 1984;252(4):487–90. Epub 1984/07/27.
20. Paffenbarger RS, Jr., Thorne MC, Wing AL. Chronic disease in former college students. VIII. Characteristics in youth predisposing to hypertension in later years. Am J Epidemiol. 1968;88(1):25–32. Epub 1968/07/01.
21. Lee IM, Hsieh CC, Paffenbarger RS, Jr. Exercise intensity and longevity in men: The Harvard alumni health study. JAMA. 1995;273(15):1179–84. Epub 1995/04/19.
22. Palatini P, Graniero GR, Mormino P, et al. Relation between physical training and ambulatory blood pressure in stage I hypertensive subjects. Results of the HARVEST Trial: Hypertension and ambulatory recording Venetia study. Circulation. 1994;90(6):2870–6. Epub 1994/12/01.
23. Sawada S, Tanaka H, Funakoshi M, et al. Five year prospective study on blood pressure and maximal oxygen uptake. Clin Exp Pharmacol Physiol. 1993;20(7–8):483–7. Epub 1993/07/01.
24. Kokkinos PF, Holland JC, Pittaras AE, et al. Cardiorespiratory fitness and coronary heart disease risk factor association in women. J Am Coll Cardiol. 1995;26(2):358–64. Epub 1995/08/01.
25. Kokkinos P, Pittaras A, Manolis A, et al. Exercise capacity and 24-h blood pressure in prehypertensive men and women. Am J Hypertens. 2006;19(3):251–8. Epub 2006/02/28.
26. Liu X, Zhang D, Liu Y, et al. Dose-response association between physical activity and incident hypertension: A systematic review and meta-analysis of cohort studies. Hypertension. 2017;69(5):813–20. Epub 2017/03/30.
27. Hagberg JM, Brown MD. Does exercise training play a role in the treatment of essential hypertension? J Cardiovasc Risk. 1995;2(4):296–302. Epub 1995/08/01.
28. Hagberg JM, Park JJ, Brown MD. The role of exercise training in the treatment of hypertension: An update. Sports Med. 2000;30(3):193–206. Epub 2000/09/22.
29. Cornelissen VA, Fagard RH. Effects of endurance training on blood pressure, blood pressure-regulating mechanisms, and cardiovascular risk factors. Hypertension. 2005;46(4):667–75. Epub 2005/09/15.
30. Fagard RH. Physical fitness and blood pressure. J Hypertens Suppl. 1993;11(5):S47–52. Epub 1993/12/01.
31. Fagard RH. Physical activity in the prevention and treatment of hypertension in the obese. Med Sci Sports Exerc. 1999;31(11 Suppl):S624–30. Epub 1999/12/11.
32. Fagard RH. Exercise characteristics and the blood pressure response to dynamic physical training. Med Sci Sports Exerc. 2001;33(6 Suppl):S484–92; discussion S93–4. Epub 2001/06/28.

33. Halbert JA, Silagy CA, Finucane P, et al. The effectiveness of exercise training in lowering blood pressure: A meta-analysis of randomised controlled trials of 4 weeks or longer. J Hum Hypertens. 1997;11(10):641–9. Epub 1997/12/24.

34. Dickinson HO, Mason JM, Nicolson DJ, et al. Lifestyle interventions to reduce raised blood pressure: A systematic review of randomized controlled trials. J Hypertens. 2006;24(2):215–33. Epub 2006/03/02.

35. Kelley GA, Kelley KA, Tran ZV. Aerobic exercise and resting blood pressure: A meta-analytic review of randomized, controlled trials. Prev Cardiol. 2001;4(2):73–80. Epub 2002/02/06.

36. Kelley GA, Kelley KS, Tran ZV. Walking and resting blood pressure in adults: A meta-analysis. Prev Med. 2001;33(2 Pt 1):120–7. Epub 2001/08/09.

37. Whelton SP, Chin A, Xin X, et al. Effect of aerobic exercise on blood pressure: A meta-analysis of randomized, controlled trials. Ann Intern Med. 2002;136(7):493–503. Epub 2002/04/03.

38. Kelley G, McClellan P. Antihypertensive effects of aerobic exercise: A brief meta-analytic review of randomized controlled trials. Am J Hypertens. 1994;7(2):115–19. Epub 1994/02/01.

39. Kelley G, Tran ZV. Aerobic exercise and normotensive adults: A meta-analysis. Med Sci Sports Exerc. 1995;27(10):1371–7. Epub 1995/10/01.

40. Kelley GA. Effects of aerobic exercise in normotensive adults: A brief meta-analytic review of controlled clinical trials. South Med J. 1995;88(1):42–6. Epub 1995/01/01.

41. Kelley GA. Aerobic exercise and resting blood pressure among women: A meta-analysis. Prev Med. 1999;28:264–75.

42. Kelley GA, Sharpe Kelley K. Aerobic exercise and resting blood pressure in older adults: A meta-analytic review of randomized controlled trials. J Gerontol A Biol Sci Med Sci. 2001;56:M298–303.

43. Börjesson M, Onerup A, Lundqvist S, Dahlöf B. Physical activity and exercise lower blood pressure in individuals with hypertension: Narrative review of 27 RCTs. Br J Sports Med. 2016;50(6):356–61. doi:10.1136/bjsports-2015-095786.

44. Fagard RH, Cornelissen VA. Effect of exercise on blood pressure control in hypertensive patients. Eur J Cardiovasc Prev Rehabil. 2007;14:12–17.

45. Pescatello LS, Franklin BA, Fagard R, et al. American College of Sports Medicine position stand: Exercise and hypertension. Med Sci Sports Exerc. 2004;36:533–53.

46. Floras JS, Sinkey CA, Aylward PE, Seals DR, Thoren PN, Mark AL. Postexercise hypotension and sympathoinhibition in borderline hypertensive men. Hypertension. 1989;14:28–35.

47. Halliwill JR, Taylor JA, Eckberg DL. Impaired sympathetic vascular regulation in humans after acute dynamic exercise. J Physiol. 1996;495 (Pt 1):279–88.

48. Pinto A, Di Raimondo D, Tuttolomondo A, Fernandez P, Arnao V, Licata G. Twenty-four hour ambulatory blood pressure monitoring to evaluate effects on blood pressure of physical activity in hypertensive patients. Clin J Sport Med. 2006;16:238–43.

49. Kelley GA, Kelley KS. Progressive resistance exercise and resting blood pressure: A meta-analysis of randomized controlled trials. Hypertension. 2000;35:838–43.

50. Appel LJ, Brands MW, Daniels SR, et al. Dietary approaches to prevent and treat hypertension: A scientific statement from the American Heart Association. Hypertension. 2006;47:296–308.

51. Appel LJ, Moore TJ, Obarzanek E, et al. A clinical trial of the effects of dietary patterns on blood pressure: DASH Collaborative Research Group. N Engl J Med. 1997;336:1117–24.

52. Ndanuko RN, Tapsell LC, Charlton KE. Dietary patterns and blood pressure in adults: A systematic review and meta-analysis of randomized controlled trials. Adv Nutr. 2016;7(1):76–89. doi:10.3945/an.115.009753.

53. Appel LJ, Sacks FM, Carey VJ, et al. Effects of protein, monounsaturated fat, and carbohydrate intake on blood pressure and serum lipids: Results of the OmniHeart randomized trial. JAMA. 2005;294:2455–64.

54. He J, Bazzano LA. Effects of lifestyle modification on treatment and prevention of hypertension. Curr Opin Nephrol Hypertens. 2000;9:267–71.

55. Vollmer WM, Sacks FM, Ard J, et al. Effects of diet and sodium intake on blood pressure: Subgroup analysis of the DASH-sodium trial. Ann Intern Med. 2001;135:1019–28.

56. Sacks FM, Svetkey LP, Vollmer WM, et al. Effects on blood pressure of reduced dietary sodium and the dietary approaches to stop hypertension (DASH) diet: DASH-sodium Collaborative Research Group. N Engl J Med. 2001;344:3–10.

57. Cutler JA, Follmann D, Elliott P, et al. An overview of randomized trials of sodium reduction and blood pressure. Hypertension. 1991;17:I27–33.

58. Geleijnse JM, Kok FJ, Grobbee DE. Blood pressure response to changes in sodium and potassium intake: A metaregression analysis of randomised trials. J Hum Hypertens. 2003;17:471–80.

59. Okubo Y, Miyamoto T, Suwazono Y, et al. Alcohol consumption and blood pressure in japanese men. Alcohol. 2001;23:149–56.

60. Okubo Y, Suwazono Y, Kobayashi E, et al. Alcohol consumption and blood pressure change: 5-year follow-up study of the association in normotensive workers. J Hum Hypertens. 2001;15:367–72.

61. Klatsky AL, Friedman GD, Siegelaub AB, Gerard MJ. Alcohol consumption and blood pressure kaiser-permanente multiphasic health examination data. N Engl J Med. 1977;296:1194–200.

62. Xin X, He J, Frontini MG, et al. Effects of alcohol reduction on blood pressure: A meta-analysis of randomized controlled trials. Hypertension. 2001;38:1112–17.

63. Geleijnse JM, Giltay EJ, Grobbee DE, et al. Blood pressure response to fish oil supplementation: Meta-regression analysis of randomized trials. J Hypertens. 2002;20:1493–9.

64. Appel LJ, Miller ER, 3rd, Seidler AJ, et al. Does supplementation of diet with 'fish oil' reduce blood pressure? A meta-analysis of controlled clinical trials. Arch Intern Med. 1993;153:1429–38.

65. Morris MC, Sacks F, Rosner B. Does fish oil lower blood pressure? A meta-analysis of controlled trials. Circulation. 1993;88:523–33.

66. Kaplan NM. Hypertension curriculum review: Lifestyle modifications for prevention and treatment of hypertension. J Clin Hypertens. 2004;6:716–19.

67. Neter JE, Stam BE, Kok FJ, et al. Influence of weight reduction on blood pressure: A meta-analysis of randomized controlled trials. Hypertension. 2003;42:878–84.

68. Staessen J, Fagard R, Lijnen P, et al. Body weight, sodium intake and blood pressure. J Hypertens Suppl. 1989;7:S19–23.

69. Gordon NF, Scott CB, Levine BD. Comparison of single versus multiple lifestyle interventions: Are the antihypertensive effects of exercise training and diet-induced weight loss additive? Am J Cardiol. 1997;79:763–7.

70. MacMahon S, Cutler J, Brittain E, et al. Obesity and hypertension: Epidemiological and clinical issues. Eur Heart J. 1987;8 Suppl B:57–70.

71. McGuire HL, Svetkey LP, Harsha DW, et al. Comprehensive lifestyle modification and blood pressure control: A review of the PREMIER trial. J Clin Hypertens. 2004;6:383–90.

72. Hinderliter AL. The ENCORE study: Examination of cardiovascular, metabolic, and autonomic changes associated with the DASH diet alone and in combination with exercise and weight reduction in hypertensive men and women. In American College of Cardiology Annuals Scientific Sessions. 2009, www.ClinicalTrials.gov.

73. Kühlmann AY, Etnel JR, Roos-Hesselink JW, Jeekel J, Bogers AJ, Takkenberg JJ. Systematic review and meta-analysis of music interventions in hypertension treatment: a quest for answers. BMC Cardiovasc Disord. 2016;16:69. Epub 2016/04/21.

14 Peripheral Artery Disease

KEY POINTS

- Peripheral artery disease (PAD) is another manifestation of systemic atherosclerosis.
- PAD is quite common in the United States with between 8 and 12 million individuals having this condition.
- PAD is not as often diagnosed or treated as either coronary heart disease or cerebrovascular disease. It is important for all clinicians to carefully assess both the history (particularly claudication) and physical examination (diminished pulses and/or bruits) of potential PAD.
- Treatment of PAD involves lowering the risk of atherosclerosis or slowing its progression and is similar to treatment for atherosclerosis of the coronary arteries or the cerebrovascular arteries.

14.1 INTRODUCTION

Peripheral artery disease (PAD) incorporates a variety of pathophysiologic conditions that can result in a variety of adverse consequences such as obstruction or aneurysmal degeneration of noncoronary arterial vasculature (1).

Atherosclerotic disease is the most common etiology. This is in common with coronary artery disease (CAD) and cerebrovascular accident (CVA) (1). While atherosclerosis is a defused disease (see also Chapter 11 on atherosclerosis), some of the other etiologies include inflammatory disorders, trauma and infectious processes that can result in similar clinical presentations. The key role for lifestyle medicine practitioners is to undertake a complete assessment of the peripheral arteries and apply the various modalities of lifestyle medicine such as lipid control, blood pressure control, weight loss (if necessary) and increased physical activity, all of which can have a positive impact on PAD.

PAD affects approximately 8–12 million Americans (2). It is often underdiagnosed and undertreated (3). Thus, it is important for all physicians, but particularly lifestyle medicine practitioners, to maintain a high level of suspicion for PAD and be familiar with the various ways it can present clinically.

Atherosclerotic PAD correlates with risk for significant cardiovascular events and is frequently associated with coronary and cerebral atherosclerosis. Patients who have PAD and concomitant cerebrovascular disease are at particularly high risk.

14.2 EPIDEMIOLOGY

The prevalence of PAD increases with age. It is present in only 2%–3% of people under the age of 50 years, but up to 29% of individuals over the age of 70 years (4).

Up to 60% of individuals with PAD will also have concomitant CHD and/or cerebrovascular disease. Patients with PAD have a two to four times increased risk of cardiovascular and total mortality. This is independent of the common symptom of intermittent claudication, since the majority of patients with PAD do not have this symptom. Typical diagnosis of significant PAD is made by employing the ankle-brachial index (ABI). There is a greater association between ABI and total mortality. Despite the increased risk for CHD and total mortality, patients with PAD are often treated less aggressively for comorbid cardiovascular conditions and are often prescribed less antiplatelet agents when compared to individuals diagnosed with CHD.

14.3   RISK FACTORS FOR PERIPHERAL ARTERY DISEASE

Atherosclerosis is the primary process for lower extremity PAD and shares common risk factors with CHD and CVD. These include age, hypertension, hyperlipidemia, type 2 diabetes mellitus (T2DM) and tobacco use (5). (See Chapter 11 on atherosclerosis.) There is also some genetic predisposition to PAD. Heritability has been determined to be 20%–45% among affected families. The role of inflammation has increasingly been understood in atherosclerosis, so inflammatory biomarkers for PAD are under active investigation (6).

There is a two- to fourfold increase in the prevalence of PAD among current smokers compared to never smokers (7,8). Importantly, smoking cessation is associated with better outcomes. Individuals with T2DM often have severe PAD. Metabolic syndrome is also associated with PAD. Diabetic patients are more likely to have critical limb ischemia requiring amputation. Abnormalities in LDL cholesterol also increase the risk of PAD. Hypertriglyceridemia also is associated with increased risk of PAD, but this may be the presence of elevated triglycerides in the context of other lipid fractions. Hypertension increases the risk of PAD by 1.3- to 2.2-fold (9,10). As with CHD, the risk of developing PAD with intermittent claudication increases substantially along with the number of risk factors.

14.4   PATHOPHYSIOLOGY OF PERIPHERAL ARTERY DISEASE

Just as patients with stable angina experience symptoms based on a mismatch of oxygen and demand, so do patients with PAD experience intermittent claudication. Blood flow may be normal at rest, but the delivery during exercise may create a situation where demand exceeds supply. It should be noted that individuals who have multiple, critical atherosclerotic lesions may have symptoms, even at rest.

14.5   CLINICAL FEATURES

The major symptom of PAD is muscle pain either with exercise (intermittent claudication) or at rest (11). The location of symptoms is typically related to the site of the most proximal stenosis. Several questionnaires are available to assess the presence and severity of claudication. These include the ROSE Questionnaire, the Edinburgh Claudication Questionnaire and the San Diego Claudication

Questionnaire. These may be used in conjunction with the physician's diagnosis of intermittent claudication based on walking distance and speed. The most frequently involved artery with intermittent claudication is the superficial femoral artery. Symptoms of claudication are usually rapidly relieved with rest or standing. However, as the atherosclerotic burden progresses, limb-threatening ischemia with rest, pain, tissue alterations and perhaps even gangrene may result. This is referred to as critical limb ischemia (CLI).

Careful physical examination is essential for all physicians treating individuals with potential PAD. To conduct a comprehensive lower extremity physical examination involves characterization of the peripheral pulses, auscultation for bruits in the abdomen and bilateral groin as well as assessment of skin changes (11,12). Signs of lower extremity arterial insufficiency include coolness, dry skin, scaling, dependent rubor, pallor worse with leg elevation, or ulcerations. Readily palpable pulses in healthy individuals include brachial, radial and ulnar arteries in the upper extremities and femoral, popliteal, posterior tibial and dorsalis pedis in the lower extremities. Bruits typically are a sign of flow disturbances at the site of a stenosis.

14.6 TESTING FOR PERIPHERAL ARTERY DISEASE

The classic way of testing for PAD is to conduct segmental systolic blood pressure along segments of both of the lower extremities. This may be beyond what a private practice physician can do, but it is a standard practice for vascular surgeons.

A more simplified version is called the ABI. This is something that private practice physicians often use with equipment that can be readily conducted at the bedside. This index is basically the ratio of the systolic blood pressure measured at the ankle to the systolic blood pressure measured at the brachial artery.

The ABI test is conducted by placing a pneumatic blood pressure cuff at the ankle and inflating it to above systolic pressure, then deflating it until the flow is detected with a Doppler ultrasound probe placed over the posterior tibial and dorsalis pedis arteries, thus denoting systolic blood pressure. Subsequently, the brachial artery SVP is assessed in a routine manner either by listening to the first Korotkoff sound or detecting with the Doppler probe.

A normal ABI is in the range of 100–140 (13,14). (Systolic blood flow is typically augmented in the ankle.) If the ABI is 0.90 or lower, it indicates a level of PAD in the lower extremities.

Another way of assessing PAD is utilizing treadmill exercise testing to provide objective evidence of the patient's walking capacity (15,16). This measurement determines the claudication onset time when claudication symptoms first appear and the peak walking time when the patient can no longer continue walking because of significant leg discomfort.

Various treadmill testing protocols may be employed to make this assessment. One standard one involves maintaining a constant grade of 12% with a speed of 1.5–2 miles per hour. Another protocol maintains a constant speed of 2 MPH, while grade is gradually increased by 2% every 2–3 minutes. In conjunction with the treadmill test, ankle and brachial systolic blood pressure is measured during resting conditions before the treadmill exercise and within 1 minute after exercise and repeated until baseline values are reestablished. A 25% or greater decrease in ABI after exercise in patients whose walking capacity is limited by claudication is diagnostic and implicates PAD as a cause of the patient's claudication symptoms.

Duplex ultrasound may be utilized at the site of suspected stenoses and can assess blood flow around stenoses. Other noninvasive procedures may include magnetic resonance angiography (MRA) or computer tomographic angiography (CTA). However, both of these tests have the disadvantage of expense and, also, the need for the use of angiographic die. However, both MRA and CTA are recognized as accurate tests by the American College of Cardiology and the American Heart Association PDA Guidelines.

14.7 PROGNOSIS

Patients with PAD are at increased risk of physical or other complications of atherosclerotic disease including cardiovascular and cerebrovascular events (4,17). Patients with PAD and an abnormal ABI are two- to fourfold more likely than those with a normal ABI to have a history of myocardial infarction (MI) (18). Worsening symptoms appear in approximately 25% of patients with claudication and over 3 years, approximately 20% of these individuals will require an intervention to improve lower extremity perfusion (5). Both smoking and T2DM independently predict progression of disease. For example, those with T2DM have at least a 12-fold higher likelihood of amputation than nondiabetic persons.

14.8 TREATMENT

As with other forms of atherosclerotic disease, medical management of PAD involves aggressive risk factor reduction. The goal of therapy is to reduce morbidity and mortality and improve quality of life by decreasing symptoms of claudication and preserving limb viability. Risk factor reduction involves multiple modalities of lifestyle medicine including lipid reduction, control of blood pressure, weight loss (if necessary), and increased physical activity, at least as much as can be tolerated in a patient who has claudication. Of course, smoking cessation is mandatory, and aggressive treatment of T2DM is also very important.

Aggressive lipid reduction may be possible with a plant-based diet. Many of the patients in the studies by Esselstyn and Ornish were able to achieve LDL cholesterol of less than 70 mg/dL. If a patient is not able to maintain the strict dietary protocols required in these studies, the addition of statins is highly appropriate.

Lipid-lowering therapy in statins in a pooled study of 17 trials reduced the risk of cerebrovascular events in patients with PAD by 26% (19). Observational evidence unequivocally shows that cigarette smoking increases the risk of PAD or other atherosclerotic disease. Individuals with PAD who discontinue smoking have approximately twice the 5-year survival rate as those who continue to smoke (19).

Aggressive treatment of T2DM is also important and lowers the risk of nephropathy and retinopathy (20). Of course, treatment of T2DM is very important for all forms of atherosclerosis, including patients with PAD.

Blood pressure control is very important in medical therapy of PAD (21,22). The HOPE (Heart Outcomes Prevention Evaluation) trial showed that blood pressure control with the angiotensin-converting enzyme inhibitor Ramipril decreased the risk of vascular death, MI or stroke by 44% in individuals with PAD (19). Of course, both weight loss and regular, moderate-intensity physical activity are cornerstone lifestyle therapies for lowering blood pressure.

Antiplatelet therapy is a key component of the treatment of PAD. The Antithrombic Trialists (ATT) collaboration meta-analysis of more than 9,000 patients with symptomatic PAD showed a 23% reduction in vascular death, MI or stroke with antiplatelet monotherapy (23).

First-line therapy has typically been aspirin. However, some randomized trials of patients with PAD found that aspirin did not reduce the risk of CV mortality or MI versus placebo. The CAPRIE trial (clopidogrel versus aspirin in patients with risk of ischemic events) showed that clopidogrel reduced ischemic events by 8.7% more compared to aspirin (24). Both aspirin and clopidogrel are potential antiplatelet agents, and one or the other should be utilized as part of the overall therapy for treating PAD.

14.9 SYMPTOMATIC TREATMENT

Exercise training is a highly effective, noninvasive intervention for limb-related symptoms (25). It is postulated that regular, moderate-intensity physical activity helps with development of collateral vessels and improves endothelium dilatation. Muscle metabolism and walking efficiency are also improved. Much of the benefit of exercise likely results from changes in the muscular function, such as increased mitochondria. The best results from exercise therapy come from supervised exercise sessions followed by home-based programs (26). The greatest benefit occurs when sessions are at least 30 minutes in duration and occur at least three times per week for a duration of 6 months.

14.10 PHARMACOTHERAPY

Several agents have been shown to be of benefit for the treatment of claudication in patients with PAD. These are pentoxifylline and cilostazol. Both have been shown to have modest therapeutic effects, largely through mechanisms such as inhibiting platelet aggregation. As already indicated, antiplatelet therapy with aspirin or clopidogrel and statins also plays a role in the medical management of PAD, as do some pharmaceutical agents for controlling blood pressure. Once again, however, lifestyle medicine modalities can play a highly efficacious role, particularly if pursued aggressively.

14.11 SURGICAL APPROACHES

Both angioplasty and stents as well as proforma surgery for treatment of symptomatic PAD are beyond the scope of this chapter and are largely in the hands of vascular surgeons.

14.12 LOWER EXTREMITY ANEURYSM

Atherosclerotic disruption of the arterial media can result in an aneurysm of the peripheral arteries such as in the aorta. Up to 70% of lower extremity aneurysms involve the popliteal arteries. The incidence of bilateral involvement of popliteal arteries is quite high (45%–68%) (27). The majority of patients (62%) with popliteal aneurysms have been reported to have concomitant abdominal aorta aneurysms (AAAs). The co-prevalence increases to over 45% in patients with femoral artery aneurysms. Thus, a patient who has a peripheral artery aneurysm in the femoral or popliteal arteries should be screened for AAA. Approximately 60% of peripheral aneurysms end up having ischemic complications. Popliteal aneurysms of greater than 2.0 centimeters and similar artery aneurysms greater than 2.0 centimeters need to be repaired for fear of ischemic events or rupture.

14.13 UPPER EXTREMITY ARTERIAL DISEASE

As in the situation of lower extremity PAD, atherosclerosis is the most common cause of upper extremity PAD, although some vasculitis syndromes and thoracic outlet syndrome as well as repetitive injury may also cause upper extremity PAD (27). Clinical symptoms include arm and hand claudication, visual alteration and neurological symptoms caused by vertebral-subclavian steal. Diagnostic mortalities are similar to those in lower extremities arterial disease. The simplest clinical maneuvers involve checking blood pressure measurements in both arms which provides an excellent screening test for upper extremity PAD. As with lower extremity PAD, risk factor reduction of atherosclerotic lesions with lipid lowering, blood pressure control and cessation of cigarette smoking are the cornerstones for treating upper extremity PAD.

14.14 SUMMARY/CONCLUSIONS

PAD is quite common in the United States, affecting 8–12 million Americans. PAD often accompanies coronary heart disease and cerebrovascular disease, although, unfortunately, PAD is less often evaluated and treated. Thus, lifestyle medicine clinicians should make a careful evaluation including detailed history and physical examination as outlined in this chapter to detect underlying PAD. Individuals who have PAD are two to four times as likely to experience other cardiovascular problems such as acute MI or stroke. The majority of individuals with PAD have underlying atherosclerosis. Thus, the treatment for PAD is similar to the treatment for CHD and CVA involving multiple aspects of risk factor reduction, most of which have a significant lifestyle component such as lipid lowering, lowering of blood pressure, smoking cessation and exercise as well as antiplatelet therapy. Pharmaceutical therapies for lipid lowering and blood pressure control may also be necessary to achieve aggressive targets.

Clinical Applications

- Clinicians should carefully evaluate peripheral pulses and look for bruits in various arteries in the upper and lower extremities.
- Individuals who have symptomatic PAD typically with claudication or intermittent claudication should be aggressively treated with risk factor

reduction such as lowering lipids, controlling blood pressure and smoking cessation as well as antiplatelet therapy.

REFERENCES

1. Gerhard-Herman MD, Gornik HL, Barrett C, et al. 2016 AHA/ACC guideline on the management of patients with lower extremity peripheral artery disease: A report of the American College of Cardiology/American Heart Association Task Force on Clinical Practice Guidelines. Circulation. 2017;135(12):e726–79. Epub 2016/11/15.
2. Fowkes FG, Rudan D, Rudan I, et al. Comparison of global estimates of prevalence and risk factors for peripheral artery disease in 2000 and 2010: A systematic review and analysis. Lancet. 2013;382(9901):1329–40. Epub 2013/08/07.
3. Pande RL, Perlstein TS, Beckman JA, et al. Secondary prevention and mortality in peripheral artery disease: National Health and Nutrition Examination Study, 1999 to 2004. Circulation. 2011;124(1):17–23. Epub 2011/06/22.
4. Criqui MH, Aboyans V. Epidemiology of peripheral artery disease. Circ Res. 2015;116(9):1509–26. Epub 2015/04/25.
5. Bonaca MP, Creager MA. Peripheral artery diseases. In Zipes, Libby, Bonow, Mann, Tomaselli, eds. Braunwald's Heart Disease. 11th ed. Amsterdam: Elsevier; 2019, pp. 1328–47.
6. Brevetti G, Giugliano G, Brevetti L, et al. Inflammation in peripheral artery disease. Circulation. 2010;122(18):1862–75. Epub 2010/11/03.
7. Conen D, Everett BM, Kurth T, et al. Smoking, smoking cessation, [corrected] and risk for symptomatic peripheral artery disease in women: A cohort study. Ann Intern Med. 2011;154(11):719–26. Epub 2011/06/08.
8. Alvarez LR, Balibrea JM, Surinach JM, et al. Smoking cessation and outcome in stable outpatients with coronary, cerebrovascular, or peripheral artery disease. Eur J Prev Cardiol. 2013;20(3):486–95. Epub 2011/10/05.
9. Criqui MH. The epidemiology of peripheral artery disease. In Creager MA, Beckman JA, Loscalzo J, eds. Vascular Medicine: A Companion to Braunwald's Heart Disease. 2nd ed. Philadelphia: Elsevier; 2013, pp. 211–22.
10. Powell TM, Glynn RJ, Buring JE, et al. The relative importance of systolic versus diastolic blood pressure control and incident symptomatic peripheral artery disease in women. Vasc Med. 2011;16(4):239–46. Epub 2011/07/07.
11. McDermott MM. Lower extremity manifestations of peripheral artery disease: The pathophysiologic and functional implications of leg ischemia. Circ Res. 2015;116(9):1540–50. Epub 2015/04/25.
12. Hiatt WR, Armstrong EJ, Larson CJ, et al. Pathogenesis of the limb manifestations and exercise limitations in peripheral artery disease. Circ Res. 2015;116(9):1527–39. Epub 2015/04/25.
13. Aboyans V, Criqui MH, Abraham P, et al. Measurement and interpretation of the ankle-brachial index: A scientific statement from the American Heart Association. Circulation. 2012;126(24):2890–909. Epub 2012/11/20.
14. Rooke TW, Hirsch AT, Misra S, et al. 2011 ACCF/AHA focused update of the guideline for the management of patients with peripheral artery disease (updating the 2005 guideline): A report of the American College of Cardiology Foundation/American Heart Association Task Force on Practice Guidelines. J Am Coll Cardiol. 2011;58(19):2020–45. Epub 2011/10/04.
15. McDermott MM, Guralnik JM, Criqui MH, et al. Six-minute walk is a better outcome measure than treadmill walking tests in therapeutic trials of patients with peripheral artery disease. Circulation. 2014;130(1):61–8. Epub 2014/07/02.

16. Hammad TA, Strefling JA, Zellers PR, et al. The effect of post-exercise ankle-brachial index on lower extremity revascularization. JACC Cardiovasc Interv. 2015;8(9):1238–44. Epub 2015/08/22.

17. Aboyans V, Ricco JB, Bartelink MEL, et al. 2017 ESC guidelines on the diagnosis and treatment of peripheral arterial diseases, in collaboration with the European Society for Vascular Surgery (ESVS): Document covering atherosclerotic disease of extracranial carotid and vertebral, mesenteric, renal, upper and lower extremity arteries. Endorsed by: The European Stroke Organization (ESO), the Task Force for the Diagnosis and Treatment of Peripheral Arterial Diseases of the European Society of Cardiology (ESC) and of the European Society for Vascular Surgery (ESVS). Eur Heart J. 2018;39(9):763–816. Epub 2017/09/10.

18. Fowkes FG, Murray GD, Butcher I, et al. Development and validation of an ankle brachial index risk model for the prediction of cardiovascular events. Eur J Prev Cardiol. 2014;21(3):310–20. Epub 2013/12/25.

19. Bonaca MP, Creager MA. Pharmacological treatment and current management of peripheral artery disease. Circ Res. 2015;116(9):1579–98. Epub 2015/04/25.

20. Inzucchi SE, Bergenstal RM, Buse JB, et al. Management of hyperglycemia in type 2 diabetes: A patient-centered approach: position statement of the American Diabetes Association (ADA) and the European Association for the Study of Diabetes (EASD). Diabetes Care. 2012;35(6):1364–79. Epub 2012/04/21.

21. Bavry AA, Anderson RD, Gong Y, et al. Outcomes Among hypertensive patients with concomitant peripheral and coronary artery disease: Findings from the International Verapamil-SR/Trandolapril Study. Hypertension. 2010;55(1):48–53. Epub 2009/12/10.

22. Sprint Research Group, Wright JT, Jr., Williamson JD, et al. A randomized trial of intensive versus standard blood-pressure control. N Engl J Med. 2015;373(22):2103–16. Epub 2015/11/10.

23. Antithrombotic Trialists Collaboration, Baigent C, Blackwell L, et al. Aspirin in the primary and secondary prevention of vascular disease: Collaborative meta-analysis of individual participant data from randomised trials. Lancet. 2009;373(9678):1849–60. Epub 2009/06/02.

24. Mora S, Ames JM, Manson JE. Low-dose aspirin in the primary prevention of cardiovascular disease: Shared decision making in clinical practice. JAMA. 2016;316(7):709–10. Epub 2016/06/21.

25. Hamburg NM, Balady GJ. Exercise rehabilitation in peripheral artery disease: Functional impact and mechanisms of benefits. Circulation. 2011;123(1):87–97. Epub 2011/01/05.

26. Fokkenrood HJ, Bendermacher BL, Lauret GJ, et al. Supervised exercise therapy versus non-supervised exercise therapy for intermittent claudication. Cochrane Database Syst Rev. 2013(8):CD005263. Epub 2013/08/24.

27. Campbell J. Peripheral arterial disease. In Griffin M, ed. Manual of Cardiovascular Disease. 5th ed. Philadelphia, PA: Wolters Kluwer; 2019, p. 407.

15 Ischemic Heart Disease

KEY POINTS

1. Ischemic heart disease (IHD) is very common in the United States. Over 15,400,000 Americans are currently living with IHD. Of these, 7,800,000 have angina and 7,600,000 have had a previous myocardial infarction.
2. Lifestyle therapies to lower the risk of developing atherosclerotic heart disease are vitally important.
3. Individuals who have an optimal risk factor profile are one-tenth as likely as individuals who have two risk factors to develop IHD.
4. Physicians should emphasize the importance of lifestyle measures in both lowering the risk of IHD and in its management.
5. The American Heart Association and American College of Cardiology have increasingly recognized and emphasized the importance of a positive lifestyle in lowering the risk of IHD.

15.1 INTRODUCTION

There are multiple different components of ischemic heart disease (IHD). The category includes individuals with chronic stable angina, asymptomatic ischemia, prior or current myocardial infarction (MI), prior coronary revascularization, as well as individuals with nonobstructive coronary atherosclerosis. IHD is typically caused by atheromatous plaque that either obstructs or gradually narrows the epicardial coronary arteries (See also Chapter 11 for a more detailed discussion of atherosclerosis.)

The key adverse consequence of atherosclerosis is that it can lead to endothelial dysfunction and microvascular and macrovascular disease. IHD sometimes has been viewed as synonymous with "obstructive coronary atherosclerosis," but it is more complicated than that (1–3).

Predisposing factors for coronary atherosclerosis ultimately result in impeded blood flow to the coronary arteries. This can result in ST segment elevation MI, non-ST segment acute coronary syndrome (ACS) and sudden cardiac death.

Multiple different symptoms may be present in individuals with IHD. Chest discomfort is usually the predominant symptom in individuals who have chronic stable, unstable angina or Prinzmetal's angina (variant) and acute MI. It is also possible that individuals who have IHD may be asymptomatic, in which case, myocardial ischemia may still be present. Heart failure (HF), cardiac arrhythmias and sudden death may also be complications of IHD. Atypical symptoms for IHD include mid-epigastric discomfort, shortness of breath, exercise intolerance and excessive fatigue. These atypical symptoms are observed more frequently in women and older adults and also in individuals with diabetes.

Myocardial ischemia may also occur in the setting of extreme myocardial oxygen demand, even in the absence of obstructive coronary artery disease (CAD). This can occur, for example, in aortic value disease or hypertrophic cardiomyopathy or pulmonary hypertension.

Lifestyle modalities such as regular physical activity, proper nutrition, weight management, not smoking cigarettes, and so on, play critical roles in not only reducing the risk of ischemic heart disease but also in its treatment. Lifestyle modalities are central to some studies that have demonstrated actual regression of atherosclerotic plaque that typically underlies ischemic heart disease (see Chapter 24).

15.2   SCOPE OF THE PROBLEM

A large number of individuals experience IHD. It has been estimated that over 50 million Americans have a history of IHD (4). About half of them present with angina pectoris, and approximately one half have experienced MI. The lifetime risk of IHD in individuals with an optimal risk factor profile is 3.6% for men and less than 1% for women. However, if individuals have two or more major risk factors, the lifetime risk rapidly accelerates to 37.5% and 18.3% for women. In 2013, IHD was responsible for 36% of all deaths caused by cardiovascular disease (CVD) and was the single most frequent cause of death in both American men and women.

Modern treatments have led to a decline in age-specific mortality from coronary heart disease (CHD) over the past several decades, yet symptoms related to IHD are a leading cause of death worldwide. It is anticipated that IHD will increase in the coming decades. The worldwide burden of risk factors for IHD has shifted to lower socioeconomic groups including increased prevalence of obesity and type 2 diabetes (T2DM). Unfortunately, this has created a rise in IHD risk factors in younger generations. The World Health Organization (WHO) has estimated that the global number of deaths from IHD will rise to 9.2 million individuals in 2030.

15.3   STABLE ANGINA PECTORIS

Individuals with angina pectoris typically present with the symptom of discomfort in the chest or adjacent areas caused by myocardial ischemia. Angina may be precipitated by exertion but can also be initiated by emotional distress. If the chest pain is prolonged or is occurring with increasing frequency, it may represent unstable IHD including unstable angina and acute MI. Epigastric discomfort alone or in association with chest pressure may be mistaken for indigestion. A typical episode of angina typically begins gradually and accelerates over a period of minutes before dissipating. Patients with angina generally should try to sit, rest or stop talking during episodes. The standard treatment for typical angina is short-acting nitroglycerin that will relieve it within minutes. This is often sublingual nitroglycerin. This can also serve as a diagnostic test.

15.4   OTHER CAUSES OF CHEST PAIN

Other causes of chest discomfort may be confused with angina. These include esophageal disorders, costochondritis or other neurological and musculoskeletal disorders. It should be noted that pulmonary embolism can also be characterized by shortness of breath, which is its cardinal symptom, but chest pain may be present. Acute pericarditis may be difficult to distinguish from angina. Pericarditis may be distinguished from angina since it is not relieved by nitroglycerin and is made worse by movement or deep inspiration or lying flat. Aortic dissection may also be confused with angina; however, it is typically more severe and radiates to the back.

Patients with stable angina will typically have normal findings on cardiac examination. Thus, the diagnosis of angina hinges on clinical history.

However, physical examination is still valuable to exclude other conditions that can mimic angina.

15.5 PATHOPHYSIOLOGY

Angina results from myocardial ischemia which is a result of imbalance between blood supply to the heart and its requirements. More detail about the process of atherosclerosis that leads to angina may be found in Chapter 11.

Angina can be caused by increased demand for myocardial oxygen occurring typically in the setting of restricted blood supply. This type of angina results from exertion, emotional duress or mental stress.

In contrast, angina caused by decrease in the blood supply to the heart is typically caused by coronary vasoconstriction that is a result of dynamic atherosclerosis plaques. This may be precipitated by decreases in the production of nitric oxide by the endothelium or by changes in the smooth muscle causing constriction to arteries distal to an atherosclerotic stenosis.

The history is very important to determine whether angina is caused by increased blood supply demand or decreased supply. For example, if episodes of angina come from increased demand (e.g., increased heart rate or emotional distress), therapeutic responses to control heart rate and blood pressure represent the most beneficial paths of treatment. While there are pharmaceutical agents that will assist in this, such lifestyle medicine techniques as stress reduction can play a very important role. Moreover, individuals who maintain a consistently active lifestyle will typically have lower heart rates both at rest and in response to exertion. This can play an important role in lessening the likelihood of demand-side myocardial ischemia.

15.6 EVALUATION AND MANAGEMENT

Lifestyle medicine modalities can play critically important roles in the ongoing management of IHD. This has been demonstrated by a variety of lifestyle medicine investigators including Caldwell Esselstyn and Dean Ornish. Lifestyle modalities will be discussed in this section along with standard medical diagnostic tests involved in the evaluation and critical management of IHD.

- Biochemical Tests—Individuals with stable ischemic heart disease (SIHD) should be evaluated for risk factors for the development of coronary heart disease (CHD). These include dyslipidemia (see also Chapter 12), insulin resistance (see also Chapter 18), overweight or obesity (see also Chapter 6) and level of physical activity (see also Chapter 4). In addition, issues related to sleep, stress levels and interactions with other individuals should be assessed in the counseling sessions.

A complete lipid profile including cholesterol, LDL cholesterol, HDL cholesterol, triglycerides and serum creatinine as well as fasting blood glucose levels and a measurement of hemoglobin A_{1C} should be measured. More detailed evaluation of other lipids related to atherosclerosis may also be appropriate (see Chapter 12).

Blood levels of cardiac troponins P and I are often used to differentiate patients who have had acute MI from those with SIHD (5,6). In particular, patients with SIHD may have small increases in high-sensitivity (hs) troponin (Tm) levels, and these individuals are at increased risk for adverse outcomes.

It is also important to evaluate inflammatory biomarkers since inflammation has now been determined to be an important component of atherosclerotic heart disease (see also Chapter 11). High-sensitivity C-reactive protein (hs-CRP) has been consistently demonstrated to relate to the risk for subsequent CVD events. Other markers of inflammation such as interleukin-6 (IL-6), cytokines and other biomarkers reflecting inflammatory pathways are currently under investigation, but hs-CRP is the most common inflammatory marker and has the most appropriate data (7). This should be routinely measured in patients with SIHD.

There is increasing interest in genetic mapping for patients with ISHD. This modality, however, is not currently available for routine testing (8) (see Chapter 3).

- Noninvasive Testing—A resting electrocardiogram ECG is appropriate for initial assessment of patients with SIHD and should also be routinely followed up every two years. Normal ECGs are found in approximately half of patients with SIHD (9,10). A resting ECG may also be helpful in determining or confirming a previous MI. The most common abnormality on the ECG in patients with SIHD, is nonspecific ST-T wave changes. This finding may correlate with severity of underlying heart disease. Obtaining periodic ECGs (at least once every few years) may also demonstrate new Q-wave MIs that have not been recognized clinically (11). During episodes of angina, ECG findings may become abnormal in 50% or more of patients with normal resting ECGs. The most common finding is ST segment depression.

A resting echocardiogram may be obtained to assess left ventricular function. Findings on this test may include wall motion abnormalities suggestive of CHD. Other findings such as aortic valve stenosis or left ventricular hypertrophy may suggest alternative diagnoses. The American College of Cardiology and American Heart Association (AHA) do not currently recommend routine echocardiography in all patients with SIHD; however, echocardiography may be appropriate for patients with a history of MI or ST-T wave abnormalities.

A chest x-ray is generally within normal limits in patients with SIHD, particularly if they have had normal findings on resting ECG. This test might be useful to individuals who have experienced a previous MI and may demonstrate cardiomegaly (increased heart size).

Noninvasive exercise stress testing can provide useful and sometimes indispensable information to follow the prognosis of patients with stable angina. However, routine use of exercise stress testing is typically not recommended, particularly as a substitute for a careful evaluation by a clinician.

Newer technologies such as cardiac computed tomography (CT) may be appropriate in some individuals (12,13). Coronary artery calcification may be present in some asymptomatic individuals; however, cost considerations must be considered before utilizing what is typically a very expensive test. The same consideration should be made for cardiac magnetic resonance imaging (MRI) (14).

- Invasive Assessment—While noninvasive technologies are very valuable in establishing a diagnosis, more precise assessment of anatomic severity of CHD still requires invasive coronary angiography. Before referring patients for an invasive assessment, however, careful consideration must be given to the utility of the likely findings. A large series of cardiac catheterization findings suggested that 50% have no significant obstructive disease in the coronary arteries (15).

Invasive assessment must be carefully considered with advice from a seasoned invasive cardiologist.

- Natural History and Risk Stratification

As many of 30% of patients with a history of stable angina experience angina one or more times per week (16). Such patients may be appropriately treated with aspirin, beta blocking agents and aggressive modification of risk factors to lower mortality risk. As discussed in Chapter 10, risk factor models are available that will help the clinician determine how aggressively to pursue risk factor reduction.

- Medical Management—Multiple lifestyle modalities have been shown to lower symptoms and improve atherosclerosis in people who have SIHD (17). The Lifestyle Heart Trial conducted by Ornish and colleagues showed that individuals who followed a low-fat diet, engaged in regular stress reduction techniques and increased their physical activity had 37% reduction in LDL, 91% reduction in angina and 5.5% reduction of stenoses (18).

The Lifestyle Modification Demonstration Project followed a somewhat similar approach utilizing a low-fat diet over a 1- and 2-year period (19). A total of 580 participants were enrolled. This project demonstrated improvement in most cardiac risk factors and improved functional cardiac capacity at the end of 12 and 24 months. This program also showed significant reductions in hospitalizations compared to either cardiac rehabilitation or noncardiac rehabilitation controls.

A 5-year study in 22 subjects was reported by Esselstyn and colleagues in individuals with several CHDs (20). These individuals followed a strict plant-based diet, with less than 10% of calories from fat and no added oils or nuts. In the initial cohort, 17 of the 22 individuals who were adherent to this strict program showed substantial reductions in their serum cholesterol levels. Eleven of the 17 individuals underwent angiographic analysis at 5 years and none showed progression, while 8 out of the 11 showed regression. There was no angina or need for angiographic procedures such as stent placement at the 5-year evaluation point.

A large study called the Lyon Diet Heart Study compared the Mediterranean diet to a prudent Western diet for secondary prevention in individuals with established atherosclerosis (21). This study also showed a significant reduction in risk of cardiac events following MI.

Other studies have dealt with risk factors for CHD. For example, the DASH diet enrolled 459 patients with systolic blood pressure <160 mm Hg and diastolic blood pressures of 80–95 mm Hg. The individuals followed the DASH diet that is high in fruits and vegetables and low in saturated fat and sodium. This diet reduced systolic blood pressure by 5.5 mm Hg and diastolic pressure by 3.0 mm Hg, thus significantly lowering the risk of CHD.

The Complete Health Improvement Program (CHIP) demonstrated substantial decreases in CVD risk factors and showed significant improvements in both total cholesterol and LDL cholesterol as well as both systolic and diastolic blood pressure (22). Thus, multiple studies have demonstrated significant improvements in risk factors in individuals who either had established IHD or were at risk for it.

Other standard approaches to medical management of IHD include treatment of associated diseases that might increase cardiac oxygen demand and reduce coronary risk factors such as hypertension, cigarette smoking and management of dyslipidemias. Approaches to increased physical activity, weight reduction (for overweight or obese individuals) and reductions in inflammation have all been utilized to lower the risk of progression of IHD.

In addition to these specific approaches, an overall approach to making multiple changes in lifestyle is important for individuals with IHD.

- Pharmacologic Management of Angina—While a detailed discussion of pharmacologic management of angina is beyond the scope of this chapter, it should be noted that both beta adrenergic blocking agents and calcium antagonists represent first-line therapies for symptom reduction. In addition, nitrates play a significant role in symptomatic management of individuals with IHD. Specific recommendations for pharmacologic agents and their use can be found in standard internal medicine or cardiology textbooks.

15.7 REVASCULARIZATION APPROACHES TO ISCHEMIC HEART DISEASE

IHD represents a continuum of disease with a variable natural history that may eventually result in periods of exertional angina or progression to accelerating angina with the culmination in unstable angina, acute MI or heart failure. Lifestyle medicine modalities may lower the risk of these complications, but at some point, revascularization may be necessary either through percutaneous coronary interventions or bypass surgery (23). The multiple options for revascularization are beyond the scope of this chapter but should be undertaken in consultation with an experienced cardiologist.

15.8 POTENTIAL COMPLICATIONS OF ISCHEMIC HEART DISEASE

Despite excellent medical management, it remains possible that individuals with ischemic heart disease will experience complications. For example, between two-thirds and three-quarters of all cases of heart failure appear to result from underlying CHD (24,25). Some individuals may start with angina and ultimately end up with symptoms of congestive heart failure, which increases the oxygen demand and will require more aggressive therapy. In addition, mitral regurgitation (MR) is a common cause of heart failure in some patients with CHD. This may be caused by ischemia or a rupture of the papillary muscles that support the mitral valve (26–28). Alternatively, chronic mitral or aortic regurgitation in individuals with CHD may result from ischemic or dilated cardiomyopathy. For this reason, it is important to do a careful physical examination including auscultation for cardiac murmurs in patients with CHD.

In addition, particularly in older patients, a degree of aortic stenosis (AS) may be present that can increase myocardial oxygen demand. This represents another reason for careful auscultation of the heart in patients with CHD. Both aortic stenosis and mitral regurgitation are beyond the scope of this chapter; however, they are handled in every major cardiac textbook.

15.9 FUTURE DIRECTIONS

Given the demonstrated benefits of multiple lifestyle therapies for IHD, it is important for practitioners in the area of lifestyle medicine to counsel their patients on these modalities and to urge other physicians including cardiologists to incorporate these procedures in the overall practice of cardiology. Both the AHA and the ACC are increasingly recognizing the role of lifestyle in multiple areas of cardiovascular disease management. These include the recent publication of "Lifestyle Management of Lipids" (29), the "Lifestyle Management of Hypertension" (30) and the "Lifestyle Management Practice Guidelines" issued by the AHA and ACC (31). Lifestyle modalities will play a critical role in the articulated vision of the AHA to emphasize primordial prevention, since lifestyle modalities can be practiced throughout the entire life span. In the future, we anticipate that we will see more emphasis on lifelong lifestyle practices to lower the likelihood of ever developing ischemic heart disease in the first place. The AHA has categorized this area as "primordial prevention" (32).

15.10 SUMMARY AND CONCLUSIONS

SIHD includes individuals with both chronic stable angina, asymptomatic ischemic and prior coronary revascularization as well as individuals who have coronary atherosclerosis that is nonobstructive.

It is estimated that over 15 million Americans currently have IHD, which includes over 7,800,000 individuals who have angina and 7,600,000 who have had a prior MI.

Lifestyle therapies can be extremely valuable both in the prevention of ischemic heart disease and also in its treatment. Individuals who have optimal risk factor profiles according to the Framingham data are one-tenth as likely to have ischemic heart disease compared to individuals who have two or more major risk factors.

IHD results in almost half of all deaths caused by all forms of CVD. This is the single most frequent cause of death for American men and women. Lifestyle modalities have been demonstrated to lower multiple risk of IHD including lowering lipids, helping to control blood pressure and assisting in long-term weight control or weight loss.

As modern understandings of atherosclerosis (the underlying condition behind the vast majority of IHD) have continued to evolve, lifestyle modalities can also play a very important role in lessening inflammation. For all of these reasons, lifestyle medicine plays an increasingly important role in both the prevention and management of IHD.

Clinical Applications

- Lifestyle therapies can lower the risk of ischemic heart disease.
- Lifestyle therapies such as increased physical activity, lipid management, control of hypertension and reduction of weight gain and lowering the likelihood of obesity can all play important roles both in reducing the risk of IHD and also in its treatment.
- All patients should be counseled in the important role of lifestyle therapies in lowering the risk of IHD and in its treatment.

REFERENCES

1. Marzilli M, Merz CN, Boden WE, et al. Obstructive coronary atherosclerosis and ischemic heart disease: An elusive link! J Am Coll Cardiol. 2012;60(11):951–6. Epub 2012/09/08.
2. Pepine CJ, Douglas PS. Rethinking stable ischemic heart disease: Is this the beginning of a new era? J Am Coll Cardiol. 2012;60(11):957–9. Epub 2012/09/08.
3. Pepine CJ. Multiple causes for ischemia without obstructive coronary artery disease: Not a short list. Circulation. 2015;131(12):1044–6. Epub 2015/02/26.
4. Writing Group Members, Mozaffarian D, Benjamin EJ, et al. Heart disease and stroke statistics—2016 update: A report from the American Heart Association. Circulation. 2016;133(4):e38–360. Epub 2015/12/18.
5. Omland T, Pfeffer MA, Solomon SD, et al. Prognostic value of cardiac troponin I measured with a highly sensitive assay in patients with stable coronary artery disease. J Am Coll Cardiol. 2013;61(12):1240–9. Epub 2013/02/19.
6. Everett BM, Brooks MM, Vlachos HE, et al. Troponin and cardiac events in stable ischemic heart disease and diabetes. N Engl J Med. 2015;373(7):610–20. Epub 2015/08/13.
7. Everett BM, Ridker PM. Biomarkers for cardiovascular screening: Progress or passe? Clin Chem. 2017;63(1):248–51. Epub 2016/12/03.
8. Weijmans M, de Bakker PI, van der Graaf Y, et al. Incremental value of a genetic risk score for the prediction of new vascular events in patients with clinically manifest vascular disease. Atherosclerosis. 2015;239(2):451–8. Epub 2015/02/18.

9. Cheng VY, Berman DS, Rozanski A, et al. Performance of the traditional age, sex, and angina typicality-based approach for estimating pretest probability of angiographically significant coronary artery disease in patients undergoing coronary computed tomographic angiography: Results from the multinational coronary CT angiography evaluation for clinical outcomes: An international multicenter registry (CONFIRM). Circulation. 2011;124(22):2423–32, 1–8. Epub 2011/10/26.

10. Douglas PS, Hoffmann U, Patel MR, et al. Outcomes of anatomical versus functional testing for coronary artery disease. N Engl J Med. 2015;372(14):1291–300. Epub 2015/03/17.

11. Task Force Members, Montalescot G, Sechtem U, et al. 2013 ESC guidelines on the management of stable coronary artery disease: The Task Force on the management of stable coronary artery disease of the European Society of Cardiology. Eur Heart J. 2013;34(38):2949–3003. Epub 2013/09/03.

12. American College of Cardiology Foundation Task Force on Expert Consensus Documents, Mark DB, Berman DS, et al. ACCF/ACR/AHA/NASCI/SAIP/SCAI/SCCT 2010 expert consensus document on coronary computed tomographic angiography: A report of the American College of Cardiology Foundation Task Force on expert consensus documents. Circulation. 2010;121(22):2509–43. Epub 2010/05/19.

13. Douglas PS, Pontone G, Hlatky MA, et al. Clinical outcomes of fractional flow reserve by computed tomographic angiography-guided diagnostic strategies vs. usual care in patients with suspected coronary artery disease: The prospective longitudinal trial of FFR (CT): Outcome and resource impacts study. Eur Heart J. 2015;36(47):3359–67. Epub 2015/09/04.

14. Chang SA, Kim RJ. The use of cardiac magnetic resonance in patients with suspected coronary artery disease: A clinical practice perspective. J Cardiovasc Ultrasound. 2016;24(2):96–103. Epub 2016/07/01.

15. Patel MR, Peterson ED, Dai D, Brennan JM, Redberg RF, Anderson HV, et al. Low diagnostic yield of elective coronary angiography. N Engl J Med. 2010;362(10):886–95. Epub 2010/03/12.

16. Morrow DA. Cardiovascular risk prediction in patients with stable and unstable coronary heart disease. Circulation. 2010;121(24):2681–91. Epub 2010/06/23.

17. Bangalore S, Maron DJ, Hochman JS. Evidence-based management of stable ischemic heart disease: Challenges and confusion. JAMA. 2015;314(18):1917–18. Epub 2015/11/10.

18. Ornish D, Scherwitz LW, Billings JH, et al. Intensive lifestyle changes for reversal of coronary heart disease. JAMA. 1998;280(23):2001–7. Epub 1998/12/24.

19. Shephard DS et al. Executive Summary: Evaluation of Lifestyle Modification and Cardiac Rehabilitation in Medicare Beneficiaries. Schneider Institutes for Health Policy, Heller School, Brandeis University; 2009 Apr. 30. Summary. brandeis.edu. Accessed February 23, 2022.

20. Esselstyn CB, Jr., Ellis SG, Medendorp SV, et al. A strategy to arrest and reverse coronary artery disease: A 5-year longitudinal study of a single physician's practice. J Fam Pract. 1995;41(6):560–8. Epub 1995/12/01.

21. de Lorgeril M, Salen P, Martin JL, et al. Mediterranean diet, traditional risk factors, and the rate of cardiovascular complications after myocardial infarction: Final report of the Lyon Diet Heart Study. Circulation. 1999;99(6):779–85. Epub 1999/02/17.

22. Appel LJ, Moore TJ, Obarzanek E, et al. A clinical trial of the effects of dietary patterns on blood pressure. DASH Collaborative Research Group. N Engl J Med. 1997;336(16):1117–24. Epub 1997/04/17.

23. Piccolo R, Giustino G, Mehran R, et al. Stable coronary artery disease: Revascularisation and invasive strategies. Lancet. 2015;386(9994):702–13. Epub 2015/09/04.

24. Phillips LM, Hachamovitch R, Berman DS, et al. Lessons learned from MPI and physiologic testing in randomized trials of stable ischemic heart disease: COURAGE, BARI 2D, FAME, and ISCHEMIA. J Nucl Cardiol. 2013;20(6):969–75. Epub 2013/08/22.

25. Mentz RJ, Fiuzat M, Shaw LK, et al. Comparison of clinical characteristics and long-term outcomes of patients with ischemic cardiomyopathy with versus without angina pectoris (from the Duke Databank for Cardiovascular Disease). Am J Cardiol. 2012;109(9):1272–7. Epub 2012/02/14.

26. Braun J, Klautz RJ. Mitral valve surgery in low ejection fraction, severe ischemic mitral regurgitation patients: Should we repair them all? Curr Opin Cardiol. 2012;27(2):111–17. Epub 2012/01/26.

27. Goldstein D, Moskowitz AJ, Gelijns AC, et al. Two-year outcomes of surgical treatment of severe ischemic mitral regurgitation. N Engl J Med. 2016;374(4):344–53. Epub 2015/11/10.

28. Michler RE, Smith PK, Parides MK, et al. Two-year outcomes of surgical treatment of moderate ischemic mitral regurgitation. N Engl J Med. 2016;374(20):1932–41. Epub 2016/04/05.

29. Grundy SM, Stone NJ, Bailey AL, Beam C, Birtcher KK, Blumenthal RS, et al. 2018 AHA/ACC/AACVPR/AAPA/ABC/ACPM/ADA/AGS/APhA/ASPC/NLA/PCNA Guideline on the management of blood cholesterol: A report of the American College of Cardiology/American Heart Association Task Force on Clinical Practice Guidelines. Circulation. 2019;139(25):e1082–143. Epub 2018/12/28.

30. Whelton PK, Carey RM, Aronow WS, et al. 2017 ACC/AHA/AAPA/ABC/ACPM/AGS/APhA/ASH/ASPC/NMA/PCNA guideline for the prevention, detection, evaluation, and management of high blood pressure in adults: Executive summary: A report of the American College of Cardiology/American Heart Association Task Force on Clinical Practice Guidelines. Circulation. 2018;138(17):e426–83. Epub 2018/10/26.

31. Stone NJ, Robinson JG, Lichtenstein AH, et al. 2013 ACC/AHA guideline on the treatment of blood cholesterol to reduce atherosclerotic cardiovascular risk in adults: A report of the American College of Cardiology/American Heart Association Task Force on Practice Guidelines. Circulation. 2014;129(25 Suppl 2):S1–45. Epub 2013/11/14.

32. Lloyd-Jones DM, Hong Y, Labarthe D, et al. Defining and setting national goals for cardiovascular health promotion and disease reduction: The American Heart Association's strategic Impact Goal through 2020 and beyond. Circulation. 2010;121(4):586–613.

16 Approach to the Patient with Chest Pain

KEY POINTS

- Chest pain is a common reason for individuals to be seen in the emergency department. Approximately 10–15% of all individuals seen in the emergency room come in with the complaint of chest pain.
- Of these, 10–15% have chest pain resulting from acute coronary syndrome.
- Lifestyle medicine physicians should be knowledgeable about how to distinguish various kinds and etiologies of chest pain.
- If clinical evaluation and diagnostic tests indicate acute coronary syndromes, the lifestyle medicine clinician will need to work with a board certified cardiologist to provide effective treatment.
- Lifestyle medicine physicians also play a critical role in lowering risk factors for acute coronary syndromes and also for supervising rehabilitation and recovery.

16.1 INTRODUCTION

Atherosclerotic heart disease, which is the underlying condition for coronary heart disease (CHD), cerebrovascular accident (CVA) and peripheral arterial disease (PAD), is a lifelong, slowly developing systemic condition of the arteries (see Chapter 11).

We know from studies of car crash victims and also autopsies of soldiers in the Korean War that there is often evidence of atherosclerosis already in the teenage years. In many instances, it appears that the process may start in early childhood or perhaps even in utero (1). For this reason, there are multiple different manifestations of atherosclerotic vascular disease. In all stages of life, lifestyle medicine modalities and techniques such as proper nutrition for lipid lowering, physical activity and weight loss for both control of hypertension and reduction of risk for overweight or obesity, smoking cessation, stress reduction and other modalities play important roles in the management of atherosclerotic heart disease.

Despite the best efforts of lifestyle medicine physicians and other physicians, it is quite possible, indeed likely, that most physicians will have to deal with patients who have underlying atherosclerotic vascular disease who ultimately develop chest discomfort. Moreover, many lifestyle medicine practitioners also work in emergency rooms where the ability to effectively evaluate patients with chest pain is critically important. Acute chest pain is one of the most common reasons for seeking care in the emergency department and accounts for approximately 10%–15% of all visits to emergency rooms nationwide or six million presentations annually in the United States (2).

While chest pain raises the possibility of acute coronary syndromes (ACS) (see later in this chapter), when chest pain in the emergency room is evaluated, only 10%–15% of individuals with acute chest pain actually have ACS. Thus, it is very important to be able to distinguish between ACS and other life-threatening conditions from those that are both noncardiac and non-life threatening but cause chest pain. Moreover, if the diagnosis of ACS is missed, as it is in approximately 2% of patients, it can lead to enormous consequences such as MI, poorly treated unstable angina and even mortality.

A variety of advances in both the accuracy and efficiency of evaluating patients with acute chest pain have occurred, along with better blood markers for myocardial injury that allows for more accurate stratification of patients (3). In addition, advances in testing such as computed tomography (CT) further make risk stratification more precise. While the role of lifestyle medicine physicians is critically important in lowering the risk of both developing atherosclerotic disease and helping to stabilize plaque leading to chronic unstable angina, it is also important that physicians have an understanding of how to diagnose acute chest pain and how to differentiate ACS from other causes of chest discomfort.

16.2   CORONARY BLOOD FLOW AND MYOCARDIAL ISCHEMIA

The coronary circulation is unique because it is required to generate consistent perfusion in blood flow even during the systolic portion of the cardiac cycle that impedes blood flow to some degree. When impedance of coronary blood flow is further exacerbated by atherosclerotic lesions, it can cause a mismatch between myocardial tissue demand and blood flow and oxygen delivery. Moreover, the heart has minimal ability to perform anaerobic metabolism and, thus, is highly dependent on a continuous and uninterrupted flow of blood.

When blood flow and oxygen delivery are not adequate for metabolic demand, the typical symptom is myocardial ischemia. In the setting of myocardial ischemia, particularly with atherosclerotic disease, a common symptom is chest discomfort or angina. The heart compensates to some degree with the process of autoregulation so that when pressure falls, coronary arterial blood flow maximally dilates. However, when atherosclerotic lesions further impede blood flow, various forms of myocardial ischemia can result and be manifested as acute chest pain.

16.3   CAUSES OF ACUTE CHEST PAIN

For patients undergoing an evaluation for acute chest pain in the emergency room, as already indicated, 10%–15% have acute myocardial infarction (AMI) or unstable angina (2). A smaller percentage may have other life-threatening problems such as a pulmonary embolism or acute aortic dissection. Most do not have a cardiac-related condition. Nonetheless, for lifestyle medicine practitioners in clinical practice, the likelihood of acute chest discomfort in a population that is currently being treated for atherosclerosis manifests in stable ischemic heart disease (IHD) or chronic angina or following an acute cardiac event. There are multiple reasons for having acute chest discomfort, as follows:

- *Myocardial ischemia or infarction*—The most common and serious cause of acute chest discomfort is myocardial ischemia or perhaps myocardial infarction. As already indicated, this occurs when the supply of myocardial oxygen consumption is inadequate for demand. This typically occurs in the setting of coronary atherosclerosis.

  The classic manifestation of myocardial ischemia is angina. This is usually described as heavy chest pressure or squeezing, a burning feeling or difficulty breathing. Perhaps the most famous sign of acute ischemia came from a Harvard cardiologist in the 1930s, Samuel Levine, where he indicated that patients would often make their hand into a fist and bring it up to their chest to decrease their symptom. This has become the "Levine sign."

  Anginal pain typically radiates either to the left shoulder, neck or arm. It will typically build over a few minutes. Patients with ACS often have chest discomfort without obvious antecedent causes, although it may occur with exercise or psychological stress. As noted by the American College of Cardiology (ACC) and the American Heart Association (AHA) (4), typical pain descriptions that are not characteristic of myocardial ischemia include the following:

  - Thoracic pain (brought on or made worse by respiratory movement or coughing),
  - Pain reproduced with movement or palpation of the chest wall or arms,
  - Primary locations in the lower or middle abdominal region,
  - Constant pain persisting for many hours,
  - Very brief episodes of pain lasting only a few seconds or less, and
  - Pain that radiates to the lower extremities.

  It is important to note that patients with ACS may also present with atypical symptoms. These are called "angina equivalents" and may be jaw pain or pain in the abdomen, nausea or vomiting, diaphoresis or fatigue. These atypical types of discomfort appear to be more common in women, older persons or individuals with diabetes.
- *Musculoskeletal or other causes*—Chest pain may also be the result of musculoskeletal disorders involving the chest wall (e.g., costochondritis) or following heavy upper arm exertion. This type of chest pain is typically elicited by direct pressure to the involved area. The pain can be fleeting or can be a dull ache at first for many hours. An unusual cause of atypical pressure or pain is panic disorder. This is often accompanied by a sense of anxiety and may last for 30 minutes or longer.
- *Gastrointestinal conditions*—Acid reflux irritating the esophagus may result in a burning discomfort. Lying down often worsens symptoms, whereas sitting upright or utilizing acid-reducing therapies typically will alleviate this symptom.
- *Pericardial disease*—Inflammation of the pericardium often involves the surrounding pleura. Patients with pericardial disease may experience worsening of this pain when coughing, taking a deep breath or changing position (5).

- *Vascular disease*—Acute dissection of the aorta causes sudden onset of excruciating pain. The location of this discomfort reflects the site and progression of the dissection. Aortic dissections are rare with an estimated annual incidence of three per 100,000. If aortic dissection is not accurately diagnosed, it can rapidly lead to mortality.
- *Pulmonary emboli*—Pulmonary emboli can cause acute onset of shortness of breath and chest pain, although some patients with PE are asymptomatic. Massive pulmonary emboli may cause severe and persistent substernal pain, whereas smaller emboli may cause lesser amounts of chest discomfort.
- *Pulmonary conditions*—Pulmonary conditions such as tracheal bronchitis may produce chest discomfort over the involved lung and are usually associated with dyspnea. Pneumothorax may occur in the setting of pulmonary disease such as chronic obstructive pulmonary disease (COPD), asthma or cystic fibrosis.

16.4   DIAGNOSTIC CONSIDERATIONS

For patients with acute chest pain, is it essential that physicians address a series of issues related to both immediate management and prognosis before trying to establish a definite diagnosis. The following three issues must be immediately addressed: clinical stability, immediate prognosis and safety of triage.

- *Initial assessment*—The evaluation of a patient with acute chest pain may begin before the physician even sees the patient. The guidelines established by the ACC and AHA emphasize that patients whose symptoms are consistent with ACS should be immediately referred to facilities that allow evaluation by a physician and a recording of a 12-lead electrocardiogram (4). These patients should be referred to an emergency department or a specialized chest pain unit if ACS is suspected and the patient has experienced chest discomfort longer than 20 minutes, hemodynamic instability or recent syncopal or near-syncopal episodes. If the patient has chest pain, pressure, tightness or heaviness that radiates to neck, jaw, shoulders or back, indigestion or heartburn, persistent shortness of breath, weakness, dizziness or lightheadedness, immediate evaluation should be made by triage nurses. This initial assessment includes taking a brief history and performing a physical examination, obtaining an ECG, obtaining a chest radiograph and measuring biomarkers for myocardial injury.
- *History*—If the patient is hemodynamically stable, the physician's assessment should include a clinical history that captures the characteristics of the pain. Patients with ACS typically describe their chest discomfort as diffuse substernal pressure that starts gradually, radiates to jaw and arms, worsens with exertion and is relieved by rest or nitroglycerine. These symptoms are fairly typical in any given patient, so reference should be made to previous episodes.

In addition, the presence of risk factors for atherosclerosis (see Chapter 11) increases the likelihood that chest pain results from myocardial ischemia. For a young patient, a history of cocaine abuse should also be obtained.

Combining the history in conjunction with the physical exam, the ECG and cardiac biomarkers are essential for the diagnostic assessment.

- *Physical examination*—The initial examination of a patient with acute chest pain focuses on potential underlying causes of myocardial ischemia, such as uncontrolled high blood pressure, mitral regurgitation or hypertension (6,7). Peripheral pulses should also be examined for diminished strength, bruits or absent pulses (see Chapter 14) for PAD features. If the clinical findings do not suggest myocardial ischemia, focus should move to other potentially life-threatening issues such as aortic dissection or PE. Myocarditis should also be evaluated and may be present in the setting of pericarditis.
- *Electrocardiography*—An electrocardiograph (ECG) should be obtained within 10 minutes of arrival if an individual is having ongoing chest discomfort (4,8). This can provide definitive data. Persistent or transient ST segment elevation that develops during a symptomatic episode at rest strongly suggests acute ischemia. Nonspecific ST segment changes are less helpful for risk stratification. It should be noted that a completely normal ECG does not exclude ACS, although a normal ECG has a negative predictive value of 80%–90%. Obtaining serial ECGs can add further diagnostic data.
- *Chest X-ray*—A chest x-ray may be useful to show pulmonary edema or may be useful to show widened mediastinum in a patient with aorta dissection.
- *Biomarkers*—If the clinical evaluation and ECG are suggestive of ACS, biomarkers for myocardial injury should be obtained (4,9). The preferred biomarker is cardiac troponin-T (cTnT). Creatine kinase MB isoenzyme (CK-MB) is less sensitive. The current guidelines from the AHA and ACC recommend measuring cTnT at presentation and then 3–6 hours after symptom onset. Normal values of these measurements have been demonstrated to yield a negative predictive value approaching 99% (10–12).
- *Testing strategy*—Biomarkers of cardiac injury are important if the history and physical exam suggest ACS. Patients who have a low probability of ACS should not undergo biomarkers because false-positive tests can lead to unnecessary hospitalizations, tests, procedures and complications (13).

16.5   IMMEDIATE MANAGEMENT

Guidelines issued by ACC and AHA suggest that if ACS is determined, the information obtained from the various diagnostic procedures should be integrated into the differential diagnoses of chronic stable angina, possible ACS and definite ACS (4). If ST segment elevations are present, these individuals fall into the different category of ST-segment elevated myocardial infarction. Patients with possible or definite ACS who do not have diagnostic ECGs and have normal initial serum cardiac markers can be observed in a chest pain unit and undergo further testing.

- *Chest pain protocols and units*—The ACC and AHA recommendations include that patients who have no further chest discomfort, have no ECG abnormalities suggesting ischemia and normal cardiac biomarkers can be discharged to home and can undergo noninvasive testing (4). However, noninvasive testing such as treadmill testing should occur within 72 hours. Such patients are eligible to receive aspirin, possibly a beta blocking agent and sublingual nitroglycerin to take with chest pain symptoms. Chest pain units in hospitals are often located adjacent to the emergency room to allow this kind of process to occur.

- *Early noninvasive testing*—A treadmill exercise, electrocardiogram should be undertaken within 72 hours. Such tests provide reliable prognostic information in low-risk patient populations. Patients who are at low risk with a normal ECG and normal biomarkers should undergo outpatient treadmill stress testing within 24 hours and no later than 72 hours.
- *Imaging tests*—If a patient cannot undergo exercise treadmill testing because of physical disability, stress echocardiography or radionuclide scans are the preferred, noninvasive testing modalities. Echocardiography may be helpful to detect wall motion abnormalities. Stress echocardiography may also be useful to detect wall motion abnormalities. Another possible test is coronary computed tomographic angiography (CTA). An advantage of CTA is that it is the test of choice for PE or aortic dissection. A disadvantage is expense and radiation exposure.

16.6 ACUTE CORONARY SYNDROMES

Ischemic heart disease may manifest itself clinically in a variety of different ways. It can be chronic stable angina or acute coronary syndrome (ACS). ACS includes ST-elevation myocardial infarction (STEMI) (see next section) and non-ST elevation acute coronary syndrome (NSTE-ACS). Non-ST elevation myocardial infarction (NSTEMI) and unstable angina (UA) have a similar clinical presentation at the initial evaluation (14).

The major differences between ACS and chronic stable angina are that in ACS there is a sudden onset of symptoms at rest or severe pain, pressure or discomfort of the chest or an accelerating pattern of angina that occurs more frequently with greater severity or awakens the patient from sleep. Twelve-lead ECGs and markers of myocardial necrosis are essential tools to distinguish between the three types of ACS, as already indicated previously in this chapter. A detailed description of non-ST elevation acute coronary syndrome is beyond the scope of this chapter and would be typically handled by a board-certified cardiologist.

Myocardial infarction (MI) requires evidence of myocardial cell death caused by ischemia. The modern approach to patients with new onset or worsening ischemic symptoms lumps all of these together in the category of acute coronary syndrome (ACS). ACS encompasses the diagnosis of unstable angina, non-ST segment elevation MI (NSTEMI) and ST-elevation MI (STEMI). The major diagnostic tool for patients with suspected ACS remains the 12-lead electrocardiogram that identifies those with ST segment elevation that are candidates for urgent revascularization. Treatment of STEMI is beyond the scope of this chapter and will be handled in almost all clinical settings by a board-certified invasive cardiologist.

16.7 THE ROLE OF LIFESTYLE MEDICINE CLINICIANS IN APPROACH TO PATIENTS WITH CHEST PAIN

As already indicated, lifestyle medicine practitioners will often see patients who have chronic ischemic heart disease. Because of the progressive nature of atherosclerosis, despite best lifestyle medicine efforts, some of these patients will move on to develop acute coronary syndromes. It is incumbent upon lifestyle medicine practitioners to be able to distinguish between acute coronary syndrome from other causes of chest pain. These were outlined previously in this chapter.

Moreover, lifestyle medicine modalities will not only lower the risk of developing ACS but will also be critically important in the rehabilitation and recovery and long-term treatment phases for atherosclerosis in these patients. Lifestyle medicine modalities in cardiac rehabilitation involve counseling, prescription for increased physical activity, lipid lowering, controlled blood pressure and counseling to cease cigarette smoking. Weight loss in overweight or obese patients is also important.

16.8 SUMMARY/CONCLUSIONS

Because of the nature of atherosclerosis, which is a lifelong, systemic disease, lifestyle medicine practitioners will often be called on to determine whether or not patients that they have with chronic ischemic heart disease are undergoing episodes where there has been an acute change. In this setting, which is often conducted in conjunction with colleagues either in the emergency department or cardiology clinic, lifestyle medicine practitioners play a critical role not only in identifying cardiac from noncardiac pain, but also in initiating prompt therapy, along with cardiologists and emergency doctors.

Clinical Applications

- Chest pain represents 10%–15% of all individuals seen in emergency rooms.
- Of these individuals, 10%–15% have chest pain resulting from acute changes in their atherosclerotic heart disease. These are called acute coronary syndromes.
- Lifestyle medicine clinicians should be aware of the potential of these complications in patients that they are treating with chronic stable coronary artery disease.
- Lifestyle physicians should also have a clear handle on how to distinguish various kinds of chest discomfort.

REFERENCES

1. Sauder KA, Dabelea D. Life course approach to prevention of chronic disease. In James Rippe MD, ed. Lifestyle Medicine. 3rd ed. Boca Raton, FL: CRC Press; 2019, chapter 74, pp. 861–72.
2. Bhuiya FA, Pitts SR, McCaig LF. Emergency department visits for chest pain and abdominal pain: United States, 1999–2008. NCHS Data Brief. 2010;(43):1–8. Epub 2010/09/22.

3. Reichlin T, Irfan A, Twerenbold R, et al. Utility of absolute and relative changes in cardiac troponin concentrations in the early diagnosis of acute myocardial infarction. Circulation. 2011;124(2):136–45. Epub 2011/06/29.

4. Amsterdam EA, Wenger NK, Brindis RG, et al. 2014 AHA/ACC guideline for the management of patients with non-ST-elevation acute coronary syndromes: Executive summary: A report of the American College of Cardiology/American Heart Association Task Force on Practice Guidelines. Circulation. 2014;130(25):2354–94. Epub 2014/09/25.

5. Dudzinski DM, Mak GS, Hung JW. Pericardial diseases. Curr Probl Cardiol. 2012;37(3):75–118. Epub 2012/02/01.

6. Fanaroff AC, Rymer JA, Goldstein SA, et al. Does this patient with chest pain have acute coronary syndrome?: The rational clinical examination systematic review. JAMA. 2015;314(18):1955–65. Epub 2015/11/10.

7. Body R, Cook G, Burrows G, et al. Can emergency physicians "rule in" and "rule out" acute myocardial infarction with clinical judgement? Emerg Med J. 2014;31(11):872–6. Epub 2014/07/14.

8. O'Gara PT, Kushner FG, Ascheim DD, et al. 2013 ACCF/AHA guideline for the management of ST-elevation myocardial infarction: A report of the American College of Cardiology Foundation/American Heart Association Task Force on Practice Guidelines. Circulation. 2013;127(4):e362–425. Epub 2012/12/19.

9. Thygesen K, Alpert JS, Jaffe AS, et al. Third universal definition of myocardial infarction. Circulation. 2012;126(16):2020–35. Epub 2012/08/28.

10. Bonaca MP, Ruff CT, Kosowsky J, et al. Evaluation of the diagnostic performance of current and next-generation assays for cardiac troponin I in the BWH-TIMI ED Chest Pain Study. Eur Heart J Acute Cardiovasc Care. 2013;2(3):195–202. Epub 2013/11/14.

11. Reiter M, Twerenbold R, Reichlin T, et al. Early diagnosis of acute myocardial infarction in patients with pre-existing coronary artery disease using more sensitive cardiac troponin assays. Eur Heart J. 2012;33(8):988–97. Epub 2011/11/03.

12. Hess EP, Jaffe AS. Evaluation of patients with possible cardiac chest pain: A way out of the jungle. J Am Coll Cardiol. 2012;59(23):2099–100. Epub 2012/06/02.

13. Amsterdam EA, Kirk JD, Bluemke DA, et al. Testing of low-risk patients presenting to the emergency department with chest pain: A scientific statement from the American Heart Association. Circulation. 2010;122(17):1756–76. Epub 2010/07/28.

14. Giugliano RP, Braunwald E. Non-ST elevation acute coronary syndromes guidelines: Unstable angina and non-ST elevation myocardial infarction. In Zipes, Libby, Bonow, Mann, Tomaselli, eds. Braunwald's Heart Disease. 11th ed. Amsterdam: Elsevier; 2019.

17 Carotid Artery Disease and Stroke

KEY POINTS

- Strokes are very common in the United States with nearly 800,000 occurring every year.
- Stroke is the third or fourth leading cause of mortality in Western societies.
- Atherosclerosis is a systemic disease and can involve the carotid arteries as well as coronary arteries and lead to stroke.
- Lifestyle medicine therapies to lower the risk of coronary heart disease are also highly appropriate to lower the risk of stroke.

17.1 INTRODUCTION

Considerable attention, particularly among lifestyle medicine practitioners, relates to ischemic heart disease and atherosclerosis. It is important to remember, however, that atherosclerosis is a systemic and dynamic process that progresses throughout an individual's life. For this reason, it is essential to consider atherosclerosis of the carotid arteries as well as the small vessels in the brain. Thus, lifestyle medicine physicians should be cognizant of and counsel all patients on prevention and management of stroke.

Each year almost 800,000 Americans have strokes (cerebrovascular accident [CVA]), and more than 150,000 die from this cause. Stroke is now the fourth leading cause of death in the United States (1). Approximately 6.6 million Americans over the age of 20 years have had a stroke. It remains the leading cause of severe long-term disability. Ischemic stroke accounts for approximately 85% of all strokes. Of these, 60% are thrombotic in nature, whereas small vessel disease and large vessel atherosclerotic lesions account for 25% and 15%, respectively (2).

The American Heart Association/American Stroke Association provides evidence-based guidelines for prevention of the first stroke as well as recurrent strokes and emergency management for patients with ischemic strokes (2).

Many of the risk factors for stroke are identical to those of coronary heart disease (CHD). For this reason, the American Heart Association/American Stroke Association have joined forces to list a Presidential Advisory on Optimal Brain Health (3). This advisory focuses on issues of cognition and lowering the risk of dementia; however, prevention of stroke is an important component of optimizing brain health.

Since lifestyle medicine physicians will often be taking care of individuals with atherosclerotic disease, it is important to have an understanding of how lifestyle

DOI: 10.1201/b23245-19

medicine modalities can play an important role in the prevention and ultimately management of ischemic stroke.

17.2   BASIC MECHANISMS FOR BRAIN HEALTH

Optimal brain health and function are highly dependent on adequate delivery of oxygen and glucose. These, of course, are delivered through cerebral blood flow. For this reason, optimal brain function depends on both cardiovascular and cerebrovascular health (4–7). Autoregulation of the cerebral vasculature is essential to maintain cerebral blood flow and independently changes in arterial pressure. This allows the brain to be protected from damaging fluctuations in cerebral perfusion. Cerebral endothelial cells, much like endothelial cells in the coronary arteries, regulate microvascular flow by releasing vasoactive substances such as nitrate oxide, which is produced in the endothelial cells (5). The collective interaction between neurons and multiple other cells constitutes what has been called the neurovascular unit (NVU). The NVU creates the blood-brain barrier through an intricate system of transporters on the endothelial cell membrane (6). In addition, the NVU is responsible for disposing unwanted products of brain activity in metabolism such as β-amyloid and tau to prevent their accumulation in the brain tissue. NVU are also involved in immune surveillance and produce growth factors to support the survival of brain cells and blood cells.

There is emerging evidence that cumulative exposure to vascular risk factors throughout life affects the risk of common neurological diseases (7,8). Thus, there is a strong relationship between stroke and dementia. Cerebrovascular risk factors include similar ones as those found for CHD including hypertension, type 2 diabetes mellitus (T2DM) and dyslipidemia, all of which have a role in atherosclerosis and impaired cerebral blood flow, including endothelial dysfunction with an end result of suboptimal brain function (see Chapter 11 for more detail).

There are strong parallels between cardiovascular and cerebrovascular health and brain health. These involve inflammation, oxidated stress, and DNA damage that contribute to epigenetic changes and abnormal proteins not only in the heart but also the brain. Thus, brain dysfunction can be damaged by a host of vascular risk factors that are similar to those in the cardiovascular system. Thus, brain health is inextricably linked to cardiovascular and cerebrovascular health, and those interventions, aimed at promoting cardiovascular health, also promote brain health, and vice versa (see also Chapter 20).

All of these issues are central to the practice of lifestyle medicine, since the same techniques involved in lowering the risk of cardiovascular health will also improve brain health and decrease the likelihood of stroke, decreases in cognition and increased likelihood of dementia.

17.3   EPIDEMIOLOGY OF STROKE

Approximately 78% of strokes are first events; thus, primary prevention is of extreme importance (1). Approximately 18% of survivors of stroke will have a second stroke within 4 years. In addition, a transient ischemic attack (TIA) creates a risk of ischemic stroke of approximately 11% over 90 days (1). The highest risk is in the first week. It is important to make an accurate diagnosis of TIA since it is often misdiagnosed. TIA is defined as a transient episode of neurological dysfunction caused by focal brain, spinal cord or retinal ischemia without acute infarction. To reduce the risk of misdiagnosis of TIAs, the American Stroke Association has developed a mantra called "ABCD2 score" (9). This involves the following factors:

- Age >60 years old
- Blood pressure >140/90 mm Hg
- Clinical features including speech deficit and no unilateral weakness
- Diabetes and duration

TIA should thus be taken seriously since it indicates a high risk of subsequent stroke.

17.4   RISK FACTORS FOR CAROTID ATHEROSCLEROSIS

The most important risk factors for carotid atherosclerosis are smoking, age and hypertension. These, of course, are similar to those risk factors for coronary atherosclerosis. Other risk factors include diabetes, gender (men more than women if younger than 75 years; women more than men if older than 75 years), and hyperlipidemia. These, of course, are risk factors that are similar to those for coronary atherosclerosis (see Chapter 11). Approximately 30%–50% of patients with peripheral artery disease (see Chapter 14) also have carotid disease, and approximately 50%–60% of patients with carotid disease have significant CHD. Conversely, only 10% of patients with CHD have severe carotid disease (1).

17.5   PATHOPHYSIOLOGY

As in both CHD and carotid disease, atherosclerotic plaque tends to develop at branch points and bends. For example, a common location for atherosclerotic plaque in the carotid artery is at the bifurcation of the common carotid artery and the origin of the internal carotid artery.

It is not completely understood why carotid stenoses becomes symptomatic; however, there is a significant increased risk of stroke as stenosis increases to greater than 70%. This may be due to the fact that carotid plaque is highly vascularized, and rupture of this vasculature or rupture of the plaque can result in plaque hemorrhage or ulceration and thrombus formation. This can lead to either obstruction of the vessel or distal emboli. This mechanism appears to account for most of the cerebrovascular events caused by carotid disease. If a plaque is large, it can cause carotid stenosis or obstruction due to obstruction of cerebral blood flow, particularly if there is inadequate collateral circulation.

17.6   THE DIAGNOSIS OF CAROTID ARTERY DISEASE

An accurate history is vitally important to localize neurological symptoms. Symptoms such as unilateral weakness, numbness, difficulty with speech or visual field defects can occur if symptoms are localized in the cerebral cortex. Dizziness may include cerebellum disturbances that may result in ataxia or brainstem symptoms such as syncope, dysphagia, dysarthria or diplopia. These symptoms (such as in a TIA) may be transient and may result in vision loss on the same side as the carotid lesion.

On physical examination, the key finding is the presence of a carotid bruit. This should not be relied on as the only marker for the presence of carotid disease. In a large study from the North American Symptomatic Carotid Endarterectomy Trial (NASCET), presence of a cerebral bruit had approximately a 60% sensitivity and specificity for high-grade carotid stenosis (10).

In the Framingham study, the presence of carotid bruit doubled the risk of stroke. The presence of a bruit may be a marker for patients who are at risk not only for cerebrovascular events but also cardiovascular events. In addition to auscultation for carotid bruits, a focused neurological exam and fundoscopic exam should be undertaken.

Any individual who reports symptoms of a TIA should have a full evaluation of the carotid arteries. The risk of stroke depends on the degree of carotid stenosis. Individuals who have greater than 70% stenosis have an 80% risk of stroke within 30 days and a 13% annual incidence of stroke, whereas asymptomatic patients with 60% or more stenosis have a stroke risk of approximately 2% per year.

Duplex ultrasound is the most widely used method for detection and quantification of carotid disease. Its sensitivity and specificity are greater than 80% among patients with over 70% stenosis. For this reason, duplex ultrasound should be the first study performed to assess carotid disease. Other modalities may also be used, such as computed tomography angiography or magnetic resonance angiography, both of which show sensitivity of greater than 75%. However, disadvantages for these procedures involve increased cost and need for contrast injection.

17.7   MANAGEMENT OF CAROTID DISEASE

Management of carotid disease and reduction of risk of stroke hinge on risk factor reduction. This involves aggressive risk factor reduction. Lifestyle medicine will play a critically important role in this. The goal is to reduce the risk of stroke and prevent progression of existing disease. This involves smoking cessation and optimally controlling various cardiac comorbidities including hypertension, hyperlipidemia, and T2DM. Lifestyle modalities play a critically important role in all of these areas. In addition, weight loss if an individual is overweight or obese and increased physical activity are very important since both of these modalities can play an important role in controlling blood pressure as well as T2DM (2,3). Weight loss and regular physical activity lower inflammatory components that play a very important role in atherosclerosis. These modalities are discussed in detail in other chapters in this book.

In addition, platelet therapy is vitally important in anyone who has had a TIA, a significant stenosis of one of the carotid arteries or a previous stroke (11,12). Aspirin is the drug of choice in this area. Current guidelines recommend starting aspirin at 75 to 325 mg per day for all patients with extracranial carotid or cerebral atherosclerosis. This is a recommendation to reduce the risk of both myocardial infarction and stroke. In individuals who cannot tolerate aspirin, or there is a relative contraindication (such as higher risk or prior higher GI bleeding), Clopidogrel 75 mg is an acceptable alternative.

In addition to lifestyle strategies for lowering lipids, there is strong evidence that there are higher stroke rates in patients with high LDL and low HDL cholesterols. To reduce LDL cholesterol to less than 70 mg/dL, in most instances it will require either very aggressive lifestyle therapies and/or the inclusion of a statin medication.

National guidelines for primary prevention of stroke recommend that all high-risk patients (e.g., people with T2DM, peripheral vascular disease and coronary artery disease should be treated with statins) (13). Recommendations for secondary prevention in patients with a history of myocardial infarction, TIA, or stroke are for them to be started on statins. More details concerning these recommendations may be found in Chapters 12 and 13.

Control of blood pressure is an absolute priority for people who are at risk for stroke. Hypertension is the single most modifiable risk for prevention of stroke. Epidemiologic data indicate that approximately 60% of all strokes may be attributed to hypertension (14–17). Multiple different medications are available to help with lowering blood pressure. However, the lifestyle techniques such as regular physical activity and weight loss have both been shown to be highly efficacious for treatment of high blood pressure.

Finally, cigarette smoking represents a significant risk factor for stroke, and all patients who smoke cigarettes should be strongly encouraged to quit. Of course, cigarette smoking creates multiple medical problems (2,3). These are discussed in more detail in Chapter 7.

Surgical management with such procedures as carotid endarterectomy is beyond the scope of this chapter but may be found in any major cardiovascular textbook or in discussions with vascular surgeons.

17.8   SUMMARY/CONCLUSIONS

Stroke is highly prevalent in the United States with approximately 800,000 strokes annually in the United States and 15 million strokes worldwide. It is the third or fourth leading cause of death around the world and the leading cause of disability in the United States.

The risks of stroke emanate typically from atherosclerosis of the carotid arteries. The same risk factor reduction strategies that are appropriate for coronary heart disease are also appropriate for lowering the risk of stroke. For this reason, the American Heart Association and American Stroke Association have joined forces and agreed that the major lifestyle factors outlined in the American Heart Associations' "Life's Seven Simple" steps are also appropriate for lowering the risk of stroke.

It is important for all practitioners of lifestyle medicine to evaluate patients not only for risk of CHD but also risk for atherosclerosis of the carotid arteries in order to reduce the risk of stroke.

Clinical Applications

- The same recommendations for reducing the risk of CHD apply to lowering the risk of carotid atherosclerosis to lower the risk of stroke.
- Patients should be counseled to employ the AHA "Life's Essential 8" steps program to lower the risk of atherosclerosis.
- Physical examination in patients with atherosclerotic heart disease should also involve careful examination of the carotid arteries.
- Individuals who have had a prior stroke or TIA are at high risk for a subsequent stroke and should be aggressively treated with aspirin or alternative platelet inhibitor, significant medication and lifestyle modifications to control lipids, and also lifestyle modification and, if appropriate, pharmacologic therapy to lower blood pressure.

REFERENCES

1. Virani SS, Alonso A, Aparicio HJ, et al. Heart disease and stroke statistics—2021 update: A report from the American Heart Association. Circulation. 2021;143(8):e254–743. Epub 2021/01/28.
2. Meschia JF, Bushnell C, Boden-Albala B, et al. Guidelines for the primary prevention of stroke: A statement for healthcare professionals from the American Heart Association/American Stroke Association. Stroke. 2014;45(12):3754–832. Epub 2014/10/31.
3. Gorelick PB, Furie KL, Iadecola C, et al. Defining optimal brain health in adults: A presidential advisory from the American Heart Association/American Stroke Association. Stroke. 2017;48(10):e284–303. Epub 2017/09/09.
4. Attwell D, Laughlin SB. An energy budget for signaling in the grey matter of the brain. J Cereb Blood Flow Metab. 2001;21(10):1133–45. Epub 2001/10/13.
5. Andresen J, Shafi NI, Bryan RM, Jr. Endothelial influences on cerebrovascular tone. J Appl Physiol. 2006;100(1):318–27. Epub 2005/12/17.
6. Zhao Z, Nelson AR, Betsholtz C, et al. Establishment and dysfunction of the blood-brain barrier. Cell. 2015;163(5):1064–78. Epub 2015/11/23.
7. Faraco G, Iadecola C. Hypertension: A harbinger of stroke and dementia. Hypertension. 2013;62(5):810–17. Epub 2013/08/28.
8. Faraci FM. Protecting against vascular disease in brain. Am J Physiol Heart Circ Physiol. 2011;300(5):H1566–82. Epub 2011/02/22.
9. Amarenco P, Lavallee PC, Labreuche J, et al. One-year risk of stroke after transient ischemic attack or minor stroke. N Engl J Med. 2016;374(16):1533–42. Epub 2016/04/21.
10. Ferguson GG, Eliasziw M, Barr HW, et al. The North American symptomatic carotid endarterectomy trial: Surgical results in 1415 patients. Stroke. 1999;30(9):1751–8. Epub 1999/09/02.
11. Kernan WN, Ovbiagele B, Black HR, et al. Guidelines for the prevention of stroke in patients with stroke and transient ischemic attack: A guideline for healthcare professionals from the American Heart Association/American Stroke Association. Stroke. 2014;45(7):2160–236. Epub 2014/05/03.
12. Johnson ES, Lanes SF, Wentworth CE, 3rd, et al. A meta-regression analysis of the dose-response effect of aspirin on stroke. Arch Intern Med. 1999;159(11):1248–53. Epub 1999/06/17.

13. Amarenco P, Labreuche J. Lipid management in the prevention of stroke: Review and updated meta-analysis of statins for stroke prevention. Lancet Neurol. 2009;8(5):453–63. Epub 2009/04/21.

14. Kivipelto M, Helkala EL, Hanninen T, et al. Midlife vascular risk factors and late-life mild cognitive impairment: A population-based study. Neurology. 2001;56(12):1683–9. Epub 2001/06/27.

15. Reitz C, Tang MX, Manly J, et al. Hypertension and the risk of mild cognitive impairment. Arch Neurol. 2007;64(12):1734–40. Epub 2007/12/12.

16. Gottesman RF, Schneider AL, Albert M, et al. Midlife hypertension and 20-year cognitive change: The atherosclerosis risk in communities neurocognitive study. JAMA Neurol. 2014;71(10):1218–27. Epub 2014/08/05.

17. Knopman D, Boland LL, Mosley T, et al. Cardiovascular risk factors and cognitive decline in middle-aged adults. Neurology. 2001;56(1):42–8. Epub 2001/01/10.

18 Diabetes, Prediabetes, Metabolic Syndrome and Cardiovascular Disease

KEY POINTS

- Type 2 diabetes mellitus (T2DM) is a significant risk factor for cardiovascular disease (CVD), in general, and coronary heart disease, in particular.
- Control of lipids and blood pressure are critically important in patients with T2DM.
- Lifestyle measures such as regular physical activity, weight loss (if necessary), healthy nutrition (increased fruits and vegetables), lower sodium and calorie control can all play important roles in managing T2DM and lowering the risk of CVD.

18.1 INTRODUCTION

Diabetes mellitus (T2DM) is an increasingly common condition in the United States and throughout the world and a significant risk factor for cardiovascular disease (CVD) (1).

Diabetes has grown rapidly worldwide in the past 30 years; consequently, death rates from CVD attributable to diabetes have increased throughout the world. According to the Global Burden of Disease Study in 2019, an estimated 346 million people worldwide have diabetes (2). The International Diabetes Foundation (IDF) definition, which added several parameters to the definition of diabetes including oral glucose tolerance and hemoglobin A_{1C} tests found that there were 356 million people with diabetes in 2011. Unfortunately, around the world, 50% of these cases were undiagnosed.

By 2030, the number of people with diabetes is expected to increase to 522 million. This rise is estimated to occur at 2.7% annually, which is faster than the total world adult population growth for a year. Over 30 million people in the United States, or approximately 10% of the population, have diabetes (3). Unfortunately, one in four people with diabetes do not know they have it. Over three-quarters of the people with diabetes ultimately die of CVD. Thus, the linkage between diabetes and CVD is quite strong, and lowering the risk of diabetes (T2DM) is a central strategy for lowering the risk of CVD, in general, and in people at risk for diabetes, in particular (4,5).

Fortunately, we have a number of powerful tools at our disposal to lower the risk of diabetes and to assist in its treatment. Most of these tools involve changes in lifestyle such as proper nutrition (in diabetes this is called "medical nutrition therapy"), weight loss (particularly for people who are obese), increased physical activity and smoking cessation. The Nurses' Health Study, which has followed over 100,000 female nurses for over 20 years, has shown that individuals who follow a cluster of lifestyle factors including regular physical activity (30 minutes of moderate physical activity per day), proper nutrition (more fruits and vegetables and whole grains), do not smoke cigarettes and maintain a healthy body weight (between 18.5 and 25 kg/m^2) can lower their risk of heart disease by 80% and diabetes by over 90% (6).

Prediabetes is diagnosed with a fasting blood sugar between 100 and 125 mg/dL and is even much more prevalent. It is estimated that over 30% of the population in the United States falls into this category.

Metabolic syndrome (MetS), which is a cluster of risk factors often found in individuals who have diabetes or prediabetes, is even more prevalent with recent estimates of 36%–38% of the adult population in the United States having MetS (7). The National Cholesterol Education Program ATP III (8) and IV (NCEP) (9) recommends that people who have MetS be treated as though they already have CVD.

For all of these reasons, it is incumbent on the medical community to utilize lifestyle measures both to reduce the risk of T2DM and assist in its treatment.

18.2   THE RELATIONSHIP BETWEEN DIABETES AND CARDIOVASCULAR DISEASE

Diabetes is associated with multiple aspects of CVD. For example, individuals with T2DM have a two- to fourfold increased risk of mortality from coronary heart disease (CHD) compared to those without T2DM (10). Diabetes is also associated with an increased risk of myocardial infarction (MI) and multiple other aspects of the acute coronary syndrome (ACS) events.

Diabetes also increases the risk of other manifestations of atherosclerotic vascular disease (ASCVD), including stroke, cerebrovascular disease and peripheral arterial disease. In addition to these aspects of ASCVD, diabetes is associated with a two- to fivefold increase in heart failure (HF). HF is a key driver of CVD morbidity and mortality (11). Finally, diabetes increases the risk of atrial fibrillation (AF). Diabetes increases the risk of both AF and stroke rate by 2%–5% per year (12). For this reason, AHA guidelines recommend anticoagulation for all patients with diabetes who have a history of AF due to the increased stroke risk in the setting of T2DM.

18.3   PATHOPHYSIOLOGIC LINKS BETWEEN CORONARY HEART DISEASE AND DIABETES

Various risk factors for CHD including hypertension, dyslipidemia and adiposity tend to be present and cluster in patients with diabetes. In addition, there are mechanisms inherent to T2DM that increase the risk of ASCVD. Included in this are hyperglycemia and insulin resistance. However, the underlying pathophysiology of this is not completely understood. Hyperglycemia may be associated with endothelial basal dysfunction as well as increased systemic inflammation (13). Multiple underlying factors such as hypertension and abnormal nitric oxide biology may contribute to endothelial dysfunction. Abnormalities in the coagulation and fibrinolytic pathways and platelet biology contribute to further thrombotic conditions, whereas increased systemic inflammation and oxidative stress may further promote CVD.

18.4   THE ROLE OF LIFESTYLE MANAGEMENT IN PREVENTION OF CORONARY HEART DISEASE AND ITS COMPLICATIONS IN DIABETES

Lifestyle interventions are the cornerstone for prevention of ASCVD complications associated with diabetes (14,15). Virtually every organization that issues guidelines for the treatment of diabetes emphasizes the importance of lifestyle interventions including 30 minutes or more of daily moderate-intensity physical activity, weight control, healthy diet and smoking cessation (14,15). In addition, pharmaceutical strategies are often used to lower CVD risk including careful management of blood pressure, treatment to lower LDL cholesterol and potential of daily aspirin. The following modalities, all of which include components of lifestyle medicine, are key components of lowering the risk of CVD associated with diabetes:

- *Therapeutic lifestyle counseling*—Therapeutic lifestyle counseling (TLC) interventions including recommendation for regular physical activity, nutritional counseling for weight management, healthy food choices and counseling for smoking cessation form the cornerstone of both primary and secondary prevention of cardiovascular disease. (See Chapters 4 and 11 for general recommendations for lipid management and increased physical activity.)
- *Lipids*—Lipids should be routinely and regularly measured in all adults with T2DM. Primary pharmacologic treatment for dyslipidemia is statin therapy (16). The goal of statin therapy is to maintain LDLC levels less than 70 mg/dL. There are currently no medical therapies recommended to target treatment of low levels of high-density cholesterol (HDLC) or high levels of triglycerides. However, lifestyle therapies for these factors are available and discussed in separate chapters in this book.
- *Blood pressure*—Maintaining a healthy blood pressure is particularly important for individuals with T2DM (17). Blood pressure should be measured in every clinical visit in individuals with T2DM. Patients with T2DM should be treated with a blood pressure target of no higher than 140/85 mm Hg and optimally a target below 130/80 mm Hg, if possible (18). Lifestyle interventions, including weight management, dietary sodium restriction and physical activity, play critical roles in the management of hypertension. (See also Chapter 13.) Primary pharmacologic therapy for people with T2DM is angiotensin-converting enzyme (ACE) inhibitors. Individuals who have symptoms such as cough, rash or angioedema alternatively can be treated with angiotensin-receptive blockers (ARBs).
- *Physical activity*—The American Heart Association (AHA) Clinical Practice Guidelines (19) and the Physical Activity Guidelines for Americans 2018 (PAGA 2018) (20) both recommend at least 150 minutes of

moderate-intensity aerobic physical activity, 75 minutes of vigorous aerobic activity per week. If weight loss is a concern, a larger amount of exercise (7 hours of moderate-intensity physical activity per week) may be appropriate.

- *Tobacco*—Individuals with T2DM should refrain from tobacco use or be advised to quit.
- *Antiplatelet agents*—Both the American Diabetes Association (ADA) and the AHA recommend aspirin therapy (75–162 mg/day) for primary prevention in patients with diabetes who are at increased risk of CVD (estimated 10-year risk greater than 10%) (15,17). This would include most individuals over the age of 50 years who have additional risk factors for CVD such as hypertension, smoking or dyslipidemia. Individuals with aspirin allergy should be treated with other antiplatelet agents.
- *Glycemic control*—The Hb_{A1C} goal for most patients with T2DM is less than 7% in the absence of CVD, although the AHA recognizes that higher targets such as 8% may be appropriate for individuals at moderate or severe risk of CVD (21).

18.5 PHARMACOTHERAPY IN PATENTS WITH DIABETES TO REDUCE THE RISK OF CVD

Beyond lifestyle, pharmacologic therapies can effectively reduce CVD risk in diabetes. In the area of lipid management, statins remain the mainstay and drug of choice. Other medicines may also be applied in certain situations, and they include Ezetimibe, PCSK9 inhibitors, fibric acid derivatives (fibrates) and omega-3 fatty acids. A complete description of the pharmacologic therapy of lipids in individuals with T2DM is beyond the scope of this chapter and is found in multiple internal medicine and endocrinology textbooks.

With regard to hypertension management, ACE inhibitors and angiotensin II receptor blockers are the cornerstones of therapy for hypertension (18). Other potential pharmacologic agents include calcium channel blockers, thiazide diuretics and, in certain instances, beta blockers, although this latter category has fallen somewhat out of favor. Again, detailed descriptions of various classes of pharmacologic agents for the treatment of high blood pressure in people with T2DM are beyond the scope of this chapter and are found in multiple internal medicine textbooks.

18.6 LIFESTYLE MEDICINE AND MANAGEMENT OF PREDIABETES

Prediabetes is diagnosed by a fasting blood glucose of 100–125 mg/dL, a 2-hour post challenge plasma glucose of 140–199 mg/dL and a hemoglobin A_{1C} of 5.7%–6.4%. Various major research trials including the Diabetes Prevention Program (22) and the Diabetes Research Trial have shown that individuals who engage in various lifestyle measures such as regular physical activity and weight loss (if necessary) on the order of 5–7 pounds may reduce their risk of prediabetes developing into diabetes by over 58%. Lifestyle interventions include healthy eating patterns, achieving and maintaining healthy weight and body composition, and regular and sufficient physical activity.

It should be noted that there is a significant overlap between prediabetes, diabetes and metabolic syndrome (MetS). Metabolic syndrome is typically diagnosed using criteria from the National Cholesterol Education Program III (NCEP III) (8). These criteria include the following:

- Blood pressure greater than 140/85 mm Hg;
- Fasting glucose greater than 100 mg/dL;
- Triglycerides greater than 150 mg/dL;
- Waist circumference in men greater than 40 inches, women greater than 35 inches; and
- HDL less than 40 mg/dL.

By these criteria, between 36% and 38% of individuals in the United States have metabolic syndrome (8). There is a strong overlap between metabolic syndrome, diabetes and prediabetes. The AHA recommends that individuals with MetS be treated with lifestyle measures that are similar to those for reducing the risk of CVD. Namely, regular physical activity, weight loss (if necessary), control of lipids and high blood pressure.

18.7   HEART FAILURE IN PATIENTS WITH DIABETES

Diabetes independently predicts heart failure risk and is associated with a two- to fivefold increase in individuals with heart failure (11). Both myocardial infarction and hypertension are also common risk factors associated with heart failure. Pharmacologic treatment of heart failure focuses largely on ACE inhibitors. Blood pressure control is particularly important in individuals with heart failure who have diabetes. Blood glucose control is also an important component of treatment of heart failure in individuals with diabetes. Lifestyle measures including weight loss (if necessary), decreased sodium in the diet and regular physical activity, as tolerated, also play important roles in the treatment of heart failure.

18.8   SECONDARY PREVENTION

Guidelines for the management of secondary CVD prevention are similar for patients with and without T2DM. In general, management of patients with diabetes and coronary syndrome is not different from those in patients without T2DM. There is ongoing debate about whether or not patients who require coronary revascularization do better with percutaneous angioplasty or coronary artery bypass grafting.

18.9   ATRIAL FIBRILLATION

T2DM is associated with an increased risk of AF, which also increases the risk of both stroke and systemic thromboembolism (12). These factors underscore the recommendation for systemic anticoagulation for patients with T2DM who also have AF. Both warfarin and direct oral anticoagulants have relatively similar benefits as anticoagulant strategies for patients with T2DM and AF.

18.10 SUMMARY/CONCLUSIONS

T2DM is a significant risk factor for CVD. In fact, over 75% of individuals with T2DM ultimately die of CVD. The large percentage of those die with CHD. Because of the significant relationship between T2DM and CVD, it is essential to aggressively utilize lifestyle and, if necessary, pharmacologic measures to treat T2DM. The cornerstone of therapy for T2DM relates to multiple lifestyle measures including increased physical activity, weight loss (if necessary), medical nutrition therapy (including more fruits and vegetables, lower sodium and whole grains), and cessation of tobacco products.

Individuals with T2DM will benefit from aggressive lipid management and control of blood pressure. As indicated in this chapter, in many instances lifestyle measures will suffice, although in some instances pharmacologic therapy, in addition to lifestyle measures, will be appropriate. Individuals with prediabetes and MetS are also at increased risk for ultimately developing CVD. Lifestyle measures for both of these entities can significantly reduce the likelihood of progression to T2DM.

Clinical Applications

- Diabetes is a significant risk factor for CVD, in general, and CHD, in particular.
- Individuals with T2DM should be carefully monitored and treated for elevated lipids and high blood pressure.
- Lifestyle measures represent the cornerstone of therapies for individuals with T2DM to help control the T2DM itself and lower the risk of CVD.
- Every clinical encounter with patients with T2DM should include discussion of the multiple lifestyle measures that are effective both for the treatment of T2DM and for lowering the risk of CVD.

REFERENCES

1. Shaw JE, Sicree RA, Zimmet PZ. Global estimates of the prevalence of diabetes for 2010 and 2030. Diabetes Res Clin Pract. 2010;87(1):4–14. Epub 2009/11/10.
2. Global Burden of Disease Collaborative Network. Global Burden of Disease Study 2019 (GBD 2019) Dietary Risk Exposure Estimates 1990–2019. Seattle, WA: Institute for Health Metrics and Evaluation (IHME); 2021.
3. N. C. D. Risk Factor Collaboration. Worldwide trends in diabetes since 1980: A pooled analysis of 751 population-based studies with 4.4 million participants. Lancet. 2016;387(10027):1513–30. Epub 2016/04/12.
4. Gregg EW, Li Y, Wang J, et al. Changes in diabetes-related complications in the United States, 1990–2010. N Engl J Med. 2014;370(16):1514–23. Epub 2014/04/18.
5. Emerging Risk Factors Collaboration, Di Angelantonio E, Kaptoge S, et al. Association of cardiometabolic multimorbidity with mortality. JAMA. 2015;314(1):52–60. Epub 2015/07/08.
6. Liu S, Stampfer MJ, Hu FB, et al. Whole-grain consumption and risk of coronary heart disease: Results from the Nurses' Health Study. Am J Clin Nutr. 1999;70:412–19.
7. Ford ES, Giles WH, Dietz WH. Prevalence of the metabolic syndrome among U.S. adults: Findings from the third National Health and Nutrition Examination Survey. JAMA. 2002;287(3):356–9. Epub 2002/01/16.

8. National Cholesterol Education Program Expert Panel on Detection Evaluation, Treatment of High Blood Cholesterol in Adults. Third report of the National Cholesterol Education Program (NCEP) expert panel on detection, evaluation, and treatment of high blood cholesterol in adults (adult treatment panel III) final report. Circulation. 2002;106(25):3143–421. Epub 2002/12/18.

9. Grundy SM, Stone NJ, Bailey AL, et al. 2018 AHA/ACC/AACVPR/AAPA/ABC/ACPM/ ADA/AGS/APhA/ASPC/NLA/PCNA Guideline on the management of blood cholesterol: A report of the American College of Cardiology/American Heart Association Task Force on Clinical Practice Guidelines. Circulation. 2019;139(25):e1082–143. Epub 2018/12/28.

10. Gore MO, Patel MJ, Kosiborod M, et al. Diabetes mellitus and trends in hospital survival after myocardial infarction, 1994 to 2006: Data from the national registry of myocardial infarction. Circ Cardiovasc Qual Outcomes. 2012;5(6):791–7. Epub 2012/11/08.

11. Standl E, Schnell O, McGuire DK. Heart failure considerations of antihyperglycemic medications for type 2 diabetes. Circ Res. 2016;118(11):1830–43. Epub 2016/05/28.

12. Lip GY, Nieuwlaat R, Pisters R, et al. Refining clinical risk stratification for predicting stroke and thromboembolism in atrial fibrillation using a novel risk factor-based approach: The Euro Heart Survey on Atrial Fibrillation. Chest. 2010;137(2):263–72. Epub 2009/09/19.

13. Hess K, Grant PJ. Inflammation and thrombosis in diabetes. Thromb Haemost. 2011;105(Suppl 1):S43–54. Epub 2011/04/12.

14. Standards of medical care in diabetes—2016: Summary of revisions. Diabetes Care. 2016;39 Suppl 1(Suppl_1):S4–5. Epub 2015/12/24.

15. Fox CS, Golden SH, Anderson C, et al. Update on prevention of cardiovascular disease in adults with type 2 diabetes mellitus in light of recent evidence: A scientific statement from the American Heart Association and the American Diabetes Association. Circulation. 2015;132(8):691–718. Epub 2015/08/08.

16. Stone NJ, Robinson JG, Lichtenstein AH, et al. 2013 ACC/AHA guideline on the treatment of blood cholesterol to reduce atherosclerotic cardiovascular risk in adults: A report of the American College of Cardiology/American Heart Association Task Force on Practice Guidelines. Circulation. 2014;129(25 Suppl 2):S1–45. Epub 2013/11/14.

17. Standards of medical care in diabetes-2016: Summary of revisions. Diabetes Care. 2015;38 Suppl 1(Supplement_1):S1–2.

18. Emdin CA, Rahimi K, Neal B, et al. Blood pressure lowering in type 2 diabetes: A systematic review and meta-analysis. JAMA. 2015;313(6):603–15. Epub 2015/02/11.

19. Eckel RH, Jakicic JM, Ard JD, et al. 2013 AHA/ACC guideline on lifestyle management to reduce cardiovascular risk: A report of the American College of Cardiology/American Heart Association Task Force on Practice Guidelines. Circulation. 2014;129(25 Suppl 2):S76–99. Epub 2013/11/14.

20. 2018 Physical Activity Guidelines Advisory Committee. 2018 Physical Activity Guidelines Advisory Committee Scientific Report. Washington, DC: U.S. Department of Health and Human Services; 2018. https://health.gov/sites/default/files/2019-09/ PAG_Advisory_Committee_Report.pdf. Accessed March 17, 2022.

21. Galaviz KI, Staimez L, Phillips LS, et al. Lifestyle medicine and the management of prediabetes. In James Rippe MD, ed. Lifestyle Medicine. 3rd ed. Boca Raton, FL: CRC Press; 2019, pp. 367–82.

22. Knowler WC, Barrett-Connor E, Fowler SE, et al. Reduction in the incidence of type 2 diabetes with lifestyle intervention or metformin. N Engl J Med. 2002;346(6):393–403. Epub 2002/02/08.

19 Sedentary Behavior and Cardiovascular Disease

KEY POINTS

- In the United States, sedentary behavior is very common and is a significant risk factor for cardiovascular disease (CVD).
- Both children and adults average greater than 7 hours sedentary behavior on a daily basis.
- Moderate or vigorous physical activity at levels recommended by the PAGA 2018 can largely ameliorate the increased risk of sedentary behavior and CVD.

19.1 INTRODUCTION

The United States has become an increasingly sedentary country. Data from the U.S. National Health and Nutrition Examination Survey (NHANES) indicate that children and adults in the United States average approximately 7.7 hours per day (55%) of monitored time being sedentary (1).

In the past decade, sedentary behavior has been clearly linked to an increased risk of cardiovascular disease (CVD) (2). In addition, sedentary behavior is linked to a variety of other adverse health consequences including multiple risk factors for CVD. Reversing the sedentary behavior trend in the United States would generate significant health improvements in multiple areas, especially in the area of reducing the risk of CVD.

While there are linkages between inactivity and sedentary behavior, the latter is significantly and independently related to increased risk of CVD. The good news is that one of the key components of lifestyle medicine, namely increased physical activity, can make a significant difference in lowering the risk of CVD, even in individuals who are otherwise sedentary (3).

19.2 SEDENTARY BEHAVIOR AND RISK OF CARDIOVASCULAR DISEASE

The risk of mortality from CVD and its relationship to sedentary behavior is documented in the Physical Activity Guidelines for Americans 2018 Scientific Report (PAGA 2018). The risk of sedentary behavior and CVD is similar to the risk of sedentary behavior and all-cause mortality. (See subsequent section in this chapter.) In addition to sedentary behavior, some studies have shown that TV viewing or screentime is also related to increased risk of CVD (4,5). The PAGA 2018

DOI: 10.1201/b23245-21

Scientific Report documented that increased physical activity can ameliorate most of the increases in sedentary behavior. (More on this in a subsequent section.) Sedentary behavior of greater than 5 hours per day significantly increases the risk of CVD, and this is further increased if sedentary behavior is greater than 7 hours per day.

19.3   SEDENTARY BEHAVIOR AND ALL-CAUSE MORTALITY

The relationship between sedentary behavior and all-cause mortality is also very strong. There appears to be a dose-response relationship between sedentary behavior and all-cause mortality. Specifically, a number of studies have shown that for every 1 hour increase in sitting time or for more than 7 hours a day sitting, there is a dose-related response to sedentary behavior and all-cause mortality (6,7). Similar relationships exist between TV viewing and all-cause mortality, where once again a dose-response relationship has been demonstrated.

> *Definition of sedentary behavior*: According to multiple research trials and the PAGA 2018, sedentary behavior has been defined as "any behavior which is characterized by an energy expenditure of 1.5 METS or less, while in a sitting, reclining or lying posture. (2,8)

Using these criteria, sedentary behavior increases the risk of coronary heart disease (CHD), type 2 diabetes mellitus (T2DM), and a variety of other adverse conditions including increased risk of cancer and weight gain (9,10).

19.4   SEDENTARY BEHAVIOR AND TYPE 2 DIABETES MELLITUS

T2DM is a significant risk factor for CVD. There is strong evidence that a significant relationship exists between the amount of sedentary behavior and risk of T2DM (11,12). Once again, similar data exist for TV viewing. However, much of the increased risk of sedentary behavior is ameliorated by physical activity. (See subsequent section.)

19.5   SEDENTARY BEHAVIOR AND CANCER MORTALITY

There are some data that suggest that there is a relationship between time spent in sedentary behavior and high mortality rates from cancer (13). Once again, moderate physical activity has been demonstrated to decrease the increased risk from sedentary behavior in breast cancer, ovarian cancer, prostate cancer and lung cancer.

19.6   SEDENTARY BEHAVIOR AND WEIGHT STATUS

Some evidence suggests that there is a relationship between sedentary behavior and weight status. However, studies in this area show considerable variabilities of the results. As already noted in multiple chapters, adult weight gain and obesity are both related to increased risks in CVD.

19.7   SEDENTARY BEHAVIOR AND MODERATE TO VIGOROUS PHYSICAL ACTIVITY

There is accumulating evidence that moderate or vigorous physical activity lowers the risk of sedentary behavior (14). Significantly, the relative reductions in risk of sedentary behavior are most prominent in those who are the most sedentary. Similar data exist related to TV viewing and risk of CVD.

An inverse relationship exists between the amount of moderate or vigorous physical activity in sedentary behavior both with respect to CVD and all-cause mortality. As demonstrated in Figure 19.1, all-cause mortality and CVD mortality from sedentary behavior are strongest for people who have low amounts of physical activity (2).

In other words, individuals who have greater than 7 hours of sedentary behavior and also low levels of moderate or vigorous physical activity substantially increase their risk of all-cause mortality. Conversely, individuals who otherwise are sedentary but accumulate between 16 and 30 MET-hours per week of moderate-intensity physical activity (the equivalent of 300 to 600 minutes of moderate physical activity per week) substantially lower their risk of CVD and all-cause mortality (2). To put this in perspective, as shown in Figure 19.1, even greater than or equal to 16 MET-hours per week substantially lowered the risk of CVD for individuals sitting even more than 7 hours a week. The PAGA 2018 recommends between 10 and 15 MET-hours per week of physical activity.

Individuals who have sedentary occupations (such as office work) will, thus, particularly benefit from following the guidelines for moderate to vigorous physical activity on a weekly basis.

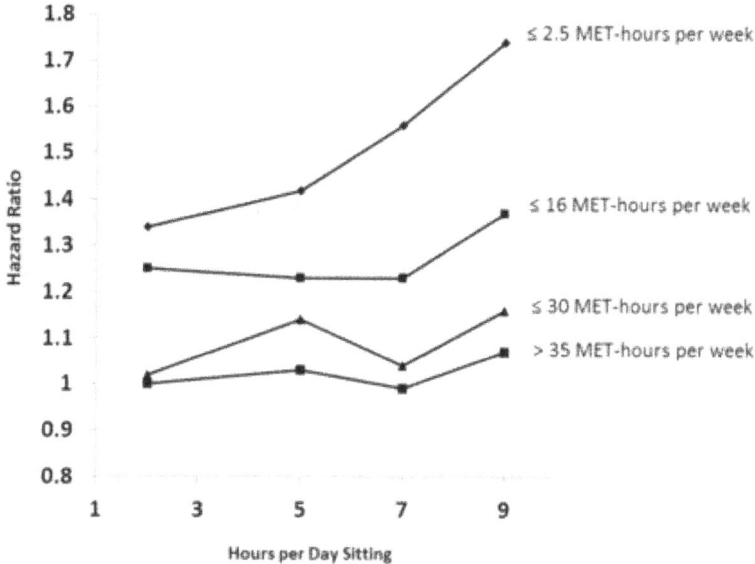

FIGURE 19.1   Relationship between sedentary behavior and periods of regular physical activity.

It has also been suggested that taking breaks from sedentary behavior may reduce adverse health effects related to both CVD and all-cause mortality. More research is needed to confirm this potential strategy.

19.8   HEALTH IMPACTS

High levels of sedentary behavior increase the risk of CVD, T2DM and all-cause mortality. The good news is that participating at recommended levels of moderate to vigorous physical activity on a weekly basis can largely ameliorate the increased risk for sedentary behavior and CVD.

19.9   SUMMARY/CONCLUSIONS

The United States has increasingly become a sedentary society. The average child or adult spends over 7 hours a day in sedentary activities. These include screen time, time watching TV, and other tasks, while sitting or lying down. These levels of sedentary behavior have clearly been demonstrated to increase morbidity and mortality from CVD and other chronic conditions.

The good news is that levels of moderate or vigorous physical activity recommended by the PAGA 2018 can largely ameliorate these increased risks. For all of these reasons, physicians should inquire of their patients the level of sedentary behavior and, if needed, emphasize the powerful role that moderate or vigorous physical activity can play in lowering the risk of CVD.

Clinical Applications

- Sedentary behavior of higher than 7 hours a day is associated with increased risk of CVD.
- Sedentary behavior is also associated with increased risk of T2DM and some cancers.
- Moderate to vigorous physical activity at levels recommended by the PAGA 2018 can largely ameliorate the adverse risks of sedentary behavior.
- Individuals who have had both sedentary behavior and are inactive significantly increase their risk of CVD.
- Physicians should assess the level of sedentary behavior and recommend increased levels of moderate or vigorous physical activity in those who are particularly sedentary.

REFERENCES

1. Matthews CE, Chen KY, Freedson PS, et al. Amount of time spent in sedentary behaviors in the United States, 2003–2004. Am J Epidemiol. 2008;167(7):875–81. Epub 2008/02/28.
2. 2018 Physical Activity Guidelines Advisory Committee. 2018 Physical Activity Guidelines Advisory Committee Scientific Report. Washington, DC: U.S. Department of Health and Human Services; 2018. Part F. Chapter 2. Sedentary Behavior.

3. Rippe JM. Lifestyle Medicine: Increasing Physical Activity: A Practical Guide. Boca Raton, FL: CRC Press; 2020.

4. George SM, Smith AW, Alfano CM, et al. The association between television watching time and all-cause mortality after breast cancer. J Cancer Surviv. 2013;7(2):247–52. Epub 2013/02/05.

5. Grontved A, Hu FB. Television viewing and risk of type 2 diabetes, cardiovascular disease, and all-cause mortality: A meta-analysis. JAMA. 2011;305(23):2448–55. Epub 2011/06/16.

6. Chau JY, Grunseit AC, Chey T, et al. Daily sitting time and all-cause mortality: A meta-analysis. PLoS One. 2013;8(11):e80000. Epub 2013/11/16.

7. Sun JW, Zhao LG, Yang Y, et al. Association between television viewing time and all-cause mortality: A meta-analysis of cohort studies. Am J Epidemiol. 2015;182(11):908–16. Epub 2015/11/17.

8. Tremblay MS, Aubert S, Barnes JD, et al. Sedentary behavior research network (SBRN): Terminology Consensus Project process and outcome. Int J Behav Nutr Phys Act. 2017;14(1):75. Epub 2017/06/11.

9. Wilmot EG, Edwardson CL, Achana FA, et al. Sedentary time in adults and the association with diabetes, cardiovascular disease and death: Systematic review and meta-analysis. Diabetologia. 2012;55(11):2895–905. Epub 2012/08/15.

10. Biswas A, Oh PI, Faulkner GE, et al. Sedentary time and its association with risk for disease incidence, mortality, and hospitalization in adults: A systematic review and meta-analysis. Ann Intern Med. 2015;162(2):123–32. Epub 2015/01/20.

11. Proper KI, Singh AS, van Mechelen W, et al. Sedentary behaviors and health outcomes among adults: A systematic review of prospective studies. Am J Prev Med. 2011;40(2):174–82. Epub 2011/01/18.

12. Thorp AA, Owen N, Neuhaus M, et al. Sedentary behaviors and subsequent health outcomes in adults a systematic review of longitudinal studies, 1996–2011. Am J Prev Med. 2011;41(2):207–15. Epub 2011/07/20.

13. Seguin R, Buchner DM, Liu J, et al. Sedentary behavior and mortality in older women: The women's health initiative. Am J Prev Med. 2014;46(2):122–35. Epub 2014/01/21.

14. Ekelund U, Steene-Johannessen J, et al. Does physical activity attenuate, or even eliminate, the detrimental association of sitting time with mortality? A harmonised meta-analysis of data from more than 1 million men and women. Lancet. 2016;388(10051):1302–10.

20 Cardiovascular Disease and Optimal Brain Health

KEY POINTS

- There are strong linkages between cardiovascular health and brain health.
- Risk factors for cardiovascular disease (CVD) and brain disorders, including dementia, are similar.
- Lifestyle measures that will lower the risk of CVD are also extremely valuable for helping to maintain brain health.
- A healthy brain is essential for a meaningful and fulfilling life.

20.1   INTRODUCTION

There is a particularly strong link between brain health and cardiovascular health (1). A healthy brain is essential for a fulfilling life. Many lifestyle measures play particularly important roles in maintaining brain health. Poor lifestyle factors may compromise brain health and are associated also with poor cardiovascular health. These include uncontrolled hypertension, type 2 diabetes mellitus (T2DM), obesity, physical inactivity, smoking and depression. The good news is that all of these conditions are potentially ameliorated to some degree by positive lifestyle measures. The linkages between heart health and brain health have been underscored by the recent release of the Presidential Advisory from the American Heart Association (AHA) and the American Stroke Association (ASA) entitled "Optimal Brain Health."

Optimal brain health is essential for maintaining quality of life and functional independence. Cognitive function, in particular, is an important component of the aging process. This has become increasingly important as life expectancy continues to increase in developed countries. The numbers of individuals over the age of 65 years have increased dramatically over the past two decades and are likely to continue to increase over the next 15–20 years. It has been estimated that there are 47 million people with dementia worldwide, and this is projected to increase to 75 million individuals by 2030 and 131 million individuals by 2050 (2).

The interaction between brain health and cardiovascular health or cardiovascular disease (CVD) has often been underestimated. This is an area where the linkages are so strong that it is imperative for clinicians to understand and counsel patients about how they can preserve brain health and cognitive function throughout life.

20.2   THE ROLE OF LIFESTYLE MEDICINE IN BRAIN HEALTH

As we emphasize in multiple chapters throughout this book, various lifestyle measures are important to lower the risk of CVD. These same measures may play

DOI: 10.1201/b23245-22

critical roles in maintaining brain health. For example, a large literature supports the positive role of regular physical activity in maintaining brain health (3–17). In addition, nutritional factors such as lowering cholesterol play an important role in both lowering the risk of CVD and in maintaining brain health. As emphasized in Chapters 4 and 5, both regular physical activity and proper nutrition play important roles in helping to control blood pressure, which is a critical component of both lowering CVD risk and maintaining brain health. In some instances, such as the area of sleep, there is a bidirectional relationship, since a healthy brain is important to maintaining healthy sleep habits, and healthy sleep habits are important components of brain health.

20.3 PARALLELS BETWEEN CARDIOVASCULAR AND CEREBROVASCULAR HEALTH AND BRAIN HEALTH

There are multiple parallels between health of the cardiovascular system and the cerebrovascular system. In particular, aging has common underlying mechanisms that include oxidative stress, DNA damage and other epigenetic changes that impact on multiple organ systems (1). In particular, aging profoundly effects the structure and function of the cerebrovascular system, which may impact vascular risk factors that can compromise brain health. Conversely, brain dysfunction and damage including vascular risk factors and aging may contribute to deleterious effects on the cardiovascular system by neurohumoral mechanisms that control heart rate, the heart blood vessels and metabolism, which may result in hypertension and other aspects of cardiovascular damage. Thus, the health of the brain is linked in significant ways to both cardiovascular and cerebrovascular health, and interactions aimed at lowering the risk of CVD would also be expected to promote brain health.

20.4 OPTIMAL BRAIN HEALTH

The brain has minimal or no energy reserves, and neurons and glia are exquisitely sensitive to minor chemical changes. Normal brain function is highly dependent on adequate delivery of energy substrates (18). These are delivered by cerebral flow, and these are dependent on both cardiovascular and cerebrovascular health.

Brain activity is strongly associated with corresponding amounts of blood flow to activated areas. These are controlled largely through cerebrovascular autoregulation that is designed to protect the brain from damaging fluctuations in cerebral profusion. The microcirculation within the brain depends on coordination between multiple cells including neurons, adipocytes, vascular endothelial cells, and so on (19). These are all components of what has been called the "neurovascular unit" (NVU). NVU is also responsible for the blood-brain barrier as well as for disposing unwanted products of brain activity such as β-amyloid and tau proteins to prevent their accumulation in the brain tissue.

There is now evidence that cumulative exposure to vascular risk factors throughout life, perhaps starting as early as in utero and certainly by the third or fourth decade, can affect common neurologic diseases such as stroke and dementia and other brain abnormalities that can diminish optimal brain function. Thus, vascular risk factors that affect not only the heart but also the cerebrovascular system such as hypertension, T2DM and dyslipidemia can adversely impact cerebral blood vessels.

While some definitions of brain health have cited the absence of overt vascular or neurodegenerative injury such as from a stroke or Alzheimer's disease (AD), the "Optimal Brain Health" statement from the AHA and ASA provides a broader prospective of the definition of brain health. In this document, optimal brain health is defined as "optimal capacity to function adaptively to the environment" (1). This definition indicates that brain function can be affected by lifestyle behavior, environment and disease and emphasizes that these changes must be detected at the earliest possible time. Quality of life functions such as sleep and appetite are affected by the brain and represent what might be considered "vital signs of the brain" and help identify adverse factors at the earliest possible stage of the impact on the brain.

20.5 COGNITIVE IMPAIRMENT AND DEMENTIA

Sustaining brain health and cognition over a lifetime is critically important to allow individuals to maximize overall functional ability and independence. Whole brain health deterioration can manifest as cognitive impairment or dementia. Underlying disorders that are classified under dementia include AD, strokes and other vascular causes of cognitive impairment, brain trauma and other neurodegenerative disorders. It has been estimated there are 2.9 million people in the United States living with dementia. This comprises the second largest number of individuals with dementia, second only to China where there are an estimated 5.4 million individuals with dementia. In addition to dementia, it has been estimated that one in eight adults over the age of 60 years will have some degree of memory loss, and 35% of individuals in this age range report functional difficulties.

Brain impairment such as dementia can have a significant adverse impact not only on the individuals but their entire family. AD is one of the most expensive conditions to treat and has direct care expenditures greater than cancer and equal to those of heart disease (20,21). For example, in 2011, over 15 million Americans spent an average of 21.9 hours per week caring for a family member with dementia (21). These costs may actually be larger than the direct cost of dementia itself.

20.6 CARDIOVASCULAR AND STROKE RISK AND BRAIN HEALTH

Multiple studies have shown that cardiovascular risk factors are major contributors to decreased cognitive health and the risk of stroke and AD. For example, high fasting glucose or T2DM have both been associated with cognitive impairment and dementia. Smoking has been implicated in the risk of cognitive decline and dementia through atherosclerosis inflammation and oxidative stress. Obesity, dyslipidemia and high blood pressure are also major contributors to vascular decrease in brain health. Nutritional strategies such as adherence to Mediterranean or DASH diets (Dietary Approach to Stop Hypertension) have also been associated with reduced cognitive decline, possibly through antioxidant components. While many of these factors occur later in life, less is known about how cardiovascular risk factor exposures on brain health in midlife or earlier impact diminished brain health. There is a suggestion that obesity, even occurring in midlife, increases the risk of cognitive impairment. Hypertension can also influence cognition and dementia and may be exacerbated by long, cumulative times of exposure. The CARDIA (Coronary Artery Disease Risk Development in Young Adults) showed that cumulative systolic and diastolic blood pressures above normal and fasting glucose were consistently related to worse cognition (22).

Multiple studies have also shown strong associations between physical activity and cognitive health function. One meta-analysis showed that physically active adults had 25% lower risk of cognitive decline than those who were physically inactive (more detail on this in a subsequent section of this chapter) (23). It has also been suggested in a number of studies that abnormalities in sleep may be associated with poorer cognition and cognitive decline. This is an area of active investigation. What should be emphasized is that virtually all of these risk factors for diminished brain health are amendable to amelioration by lifestyle interventions.

20.7 RELATIONSHIP BETWEEN CARDIOVASCULAR HEALTH AND BRAIN HEALTH

There are multiple risk factors for cognitive decline, as outlined in the previous section. In order to combat this risk, the AHA and the ASA have advocated a plan that is based on the strong relationship between cardiovascular health and brain health. In particular, the AHA and the ASA have recommended that individuals follow what has been called "Life's Simple 7" by the AHA (23). This involves the following factors as articulated by the AHA:

- *Manage blood pressure*—High blood pressure is a major risk factor for heart disease and stroke. When blood pressure stays within healthy ranges, individuals reduce strain on their heart, arteries and kidneys which keeps individuals healthier longer.
- *Control cholesterol*—High cholesterol contributes to plaque that can clog arteries and lead to heart disease and stroke. When cholesterol is controlled, this lowers the risk that arteries will experience blockages.
- *Reduce blood sugar*—Most of the food that is consumed is turned into glucose that is used for energy. Over time, high levels of blood sugars, unfortunately, can damage the heart, kidneys, eyes and nerves.
- *Get active*—Living an active lifestyle is one of the most rewarding gifts that individuals can give themselves. Numerous studies show that daily physical activity increases both length and quality of life. This is so important that we focus on this in the next section. There are abundant, new data available in the PAGA 2018.
- *Improved nutrition*—A healthy diet is an important weapon for fighting both cardiovascular disease and stroke. When eating a heart healthy diet, you lower your risk of CVD and help lower your risk of decreased brain function. This key contributor to cardiovascular health and CVD is discussed in detail in Chapter 5.

- *Lose weight*—Overweight and obesity create an added burden on the heart, lungs, blood vessels and skeleton. If an individual is overweight or obese, weight loss will also help lower blood pressure and improve quality of life. The issue of weight loss and its important role in CVD is discussed in detail in Chapter 6.
- *Stop smoking*—Cigarette smokers have a significantly increased risk for all forms of cardiovascular disease including coronary heart disease (CHD) and cerebrovascular disease. Cessation of cigarette smoking is a powerful way for individuals to lower their risk of all forms of cardiovascular disease.

All of these recommendations can be found at https://playbook.heart.org/lifes-simple-7/. Many other factors impact brain health. The key component of Life's Simple 7 all relate to lifestyle habits and practices, which adds further impulse to the powerful role that lifestyle medicine modalities can play in both cardiovascular health and brain health.

20.8 PHYSICAL ACTIVITY AND BRAIN HEALTH

As outlined in Chapter 4, regular physical activity plays a very important role in lowering the risk of CVD. Many physicians are not aware of the strong impact of regular physical activity on both cognition and brain health. According to the PAGA 2018 Scientific Report, moderate evidence exists associating greater amounts of physical activity with improvements in cognition (24). This includes components such as academic achievement, tests involving processing speed, memory and executive function, as well as decreased risk of dementia. In addition, physical activity has been demonstrated to improve a variety of biomarkers in brain health including neurotropic factors, task-evoked brain activity, volume and connectivity. According to Framingham data, physical activity was associated with increased total brain volume in individuals over the age of 60 years. In contrast, individuals in the lower quartile for physical activity increased the risk of dementia compared to those in higher quartiles by approximately 50% (25).

Physical activity improves quality of life, which relates to the way individuals perceive and react to their health status and nonmedical aspects of their life. In addition, physical activity has been shown in many studies to improve effect by lowering anxiety and depression as well as lowering both acute and chronic CVD responses to stress. Finally, physical activity has a bidirectional relation with improved sleep and can contribute to a concept that has been called "cognitive reserve." These topics are discussed in subsequent sections in this chapter.

20.9 NUTRITION AND BRAIN HEALTH

For all of the reasons that heart healthy nutrition is important to lower the risk of CVD, it is also important to lower the risk of deterioration in brain function. As already indicated, studies conducted in individuals who followed the Mediterranean diet or the DASH diet have a significantly reduced risk of developing dementia (26). It is thought that the components of this diet lower the risk of inflammation. More details about nutrition and cardiovascular disease may be found in Chapter 5.

20.10   BRAIN HEALTH ACROSS THE LIFE SPAN

While many brain disorders become manifested later in life, risk factors for CVD are established through the life course, as are risk factors for brain disorders. For example, the risk of stroke, which becomes more prevalent after the sixth decade in life, depends not only on the blood pressure at the time of these strokes, but also the accumulated levels of blood pressure throughout a life. This makes lifestyle interventions focused on modifiable risk factors important, even in young adults and perhaps even back into childhood.

20.11   MAINTENANCE OF BRAIN HEALTH

It is important to emphasize that health-related behaviors, such as those outlined in this chapter, lower the risk of both cardiovascular disease and brain disorders throughout a lifetime. There appears to be a significant role for primordial prevention throughout a lifetime that involves lowering the likelihood of developing risk factors in the first place. For example, controlled blood pressure throughout a lifetime is important to lower the risk of stroke, but those who have maintained a blood pressure of <120/80 mm Hg have an even lower risk of stroke. Individuals who followed a Mediterranean diet had better cognition after 40 years, as did individuals in the FINGER Study (Finnish Geriatric Intervention Study to Prevent Cognitive Impairment and Disability), who had not only better cognitive performance at 2 years, but improvement in executive function and processing speed. Maintaining brain health adds to a number of important, positive aspects of maintaining positive lifestyle measures throughout a life. This is another point for clinicians to raise during counseling sessions with their patients.

20.12   MENTAL HEALTH, CARDIOVASCULAR DISEASE AND BRAIN HEALTH

As discussed in Chapter 8, there are multiple interactions between issues related to mental health and cardiovascular disease. These certainly apply, as well, to brain health. Such issues as anxiety, depression and stress that may impact in multiple ways on cardiovascular disease can also impact brain health. Moreover, brain health is important in lowering the risk of all of these conditions. As discussed in Chapter 20, multiple lifestyle interventions including physical activity and mind-body therapies can play a significant role in all of these mental health issues.

20.13   SLEEP

Healthful sleep is one of the main pillars of lifestyle medicine. Sleep not only impacts CVD but is a significantly underestimated component of brain health across the life span (24,27,28). There are multiple interactions between sleep and other components of lifestyle medicine, including physical activity. These issues are discussed in detail in Chapter 9. As indicated in this chapter, sleep problems are associated with multiple health issues including CVD risk, obesity, stroke and all-cause mortality. There is a bidirectional relationship between brain health and sleep. A healthy brain is essential for healthy sleep, and vice versa. (Issues related to healthy sleep are discussed in Chapter 9.)

20.14   COGNITIVE RESERVE

An important and emerging component of brain health is an area that researchers have called "cognitive reserve." It has been argued that lifestyle measures such as increased physical activity help the brain build cognitive reserve (29). Physical activity is hypothesized to enhance the capacity of the mature brain to maintain function and resist affective disease, rendering it significant enough to cause decline in cognition or clinical dementia. It has been suggested that individuals who experience these difficulties have less cognitive reserve than those who do not, and lifestyle measures such as regular physical activity are associated with increased cognitive reserve.

Cognitive reserve is further classified as either "active reserve" or "passive reserve." "Active" reserve refers to the adaptability of neural circuits to respond to cognitive challenge. This is exemplified by compensation and use of other parts of the brain. "Passive" reserve refers to structural anatomical processes such as density of brain tissue, white matter integrity and vascularity. All of these components can be impacted both by regular physical activity and proper nutrition.

20.15   SUMMARY/CONCLUSIONS

There are profound linkages between cardiovascular health and brain health. This is an area that clinicians often fail to recognize. The recent Presidential Advisory from the AHA and ASA points to the intimate linkage between cardiovascular health and brain health. This involves not only risk factors for atherosclerosis but also various risk factors that are held in common by the cardiovascular system and the brain. For these reasons, the AHA and ASA have recommended that individuals follow the AHA "Life's Simple 7" program not only to lower their risk of CVD but also to lower the risk of dementia. Cognition is vital to a healthy and fulfilling life. The lifestyle components that are relevant to cardiovascular health are also highly relevant to brain health. This is a topic that clinicians should discuss in detail with every patient. These topics are particularly important in a society where the number of people over the age of 60 years has dramatically increased. However, it is important to emphasize that risk factors for cognitive decline may occur over many decades. Thus, even younger individuals should be counseled that their daily habits and actions profoundly impact every aspect of their health, including brain health and cognition.

Clinical Applications

- The linkage between cardiovascular health and brain health is strong.
- Risk factors for increases to CVD and decreased brain health are similar.

- Multiple lifestyle interventions such as regular physical activity, healthy nutrition, blood pressure control, healthy sleep, stress reduction and others can lower the risk of adverse brain conditions and dementia.

REFERENCES

1. Gorelick PB, Furie KL, Iadecola C, et al. Defining optimal brain health in adults: A presidential advisory from the American Heart Association/American Stroke Association. Stroke. 2017;48(10):e284–303. Epub 2017/09/09.
2. Winblad B, Amouyel P, Andrieu S, et al. Defeating Alzheimer's disease and other dementias: A priority for European science and society. Lancet Neurol. 2016;15(5):455–532. Epub 2016/03/19.
3. Etnier JL, Nowell PM, Landers DM, et al. A meta-regression to examine the relationship between aerobic fitness and cognitive performance. Brain Res Rev. 2006;52(1):119–30. Epub 2006/02/24.
4. Smith PJ, Blumenthal JA, Hoffman BM, et al. Aerobic exercise and neurocognitive performance: A meta-analytic review of randomized controlled trials. Psychosom Med. 2010;72(3):239–52. Epub 2010/03/13.
5. Colcombe S, Kramer AF. Fitness effects on the cognitive function of older adults: A meta-analytic study. Psychol Sci. 2003;14(2):125–30. Epub 2003/03/29.
6. Kelly ME, Loughrey D, Lawlor BA, et al. The impact of exercise on the cognitive functioning of healthy older adults: A systematic review and meta-analysis. Ageing Res Rev. 2014;16:12–31. Epub 2014/05/28.
7. Bustamante EE, Williams CF, Davis CL. Physical activity interventions for neurocognitive and academic performance in overweight and obese youth: A systematic review. Pediatr Clin North Am. 2016;63(3):459–80. Epub 2016/06/05.
8. Carson V, Hunter S, Kuzik N, et al. Systematic review of physical activity and cognitive development in early childhood. J Sci Med Sport. 2016;19(7):573–8. Epub 2015/07/23.
9. Donnelly JE, Hillman CH, Castelli D, et al. Physical activity, fitness, cognitive function, and academic achievement in children: A systematic review. Med Sci Sports Exerc. 2016;48(6):1197–222. Epub 2016/05/18.
10. Esteban-Cornejo I, Tejero-Gonzalez CM, Sallis JF, et al. Physical activity and cognition in adolescents: A systematic review. J Sci Med Sport. 2015;18(5):534–9. Epub 2014/08/12.
11. Tan BW, Pooley JA, Speelman CP. A meta-analytic review of the efficacy of physical exercise interventions on cognition in individuals with autism spectrum disorder and ADHD. J Autism Dev Disord. 2016;46(9):3126–43. Epub 2016/07/15.
12. Beckett MW, Ardern CI, Rotondi MA. A meta-analysis of prospective studies on the role of physical activity and the prevention of Alzheimer's disease in older adults. BMC Geriatr. 2015;15:9. Epub 2015/04/19.
13. Sofi F, Valecchi D, Bacci D, et al. Physical activity and risk of cognitive decline: A meta-analysis of prospective studies. J Intern Med. 2011;269(1):107–17. Epub 2010/09/14.
14. Zheng G, Xia R, Zhou W, et al. Aerobic exercise ameliorates cognitive function in older adults with mild cognitive impairment: A systematic review and meta-analysis of randomised controlled trials. Br J Sports Med. 2016;50(23):1443–50. Epub 2016/04/21.
15. Chang YK, Labban JD, Gapin JI, et al. The effects of acute exercise on cognitive performance: A meta-analysis. Brain Res. 2012;1453:87–101. Epub 2012/04/07.
16. Lambourne K, Tomporowski P. The effect of exercise-induced arousal on cognitive task performance: A meta-regression analysis. Brain Res. 2010;1341:12–24. Epub 2010/04/13.

17. Ludyga S, Gerber M, Brand S, et al. Acute effects of moderate aerobic exercise on specific aspects of executive function in different age and fitness groups: A meta-analysis. Psychophysiology. 2016;53(11):1611–26. Epub 2016/08/25.

18. Attwell D, Laughlin SB. An energy budget for signaling in the grey matter of the brain. J Cereb Blood Flow Metab. 2001;21(10):1133–45. Epub 2001/10/13.

19. Cipolla MJ. The Cerebral Circulation. San Rafael (CA): Morgan & Claypool Life Sciences; 2009, pp. 1–59.

20. World Health Organization and Alzheimer's Disease International. Dementia: A public health priority. Paper presented at: World Health Organization; April 11, 2012; Geneva, Switzerland. Dementia: A public health priority (who.int). Accessed December 29, 2021.

21. Alzheimer's Association. 2013 Alzheimer's disease facts and figures. Alzheimers Dement. 2013;9(2):208–45. Epub 2013/03/20.

22. Yaffe K, Vittinghoff E, Pletcher MJ, et al. Early adult to midlife cardiovascular risk factors and cognitive function. Circulation. 2014;129(15):1560–7. Epub 2014/04/02.

23. Blondell SJ, Hammersley-Mather R, Veerman JL. Does physical activity prevent cognitive decline and dementia? A systematic review and meta-analysis of longitudinal studies. BMC Public Health. 2014;14(1):510. Epub 2014/06/03.

24. Physical Activity Guidelines Advisory Committee. 2018 Physical Activity Guidelines Advisory Committee. 2018 Physical Activity Guidelines Advisory Committee Scientific Report. Washington, DC: U.S. Department of Health and Human Services; 2018.

25. Tan ZS, Spartano NL, Beiser AS, et al. Physical activity, brain volume, and dementia risk: The Framingham study. J Gerontol A Biol Sci. 2017;72(6):789–95. Epub 2016/07/17.

26. Scarmeas N, Stern Y, Mayeux R, et al. Mediterranean diet and mild cognitive impairment. Arch Neurol. 2009;66(2):216–25. Epub 2009/02/11.

27. Lo JC, Groeger JA, Cheng GH, et al. Self-reported sleep duration and cognitive performance in older adults: A systematic review and meta-analysis. Sleep Med. 2016;17:87–98. Epub 2016/02/06.

28. Wu L, Sun D, Tan Y. A systematic review and dose-response meta-analysis of sleep duration and the occurrence of cognitive disorders. Sleep Breath. 2018;22(3):805–14. Epub 2017/06/08.

29. Kayes M, Hatfield B. Influence of physical activity on brain aging and cognition: The role of cognitive reserve, thresholds for decline, genetic influence, and the investment hypothesis. In Rippe JM, ed. Lifestyle Medicine. 3rd ed. Boca Raton, FL: CRC Press; 2019.

Part III

Specialized Topics

21 Women and Cardiovascular Disease

KEY POINTS

- Cardiovascular disease (CVD) is the leading cause of morbidity and mortality in both men and women.
- Lifestyle factors such as increased physical activity, not smoking cigarettes, maintaining a healthy body weight and following healthy nutritional practices can significantly lower the risk of CVD in women.
- The impact of lifestyle factors can be significant. In one longitudinal study, over 83% of all CVD in women could be eliminated if women followed a cluster of positive lifestyle factors.
- Physicians should counsel women on the use of lifestyle factors to lower the risk of CVD and CHD.

21.1 INTRODUCTION

Cardiovascular disease (CVD) is the leading cause of death in women. Coronary heart disease (CHD) accounted for almost 400,000 deaths in women in 2014 and accounts for one in every four female deaths in the United States (1). CHD tends to appear later in women than in men, 10 years later for total CHD and 20 years later for its most serious manifestations such as myocardial infarction (MI) and sudden cardiac death. Once women develop CHD, they have a worse prognosis than men. Among women over the age of 40 years, 42% die within 5 years after the first MI, but only 32% of men experience this.

There are multiple interactions between daily habits and actions and both the prevention and treatment of CVD in women (2). Thus, it is incumbent upon all physicians to focus on the importance of lifestyle habits and actions in every clinical encounter with women.

Unfortunately, the early rate of decline in CHD and deaths in women has been less pronounced than among men. In fact, between 1980 and 1989, there was a decline of 5.4% per year in the CHD test rate in women, and yet, between 2000 and 2002, there was an increase of 1.5% per year. Unfortunately, physicians tend to underestimate the impact of CVD in women. In one national survey, fewer than one in five physicians knew that more women than men die each year from CVD.

This chapter focuses on the key lifestyle factors that link habits and practices in daily lives to both prevention and treatment of all forms of CVD, in general, and CHD, in particular.

DOI: 10.1201/b23245-24

21.2   THE ROLE OF LIFESTYLE FACTORS IN THE PREVENTION AND TREATMENT OF HEART DISEASE IN WOMEN

Multiple studies have shown that various lifestyle factors such as level of physical activity, cigarette smoking, obesity and nutrition all play significant roles in the prevention and treatment of heart disease in women. One study that demonstrates the power of these factors was the Nurses' Health Study (3) that showed that women who engaged in the following five lifestyle factors reduce their risk of CHD by 83% and diabetes by 91%:

- Engage in moderate physical activity of 30 minutes or more each day;
- Maintain a proper body weight (body mass index [BMI] ≥19 or ≤25);
- Follow healthy nutritional practices;
- Do not smoke cigarettes; and
- If consuming alcohol, consume only one alcoholic beverage/day.

Thus, the power of lifestyle factors impacting the likelihood of CHD is very high.

21.3   RISK FACTORS FOR CARDIOVASCULAR DISEASE IN WOMEN

There are multiple risk factors for CVD in women. These are similar to the ones found in men. However, the degree to which they are found in women and the level of risk may be somewhat different.

- *Age*—Age is a substantial risk factor for risk for CVD and, specifically, for CHD. While the prevalence of CVD increases with age in both men and women, CHD events lag by at least 10 years in women compared to men. CHD in women over the age of 60 years occurs in one in three women (4). The risk of atherosclerotic CVD also increases with increasing age.
- *Family history*—A history of CHD in a first-degree relative increases the risk for an individual. Premature CHD is defined as a first-degree relative with CHD before the age of 65 years for women and age 55 years for men (5). Premature CHD in a first-degree female relative is a more potent family history risk factor than for a male relative. The Practice Guidelines issued in 2013 by the American College of Cardiology (ACC) and the American Heart Association (AHA) recommend consideration of premature family history of CVD as a component of risk assessment in asymptomatic adults.
- *Hypertension*—Women experience a higher overall prevalence of hypertension compared to men (6). This is true for women under the age of 62 years and for men under the age of 60 years and is particularly strong after the age of 60 years. Hypertension is associated with increased risk of CHD and heart failure, and this risk is greater in women than in men.
- *Dyslipidemia*—Dyslipidemia is very common in women. More than half of American women have total cholesterol levels greater than 200 mg/dL, and 36% have low-density lipoprotein cholesterol (LDL-C) greater than 130 mg/dL (7). Adverse changes in lipid profiles accompany menopause and include

increased levels of total cholesterol, LDL-C and triglycerides, as well as decreased level of high-density lipoprotein cholesterol (HDL-C) (8). CVD risk assessment focuses on LDL-C as a primary target for lipid-lowering therapy.

- *Diabetes*—Diabetes is a significant risk factor for CHD in both men and women. Diabetes increases a women's risk of CHD by between three- and sevenfold in comparison to a two- to threefold increase in men with diabetes. The American Diabetes Association (ADA) suggests consideration of diabetes screening for women and men over the age of 45 years and thereafter every 3 years if results are normal (9). Women who have a history of gestational diabetes should be screened 6–12 weeks' postpartum and every 1–2 years thereafter.
- *Obesity*—Obesity is a significant risk factor for both CVD and diabetes. A rising incidence of diabetes is closely associated with obesity (10). Central accumulation of body fat is also associated with increased risk of CVD. In women, a waist circumference of greater than 35 inches is particularly associated with increased risk of CVD (11).
- *Smoking*—Unfortunately, 14.8% of women still report tobacco use, which makes them at an increased risk for CVD (12). Female smokers die 14.5 years earlier than female nonsmokers (13). Cessation of smoking substantially reduces the risk for women in very short periods of time. (See subsequent section.)
- *Inactivity*—Inactivity is more common in women than men (31.7% versus 29.9%) and increases with age. Women who are inactive increase their risk of CVD 150%–240% compared to active women (14). (See subsequent section.)
- *Inflammation*—CVD, diabetes (T2DM) and obesity are all associated with increased incidence of inflammation. This may be routinely measured in clinical practice with C-reactive protein (hs-CRP) (15).
- *Metabolic syndrome*—According to NHANES data from 2003 to 2012, 35.6% of women meet the criteria for metabolic syndrome (16). Individuals with metabolic syndrome have an increased risk of developing CVD. In women, the relative risk of CHD is over 2.6 times compared to females without the metabolic syndrome.

21.4   ISCHEMIC HEART DISEASE IN WOMEN

Both men and women may experience typical symptoms of myocardial ischemia. However, there may be a difference in symptom perception between men and women. More women report symptoms that have been called "atypical." For example, in individuals with acute coronary syndrome (ACS), the absence of chest pain or chest discomfort occurred more often in women than in men (37% versus 27%) (17). Moreover, data from the National Registry of Myocardial Infarction showed that women were more likely than men to present with MI without any chest pain (42% versus 31%). In women, myocardial ischemia may present with symptoms that are specific and less severe and can include shortness of breath, pain or discomfort in other locations such as located to the shoulder or middle back, indigestion, nausea or vomiting, dizziness or syncope, fatigue or generalized weakness or palpitations (18). Because of the central differences in presentation of women with myocardial ischemia, it is important for clinicians to be particularly aware of these differences in presentation between men and women.

21.5 PHYSICAL ACTIVITY AND CVD IN WOMEN

Multiple organizations have consistently recommended increased physical activity to lower the risk of CVD in both men and women. These include the Physical Activity Guidelines for Americans 2018 (PAGA 2018) (19), AHA (20), the American College of Sports Medicine (ACSM) and the U.S. Surgeon General (21).

The most recent guidelines from the PAGA 2018 recommend that individuals accumulate 150 minutes of moderate-intensity physical activity every week or 75 minutes of vigorous physical activity per week and two sessions of muscle-strengthening exercise. Unfortunately, only 28% of U.S. women and 31% of U.S. men meet these guidelines. Furthermore, 41% of women and 39% of men are entirely sedentary (19).

There is strong support for the PAGA 2018 recommendations. For example, among 73,000 postmenopausal women, aged 50–79 years, in the Women's Health Initiative Study, walking briskly at least 2.5 hours per week (e.g., ½ hour five times per week) was associated with a 30% reduction in CVD events at over 3 years of follow-up (22). Numerous other studies have demonstrated CVD benefits for walking. In an 8-year follow-up of 72,000 healthy, middle-aged, female nurses in the Nurses' Health Study, 3 hours per week of brisk walking or 1.5 hours per week in vigorous exercise resulted in a 30%–40% lower risk of heart attack compared to sedentary peers (23). Previous research has suggested that physical activity lasting over 10 minutes favorably affects the CVD risk profile in otherwise healthy individuals. However, the PAGA 2018 citing new evidence indicated that the bouts of moderate activity can be less than 10 minutes and still result in significant reductions in CVD. Both the PAGA 2018 guidelines and numerous AHA documents conclude that "some is better than none." It is important to note that even 30 minutes of moderate-intensity exercise per week results in a 20% decrease in risk of CVD. In addition, prospective studies have shown that regular physical activity results in a 17%–25% decrease in stroke.

21.6 OBESITY AND ADULT WEIGHT GAIN

Obesity, as measured by BMI, is extremely common in the United States in both men and women. Between 1980 and 2004, the prevalence of obesity doubled among U.S. adults. Recent data suggest that between 2003 and 2010, obesity has continued to increase. The current level of obesity in the United States is 37.7%, while 68.8% of adults in the United States are considered overweight or obese. More men than woman were considered overweight or obese (72.9% versus 63.7%) in 2009–2010 (24). There is a strong correlation between BMI and multiple risk factors for CHD including high blood pressure, T2DM, ischemic stroke and CHD. These increases in risks are quite dramatic and are indicated in Figure 21.1.

Even women in the upper limits of healthy weight range with a BMI of greater than 22 increase their risk of CVD. For example, in the Nurses' Health Study, the

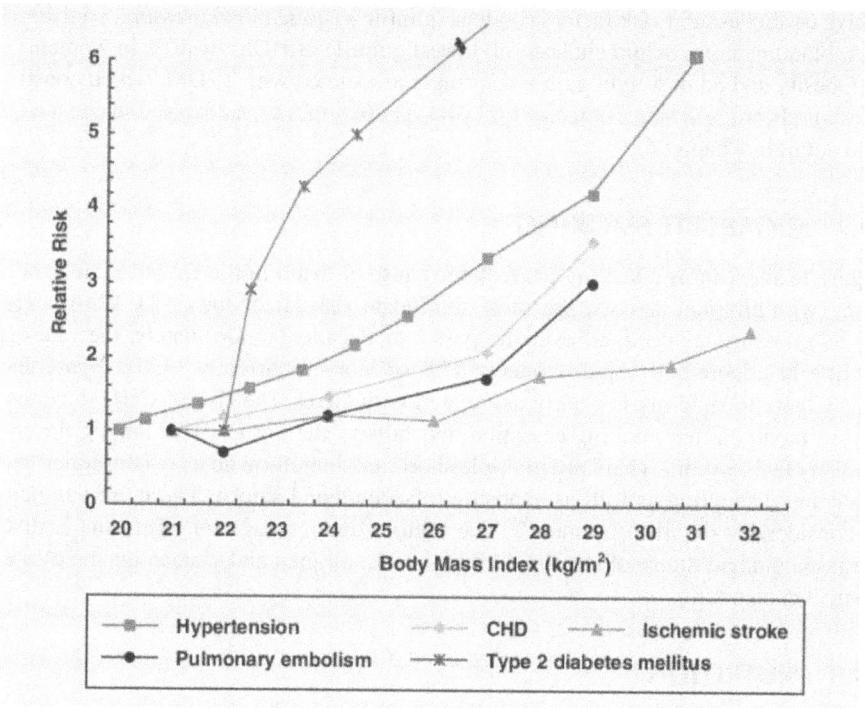

FIGURE 21.1   Relative risks for hypertension, CHD, ischemic stroke, pulmonary embolism, and T2DM, according to BMI up to 32 kg/m², after 14–16 years of follow-up, among women in the Nurses' Health Study. Relative risks for T2DM are age adjusted. Relative risks for other conditions are adjusted for age, smoking status, menopausal status, postmenopausal hormone use, parental history of MI, oral contraceptive use (for the outcomes of hypertension, ischemic stroke, and pulmonary embolism), and parity (for the outcomes of hypertension and pulmonary embolism). (Adapted from Bassuk S, Manson J. Lifestyle and risk of cardiovascular disease and type 2 diabetes in women: A review of the epidemiologic evidence. *Am J Lifestyle Med.* Vol. 2, 3: pp. 191–213. 2008. Used with permission of the Editor of AJLM, Dr. James M. Rippe.)

risk of hypertension increased by 80% in individuals with a BMI between 22.0 and 22.9 kg/m² (25). Individuals who have a BMI of greater than 31 kg/m² are six times as likely to have risk for CVD compared to individuals in the healthy weight range. It appears that excess weight and risk of CHD are linear starting as low as a BMI of 21.

In addition, weight gain during adult years was associated in women with increased risk of CHD. Compared to women of stable weight, women who gain 5–7.9 kg older than the age of 18 years through middle age were 25% more likely to develop CHD, and individuals who gained ≥20 kg were over two and one-half times more likely to develop CHD (26). There are relatively few data concerning long-term benefits of intentional weight loss on CVD risk. However, the small trials that are available suggest there is benefit for intentional weight loss. For example, in the Framingham Heart Study, a 5 pound weight loss over 16 years lowered the sum of five cardiovascular risk factors (highest quintile systolic blood pressure, triglycerides, blood glucose, serum cholesterol; lowest quintile of HDL) by 40% in women.

Obesity and adult weight gain are strongly associated with T2DM, which constitutes another significant risk factor for CHD. These topics are addressed in considerable detail in Chapter 6.

21.7   CIGARETTE SMOKING

Cigarette smoking is a leading preventable cause of death in the United States and, along with physical activity, the most significant risk factor for CVD. While cigarette smoking has declined over the past four decades, unfortunately, the rate of decline has decreased. Approximately 15% of women currently smoke cigarettes (12). Cigarette smoking is clearly associated with CHD. The risk of CHD declines within months after smoking cessation and falls to the level of risk among never-smokers in 3–5 years. There are multiple short- and long-term adverse consequences of cigarette smoking as well as exposure to secondhand smoke. These are handled in considerable detail in Chapter 7. The bottom-line message for clinicians is that the issue of cigarette smoking should be raised in all men and women during every clinical encounter.

21.8   NUTRITION

Multiple organizations have developed guidelines related to nutrition and the interaction between dietary factors and CVD. The recommendations from the AHA (27) and the Dietary Guidelines for Americans 2020–2025 (DGA 2020–2025) are consistent and recommend focus on the whole diet emphasizing whole grains, unsaturated fats, an abundance of fruits and vegetables and minimal intake of refined grains, sugar-sweetened beverages and red meat (28). All of these factors are associated with lower risk of both cardiovascular and metabolic risk factors including CVD and T2DM in both men and women. Nutrition has been a cornerstone of reducing the risk of CVD for many years. These issues are discussed in detail in Chapter 5. There are no significant differences between nutritional recommendations for women and men. Diets within the parameters outlined by the AHA and DGA 2020–2025 include the Mediterranean diet, the Healthy U.S.-Style Dietary Pattern and the DASH diet.

21.9   THE ROLE OF PHYSICIANS IN PROMOTING HEALTHY LIFESTYLES

As discussed in this chapter, CVD is the leading cause of morbidity and mortality for women. As already indicated, lifestyle measures can play a major role in lowering the risk of CVD in both men and women. Unfortunately, a minority of physicians are counseling patients in these areas. A number of studies have shown that less than 40% of physicians counsel patients in the areas of weight gain and obesity, physical activity and even cigarette smoking. This represents a significant wasted opportunity since over 70% of both men and women see their primary care physician (or, in the case of women, their obstetrician/gynecologist) on an annual basis.

The key message for physicians should be that lifestyle factors impact in significant ways on CVD and that CVD is the leading cause of morbidity and mortality in women (29). There are multiple resources available to physicians to help in these counseling areas. These include the Exercise is Medicine Movement (30) sponsored by the ACSM and AHA, Executive Summaries of the PAGA 2018 and DGA's 2020–2025. These documents should be part of every physician's toolbox.

In addition, the American College of Lifestyle Medicine (ACLM) provides numerous educational materials, webinars and even a certification for clinicians to become more knowledgeable and effective as counselors in the area of lifestyle and CVD. In addition to counseling individual patients, clinicians should hopefully become involved in playing a significant role in the community and endorsing government and workplace policies to promote healthy weight, increased physical activity and disease prevention. There is no question that lifestyle factors play a significant role in multiple chronic diseases. This is probably not true more than in the areas of CVD and CHD.

21.10 SUMMARY/CONCLUSIONS

Physicians should recognize that heart disease is the leading cause of death in women. While symptomatic heart disease typically occurs 10 years later in women than in men, it is still highly prevalent. It should be noted that heart disease in women may present with different symptoms than in men. Abdominal discomfort, shortness of breath and nausea are more common in women than in men, although chest discomfort may also be a symptom of heart disease in women. It is important for physicians to counsel patients on the importance of lowering risk factors for heart disease. This includes increasing physical activity, not smoking cigarettes, maintaining a healthy body weight and following healthy nutritional practices (more fruits and vegetables, whole grains, etc.). Lifestyle factors have been shown to be significant in reducing the risk of heart disease in women. In the Nurses' Health Trial, over 83% of all cardiovascular disease in women could be eliminated if women followed a cluster of positive lifestyle factors.

Clinical Applications

- CVD remains the leading cause of morbidity and mortality in women.
- Less than one physician out of five recognize CVD is more prevalent in women than in men.
- Lifestyle factors significantly lower the risk of CVD in women.
- Clinicians should address lifestyle issues such as cigarette smoking, weight management and adult weight gain, and physical activity in every clinical encounter.

REFERENCES

1. Tsao CW, Aday AW, Almarzooq ZI, et al. Heart disease and stroke statistics—2022 update: A report from the American Heart Association. Circulation. 2022;145(8).
2. Wilmot KA, O'Flaherty M, Capewell S, et al. Coronary heart disease mortality declines in the United States from 1979 through 2011: Evidence for stagnation in young adults, especially women. Circulation. 2015;132(11):997–1002. Epub 2015/08/26.

3. Liu S, Stampfer MJ, Hu FB, et al. Whole-grain consumption and risk of coronary heart disease: Results from the Nurses' Health Study. Am J Clin Nutr. 1999;70:412–9.
4. Stone NJ, Robinson JG, Lichtenstein AH, et al. 2013 ACC/AHA guideline on the treatment of blood cholesterol to reduce atherosclerotic cardiovascular risk in adults: A report of the American College of Cardiology/American Heart Association Task Force on Practice Guidelines. Circulation. 2014;129(25 Suppl 2):S1–45. Epub 2013/11/14.
5. Mosca L, Benjamin EJ, Berra K, et al. Effectiveness-based guidelines for the prevention of cardiovascular disease in women—2011 update: A guideline from the American Heart Association. Circulation. 2011;123(11):1243–62. Epub 2011/02/18.
6. Yoon SS, Carroll MD, Fryar CD. Hypertension prevalence and control among adults: United States, 2011–2014. NCHS Data Brief. 2015(220):1–8. Epub 2015/12/04.
7. Polotsky HN, Polotsky AJ. Metabolic implications of menopause. Semin Reprod Med. 2010;28(5):426–34. Epub 2010/09/25.
8. Mora S, Otvos JD, Rifai N, et al. Lipoprotein particle profiles by nuclear magnetic resonance compared with standard lipids and apolipoproteins in predicting incident cardiovascular disease in women. Circulation. 2009;119(7):931–9. Epub 2009/02/11.
9. Standards of Medical Care in Diabetes—2016: Summary of revisions. Diabetes Care. 2016;39 Suppl 1(Supplement_1):S4–5. Epub 2015/12/24.
10. Ogden CL, Carroll MD, Fryar CD, et al. Prevalence of obesity among adults and youth: United States, 2011–2014. NCHS Data Brief. 2015(219):1–8. Epub 2015/12/04.
11. Olson MB, Shaw LJ, Kaizar EE, et al. Obesity distribution and reproductive hormone levels in women: A report from the NHLBI-sponsored WISE Study. J Womens Health (Larchmt). 2006;15(7):836–42. Epub 2006/09/27.
12. Jamal A, Homa DM, O'Connor E, et al. Current cigarette smoking among adults—United States, 2005–2014. MMWR Morb Mortal Wkly Rep. 2015;64(44):1233–40. Epub 2015/11/13.
13. The 2004 United States surgeon general's report: The health consequences of smoking. N S W Public Health Bull. 2004;15(5–6):107. Epub 2004/11/16.
14. Chomistek AK, Manson JE, Stefanick ML, et al. Relationship of sedentary behavior and physical activity to incident cardiovascular disease: Results from the Women's Health Initiative. J Am Coll Cardiol. 2013;61(23):2346–54. Epub 2013/04/16.
15. Cook NR, Buring JE, Ridker PM. The effect of including C-reactive protein in cardiovascular risk prediction models for women. Ann Intern Med. 2006;145(1):21–9. Epub 2006/07/05.
16. Gami AS, Witt BJ, Howard DE, et al. Metabolic syndrome and risk of incident cardiovascular events and death: A systematic review and meta-analysis of longitudinal studies. J Am Coll Cardiol. 2007;49(4):403–14. Epub 2007/01/30.
17. Canto JG, Goldberg RJ, Hand MM, et al. Symptom presentation of women with acute coronary syndromes: Myth vs reality. Arch Intern Med. 2007;167(22):2405–13. Epub 2007/12/12.
18. McSweeney JC, Rosenfeld AG, Abel WM, et al. Preventing and experiencing ischemic heart disease as a woman: State of the science: A scientific statement from the American Heart Association. Circulation. 2016;133(13):1302–31. Epub 2016/03/02.
19. 2018 Physical Activity Guidelines Advisory Committee. 2018 Physical Activity Guidelines Advisory Committee Scientific Report. Washington, DC: U.S. Department of Health and Human Services; 2018.
20. American Heart Association. Life's Simple 7. My Life Check. Life's Simple 7. American Heart Association. Accessed March 28, 2022.
21. Surgeon General's Report on Physical Activity and Health. Washington, DC: US Department of Health and Human Services, Centers for Disease Control; 1999.

22. Manson JE, Greenland P, LaCroix AZ, et al. Walking compared with vigorous exercise for the prevention of cardiovascular events in women. N Engl J Med. 2002;347(10):716–25. Epub 2002/09/06.

23. Sesso HD, Paffenbarger RS, Ha T, et al. Physical activity and cardiovascular disease risk in middle-aged and older women. Am J Epidemiol. 1999;150(4):408–16. Epub 1999/08/24.

24. Rippe J, Foreyt JP. COVID-19 and obesity: A pandemic wrapped in an epidemic. Am J Lifestyle Med. 2021;15(4):364–5. Epub 2021/08/10.

25. Ashton WD, Nanchahal K, Wood DA. Body mass index and metabolic risk factors for coronary heart disease in women. Eur Heart J. 2001;22(1):46–55. Epub 2001/01/03.

26. Field AE, Coakley EH, Must A, et al. Impact of overweight on the risk of developing common chronic diseases during a 10-year period. Arch Intern Med. 2001;161(13):1581–6. Epub 2001/07/24.

27. American Heart Association Nutrition Committee, Lichtenstein AH, Appel LJ, et al. Diet and lifestyle recommendations revision 2006: A scientific statement from the American Heart Association Nutrition Committee. Circulation. 2006;114(1):82–96. Epub 2006/06/21.

28. U.S. Department of Agriculture and U.S. Department of Health and Human Services. Dietary Guidelines for Americans, 2020–2025. 9th ed. December 2020. DietaryGuidelines. gov. www.dietaryguidelines.gov/resources/2020-2025-dietary-guidelines-online-materials. Accessed March 23, 2022.

29. Berra K, Rippe J, Manson JE. Making physical activity counseling a priority in clinical practice: The time for action is now. JAMA. 2015;314(24):2617–8. Epub 2015/12/15.

30. Exercise Is Medicine. American College of Sports Medicine. Exercise Is Medicine-Exercise Is Medicine. https://www.exerciseismedicine.org/. Accessed March 23, 2022.

22 Risk Factor Reduction in Children

KEY POINTS

- Recently, there has been a significant increase in cardiovascular disease (CVD) risk factors in children.
- Over one-third of U.S. children between the ages of 2 and 19 are overweight, and 17% are obese.
- An association exists between pediatric obesity and other cardiovascular risk factors such as dyslipidemia and hypertension.
- Pediatric CVD risk factors often track into adulthood.
- Front-line therapies for virtually all CVD risk factors in children emphasize lifestyle modalities.
- Family counseling to establish a healthy environment to lower CVD risk factors can play a very important role in helping children lower their risk of CVD.
- While CVD manifestations typically occur in adulthood, the roots of CVD are often found in childhood.

22.1 INTRODUCTION

Although this book is largely devoted to heart disease in adults, it is important to recognize that the roots of cardiovascular disease (CVD) and coronary heart disease (CHD) are typically found in childhood (1–4). In fact, evidence has emerged recently that many cardiovascular risk factors may occur as early as in utero.

Compelling evidence exists that atherosclerosis (ASCVD) begins in childhood and then progresses slowly into adulthood. Multiple risk factors, some of which may emerge in childhood, are important for development of CVD. These include obesity, elevated blood pressure, dyslipidemias, diabetes and sometimes smoking. Diets that are low in fruits and vegetables and high in saturated and trans fats as well as excessive energy intake and physical inactivity are lifestyle-related behaviors increasingly being found in children, which can increase the risk of CVD.

Unfortunately, there is a tendency for risk factors in children to cluster. It is well known that the majority of CVD in adults occurs in people who have more than one risk factor. At the current time, approximately one-third of children and adults in the United States are overweight or obese, 15% have diabetes or prediabetes and 13% have hypertension or prehypertension (5,6). As discussed in detail in multiple other chapters in this book, lifestyle modalities are highly relevant components of reducing risk factors for CVD that are often applied to adults. Increasingly, the risk factors found in children mandate that these lifestyle medicine approaches also be applied to children.

DOI: 10.1201/b23245-25

22.2 LIFE COURSE OF RISK FACTORS FOR CARDIOVASCULAR DISEASE

The Developmental Origins of Health and Disease Theory suggests that there are critical periods of development during which environmental exposures have lasting effects. This association was initially described with respect to fetal undernutrition and the likelihood that adults would develop CHD. This theory has now been expanded to include a variety of health outcomes such as obesity, diabetes and psychiatric diseases. It is important to understand that transgenerational factors may impact the risk of chronic diseases, such as pregnant women with risk factors for these conditions. Thus, young women who have early signs of chronic disease may have already established risk factors for CVD and CHD when they are pregnant. This may, in fact, increase the likelihood in utero that their babies will have risk factors for chronic disease. Both undernutrition and overnutrition during pregnancy can increase risk factors for CVD. In addition, level of maternal physical activity has been shown to influence fetal outcomes. Finally, there is substantial evidence that maternal smoking during pregnancy is associated with fetal overweight, obesity and high blood pressure. Thus, lifestyle factors during pregnancy are critically important and may have a significant relationship to cardiovascular disease in children.

22.3 CHILDHOOD OBESITY AND CARDIOVASCULAR DISEASE

As already indicated, 31% of children between the ages of 2 and 19 are overweight or obese, and 17% of these (12.7 million) children in the United States are obese (7). Just as in adults, fat accumulates in excess during childhood and adolescence if total energy intake exceeds energy expenditure. Pediatric obesity is associated with multiple health problems including hypertension, dyslipidemias (including elevated cholesterol and LDL cholesterol and low HDL) and diabetes (8–10). Overweight and obesity in childhood are strongly associated with increased mortality from CVD in adulthood.

The good news is that weight loss in children is associated with significant improvement in cardiometabolic outcomes including high-density lipoprotein cholesterol (HDL-C), triglycerides (TG), and systolic blood pressure (11). A 1 kg weight loss may reduce serum TG by 5 mg/dL. A decrease of body mass index (BMI) of one unit in adolescents may decrease systolic blood pressure by 6 mm Hg. Multiple positive behaviors such as increased intakes of fruits and vegetables, regular physical activity, positive family food-related dynamics at meals and eating meals together have all been shown to lower the risk of childhood overweight or obesity. Eating breakfast has also been associated with both weight loss or weight maintenance and improved nutrient intake.

Increasing physical activity may decrease the risk of development of obesity in children. Shorter sleep duration and poor sleep quality can also increase the risk of obesity. Screen time including television viewing and recreational use of computers are all sedentary behaviors (12). Screen time greater than 2 hours per day increases the likelihood of childhood obesity.

Finally, family factors such as lack of support or overconcern about a child's weight may also stimulate an increased risk of obesity. Food insecurity may possibly be related to pediatric overweight or obesity, although this relationship has not been completely proven.

22.4 DYSLIPIDEMIAS

There are a variety of potential causes for dyslipidemia in children. As in adults, elevated cholesterol and LDL cholesterol carried by circulating lipoproteins are primary risk factors for ASCVD (13,14). Acceptable borderline and high plasma lipoprotein concentrations for children and adolescents are found in Table 22.1.

Reducing atherogenic lipoproteins with a healthy diet and lifestyle is the primary intervention for youth in order to lower the lifetime risk of ASCVD.

The current pediatric recommendations for treating identified dyslipidemia involve a two-step approach called the "Cardiovascular Health Integrated Lifestyle Diet" (CHILD-1 or CHILD-2) (15). These are both consistent with the 2020–2025 Dietary Guidelines for Americans (DGA) (16). CHILD-1 is the first-line approach for managing elevated LDL-C and non-LDL-C. After 3–6 months of compliance with CHILD-1, if there are still persistently elevated LDL-C, CHILD-2 is recommended. These diets are appropriate for children and adolescents over the age of 2 years. The nutritional components of CHILD-1 and CHILD-2 are found in Table 22.2.

Of note, the Dietary Approaches to Stop Hypertension (DASH) diet is comparable to the CHILD-1 food plan (see also Chapter 13). CHILD-2 has similar components to CHILD-1, although saturated fat is further reduced from less than 10% of daily calories to less than 7% of daily calories, and dietary cholesterol is reduced from 300 milligrams or less to 200 milligrams or less. The CHILD-2 diet is recommended for children whose dyslipidemia is characterized by high triglycerides and/or low HDL cholesterol.

TABLE 22.1
Acceptable, Borderline and High Plasma Lipoproteins and Lipid Concentrations for Children and Adolescents

Lipid/lipoprotein	Low, mg/dL	Acceptable, mg/dL	Borderline, mg/dL	High, mg/dL
TC	—	<170	170–199	≥200
LDL-C	—	<110	110–129	≥130
Non-HDL-C	—	<120	120–144	≥145
Triglyceride				
0–9 y	—	<75	75–99	≥100
10–19 y	—	<90	90–129	≥130
HDL-C	40	>45	40–45	—

Note: TC, total cholesterol; LDL-C, low-density lipoprotein cholesterol; non-HDL-C, non-high-density lipoprotein cholesterol, which is TC-HDL-C (Jacobson TA et al. 2015).

TABLE 22.2

Comparing the Nutritional Intervention Approaches in the Cardiovascular Health Integrated Lifestyle Diet 1 and 2 for LDL-Cholesterol and Non-HDL-Cholesterol Lowering in Children Younger than 2 Years of Age

Nutrient target for LDL lowering	CHILD-1	CHILD-2
Total dietary fat*	25%–30% of calories	25%–30% of calories
Saturated fat	<10% of daily calories	<7% of daily calories
Trans fat	Avoided	Avoided
Monounsaturated fat	Up to 10%–15% of calories	Up to 10%–15% of calories
Polyunsaturated fat	Up to 10% of calories	Up to 10% of calories
Cholesterol	300 mg or less	200 mg or less
Dietary fiber	Child's age + 5 g up to 14 g/1,000 calories	Child's age + 5 g up to 14 g/1,000 calories
Simple carbohydrates	Reduction of sugar-sweetened beverages	Reduction of sugar-sweetened beverages

TABLE 22.2

(continued). Top 10 Sources of Saturated Fat among U.S. Children 2–18 Years

Ranking	Food group
1	Cheese
2	Milk
3	Frankfurters, sausages, luncheon meats
4	Beef
5	Other fats and oils
6	Milk desserts
7	Cakes, cookies, quick breads, pastry, pie
8	Crackers, popcorn, pretzels, chips
9	Poultry
10	Margarine and butter

Source: Keast DR, Fulgoni VL, Nicklas TA et al. Food sources of energy and nutrients among children in the United States: National Health and Nutrition Examination Survey 2003–2006. *Nutrients.* 2013;5:283.

22.5 PHYSICAL ACTIVITY

The Physical Activity Guidelines for Americans 2018 (PAGA 2018) (17) and multiple documents from the American Heart Association recommend that children obtain at least 60 minutes of physical activity (PA) on most, if not all days (18). In fact, the PAGA 2018 document recommends 60 minutes of moderate-intensity physical activity on most days. Unfortunately, less than 20% of adolescents are achieving this level.

Conversely, it has been shown that inactivity is associated with CVD, type 2 diabetes and many other diseases in children (19). It should be noted that physical activity or sports participation in childhood has been shown to influence physical activity levels in adulthood. Thus, it is very important to establish the lifetime healthy habit of regular physical activity during childhood.

The focus on physical activity in children has been approached either from habitual physical activity or PA interventions. Interventions for PA in children have often focused on school settings, both during and after school.

Risk factors for CVD cluster in some children (20). Thus, an inactive lifestyle is likely to involve other risk factors for CVD. This clustering of risk factors may be associated with other metabolic abnormalities such as high levels of fasting insulin often found in overweight or obese children. This represents another strong reason for children to adopt a healthy lifestyle.

A sedentary lifestyle in children, in contrast, has been shown to increase risk factors for CVD. This carries additional importance since sedentary behavior established during childhood has been demonstrated to track into adulthood. Thus, for multiple reasons, it is important to emphasize the high value of physical activity in children.

22.6 HYPERTENSION

High blood pressure has become increasingly common in children and adolescents. Because blood pressure increases with age and body size, in contrast to adults, there is not a single blood pressure level that defines hypertension in children. Instead, the diagnosis of elevated blood pressure in children is based on a percentile distribution according to gender, age and height (21).

It is important to understand that lifestyle therapies are the first line of treatment of high blood pressure in children. Definitions for blood pressure categories and stages in children and adolescents are found in Table 22.3.

TABLE 22.3

Definitions of Blood Pressure Categories and Stages in Children and Adolescents

Blood pressure category	For children ages 1 to <13 years of age	For children >13 years of age
Normal	<90th percentile	<120/<80 mm Hg
Elevated	≥90th percentile to <95th percentile or 120/80 mm Hg to <95th percentile, whichever is lower	120/<80 to 129/<80 mm Hg
Stage 1 Hypertension	≥95th percentile to <95th percentile +12 mm Hg, or 130/80 to 139/89 mm Hg, whichever is lower	130/80 to 139/89 mm Hg
Stage 2 Hypertension	≥95th percentile + 12 mm Hg, or ≥140/90 mm Hg, whichever is lower	≥140/90 mm Hg

Diagnosis of elevated blood pressure and hypertension in children should be confirmed with a minimum of three blood pressure measurements taken on three separate occasions utilizing standardized techniques and age-appropriate equipment.

It is currently estimated that consistently elevated blood pressure occurs in between 2.2% and 3.5% of children (7). Prevalence of pediatric hypertension is also about 3.5% (22,23). There is a considerably higher rate of hypertension in overweight or obese children (22,23). As in adults, hypertension is either categorized as not having an identifiable cause (essential hypertension) or secondary hypertension results from another medical condition such as chronic renal disease or obstructive sleep apnea. Secondary hypertension is more common early in life, while primary hypertension (essential hypertension) is more prevalent after the age of 6 years.

Weight management and nutritional counseling are recommended in the majority of children with hypertension. Obesity and overweight are strong predicters of elevated blood pressure in children accounting for more than half of the cases of primary pediatric hypertension (24,25). Lifestyle interventions for weight loss have been consistently demonstrated to exert a favorable impact on pediatric blood pressure as well as other risks for CVD (26). Given the regular benefits of weight loss on CVD risk factors, weight reduction is the primary intervention for blood pressure lowering in hypertensive, overweight or obese children. It should be emphasized that the goal for children who are overweight is to reduce the rate of weight gain while allowing normal growth and development (27). Referral to a registered dietitian may be helpful in educating families about how to plan meals and select foods to provide adequate nutrition and appropriate caloric levels for children.

As in adults, current dietary recommendations for blood pressure management in children emphasize dietary plans high in fruits and vegetables and limited in sugar, fat and sodium (21). Both the Dietary Approaches to Stop Hypertension (DASH) eating plan and also the DASH dietary approach with lower sodium have been shown to be effective in lowering blood pressure in both children and adults. (See Chapter 13 for detailed description of the DASH diet.) The use of a DASH-type dietary pattern as the means for lowering blood pressure in adolescents also, in general, lowers CVD risk (28).

As in adults, there is a significant relationship between salt intake and hypertension in children. For this reason, lowering sodium intake is highly recommended, particularly in children with hypertension who are overweight or obese. The Clinical Practice Guidelines for Screening and Management of High Blood Pressure in Children and Adolescents recommends a sodium intake of less than 2,300 mg/day in conjunction with a DASH dietary pattern (21). It is important to note that in the United States, an average of 83% of total sodium consumption comes from prepackaged foods purchased either in grocery stores (65%) or restaurants (18%) (29). Pizza and bread rolls are the greatest source of sodium in the diets of children 2–18 years old.

22.7   METABOLIC SYNDROME

Because there is a tendency for risk factors for CVD to cluster in children, there has been some recent interest in defining and perhaps treating the metabolic syndrome (MetS) in children and adolescents.

In adults, the metabolic syndrome is typically defined as a cluster of abnormalities including elevated blood pressure, elevated fasting blood glucose, elevated waist circumference, elevated triglycerides and depressed HDL (20). The difficulty in defining and measuring metabolic syndrome in children is that some of the cut points for adults are not appropriate for children. In addition, some organizations have recommended that a measure of inflammation and insulin resistance should be added to the definition of MetS. Using ATP-III World Health Organization criteria, in one study of 1,513 North American adolescents, 4.2% prevalence of MetS was found (30,31). A study of 955 Mexican children and adolescents found 6.5% and 4.5% of MetS prevalence, respectively. Other studies have found somewhat similar findings. It is clear that as the degree of obesity increases, the prevalence of MetS increases (32,33). In one study of obese children, 38.7% of moderately obese children (mean BMI 33.4 kg/m^2) and 49.7% of severely obese children (mean BMI 40.6 kg/m^2) met the criteria for MetS (34). Diagnosing metabolic syndrome in children is of great importance since we know that the roots of adult CVD are often found in children, and clustering of risk factors has been clearly shown to substantially increase the risk of CVD.

22.8 SUMMARY/CONCLUSIONS

While the manifestations of CVD typically occur in adulthood, numerous studies have now shown that the roots of CVD risk factors are found in childhood. In the past 20 years, there has been a significant increase in multiple risk factors for CVD in children including obesity, dyslipidemia, hypertension and an inactive lifestyle.

Fortunately, we have tools to combat all these risk factors for CVD in childhood. These tools include the typical lifestyle medicine modalities used in adults including increased physical activity, weight management, a healthy diet including more fruits and vegetables and whole grains and less saturated fat and sugar, as well as nutritional and physical activity strategies for lowering blood pressure.

Unfortunately, risk factors in children tend to cluster, creating significant increases in CVD. Clustering of risk factors particularly occurs in children who are overweight or obese. Guidelines for what constitutes overweight or obesity or elevated blood pressure, as well as recommendations for proper nutrition for childhood are found in various guidelines put out by the American Heart Association and the Dietary Guidelines for Americans 2020–2025. Lifestyle strategies are particularly important in this age group not only because they carry few adverse side effects but also because CVD risk factors in children tend to carry on to adulthood. Family counseling is also very appropriate in many of these areas.

It is clear that multiple lifestyle factors including physical activity and sleep, proper nutrition and weight management are vital strategies for lowering CVD risk factors in children. Unfortunately, children and adolescents often do not live in environments that encourage healthy choices. Often the best approach is to encourage the entire family to make healthy choices. This is a strategy that lifestyle medicine practitioners should adopt.

Clinical Applications

- Body weight and dyslipidemia and elevated blood pressure should be assessed in all children, particularly those who are overweight or obese.
- Lifestyle management of CVD risk factors in children is particularly important.
- Counseling of the entire family may be valuable to create a healthy home environment such as healthy eating habits and regular physical activity.

REFERENCES

1. Berenson GS, Srinivasan SR, Bao W, et al. Association between multiple cardiovascular risk factors and atherosclerosis in children and young adults: The Bogalusa Heart Study. N Engl J Med. 1998;338(23):1650–6. Epub 1998/06/06.
2. McMahan CA, Gidding SS, Malcom GT, et al. Pathobiological determinants of atherosclerosis in youth risk scores are associated with early and advanced atherosclerosis. Pediatrics. 2006;118(4):1447–55. Epub 2006/10/04.
3. Newman WP, 3rd, Freedman DS, Voors AW, et al. Relation of serum lipoprotein levels and systolic blood pressure to early atherosclerosis: The Bogalusa Heart Study. N Engl J Med. 1986;314(3):138–44. Epub 1986/01/16.
4. Raitakari OT, Juonala M, Kahonen M, et al. Cardiovascular risk factors in childhood and carotid artery intima-media thickness in adulthood: The Cardiovascular Risk in Young Finns Study. JAMA. 2003;290(17):2277–83. Epub 2003/11/06.
5. Nguyen DT, Kit BK, Carroll MD. Abnormal Cholesterol among Children and Adolescents in the United States, 2011–2014. NCHS data brief, no 228. Hyattsville, MD: National Center for Health Statistics; 2015.
6. Kit BK, Kuklina E, Carroll MD, et al. Prevalence of and trends in dyslipidemia and blood pressure among US children and adolescents, 1999–2012. JAMA Pediatr. 2015;169(3):272–9. Epub 2015/01/20.
7. Expert Panel on Integrated Guidelines for Cardiovascular Health, Risk Reduction in Children, Adolescents, National Heart Lung Blood Institute. Expert panel on integrated guidelines for cardiovascular health and risk reduction in children and adolescents: Summary report. Pediatrics. 2011;128 Suppl 5(Suppl 5):S213–56. Epub 2011/11/16.
8. Freedman DS, Khan LK, Dietz WH, et al. Relationship of childhood obesity to coronary heart disease risk factors in adulthood: The Bogalusa Heart Study. Pediatrics. 2001;108(3):712–18. Epub 2001/09/05.
9. Weiss R, Dziura J, Burgert TS, et al. Obesity and the metabolic syndrome in children and adolescents. N Engl J Med. 2004;350(23):2362–74. Epub 2004/06/04.
10. Freedman DS, Dietz WH, Srinivasan SR, et al. The relation of overweight to cardiovascular risk factors among children and adolescents: The Bogalusa Heart Study. Pediatrics. 1999;103(6 Pt 1):1175–82. Epub 1999/06/03.
11. Rajjo T, Almasri J, Al Nofal A, et al. The association of weight loss and cardiometabolic outcomes in obese children: Systematic review and meta-regression. J Clin Endocrinol Metabol. 2017;102(3):758–62. Epub 2017/03/31.
12. Hildebrant J, Couch S. Cardiovascular risk and diet in children. In James Rippe MD, ed. Lifestyle Medicine. 3rd ed. Boca Raton, FL: CRC Press; 2019.
13. Hegele RA. Plasma lipoproteins: Genetic influences and clinical implications. Nat Rev Genet. 2009;10(2):109–21. Epub 2009/01/14.

14. Benn M. Apolipoprotein B levels, APOB alleles, and risk of ischemic cardiovascular disease in the general population, a review. Atherosclerosis. 2009;206(1):17–30. Epub 2009/02/10.

15. Jacobson TA, Maki KC, Orringer CE, et al. National lipid association recommendations for patient-centered management of dyslipidemia: Part 2. J Clin Lipidol. 2015;9(6 Suppl):S1–122 e1. Epub 2015/12/25.

16. U.S. Department of Agriculture and U.S. Department of Health and Human Services. Dietary Guidelines for Americans, 2020–2025. 9th ed. December 2020. DietaryGuidelines.gov. www.dietaryguidelines.gov/resources/2020-2025-dietary-guidelines-online-materials.

17. Physical Activity Guidelines Advisory Committee. 2018 Physical Activity Guidelines Advisory Committee. 2018 Physical Activity Guidelines Advisory Committee Scientific Report. Washington, DC: U.S. Department of Health and Human Services; 2018.

18. American Heart Association. American Heart Association Recommendation for Physical Activity in Adults and Kids. American Heart Association. Accessed March 31, 2022.

19. Rippe JM. Overcoming Sedentary Behavior. Ch 14. In James Rippe MD, ed. Increasing Physical Activity. Boca Raton, FL: CRC Press; 2021.

20. Steinberger J, Daniels SR, Eckel RH, et al. Progress and challenges in metabolic syndrome in children and adolescents: A scientific statement from the American Heart Association Atherosclerosis, Hypertension, and Obesity in the Young Committee of the Council on Cardiovascular Disease in the Young; Council on Cardiovascular Nursing; and Council on Nutrition, Physical Activity, and Metabolism. Circulation. 2009;119(4):628–47. Epub 2009/01/14.

21. Flynn JT, Kaelber DC, Baker-Smith CM, et al. Clinical practice guideline for screening and management of high blood pressure in children and adolescents. Pediatrics. 2017;140(3). Epub 2017/08/23.

22. Hansen ML, Gunn PW, Kaelber DC. Underdiagnosis of hypertension in children and adolescents. JAMA. 2007;298(8):874–9. Epub 2007/08/23.

23. Chiolero A, Cachat F, Burnier M, et al. Prevalence of hypertension in schoolchildren based on repeated measurements and association with overweight. J Hypertens. 2007;25(11):2209–17. Epub 2007/10/09.

24. Ho M, Garnett SP, Baur L, et al. Effectiveness of lifestyle interventions in child obesity: Systematic review with meta-analysis. Pediatrics. 2012;130(6):e1647–71. Epub 2012/11/21.

25. Tu W, Eckert GJ, DiMeglio LA, et al. Intensified effect of adiposity on blood pressure in overweight and obese children. Hypertension. 2011;58(5):818–24. Epub 2011/10/05.

26. Reinehr T, Lass N, Toschke C, Rothermel J, et al. Which amount of BMI-SDS reduction is necessary to improve cardiovascular risk factors in overweight children? J Clin Endocrinol Metabol. 2016;101(8):3171–9. Epub 2016/06/11.

27. Moore J, Haemer M. Childhood obesity. In James Rippe, ed. Lifestyle Medicine. 4th ed. CRC Press, in press.

28. Couch SC, Saelens BE, Levin L, et al. The efficacy of a clinic-based behavioral nutrition intervention emphasizing a DASH-type diet for adolescents with elevated blood pressure. J Pediatr. 2008;152(4):494–501. Epub 2008/03/19.

29. Centers for Disease Control Prevention. Trends in the prevalence of excess dietary sodium intake—United States, 2003–2010. MMWR Morb Mortal Wkly Rep. 2013;62(50):1021–5. Epub 2013/12/20.

30. World Health Organization. Definition, Diagnosis and Classification of Diabetes Mellitus and Its Complications: Report of a WHO Consultation. Part 1, Diagnosis and Classification of Diabetes Mellitus. Geneva: World Health Organization; 1999.

31. Rodriguez-Moran M, Salazar-Vazquez B, Violante R, et al. Metabolic syndrome among children and adolescents aged 10–18 years. Diabetes Care. 2004;27(10):2516–17. Epub 2004/09/29.
32. Goodman E, Daniels SR, Morrison JA, et al. Contrasting prevalence of and demographic disparities in the World Health Organization and National Cholesterol Education Program Adult Treatment Panel III definitions of metabolic syndrome among adolescents. J Pediatr. 2004;145(4):445–51. Epub 2004/10/14.
33. Sinaiko AR, Steinberger J, Moran A, et al. Relation of body mass index and insulin resistance to cardiovascular risk factors, inflammatory factors, and oxidative stress during adolescence. Circulation. 2005;111(15):1985–91. Epub 2005/04/20.
34. Jones KL. The dilemma of the metabolic syndrome in children and adolescents: Disease or distraction? Pediatr Diabetes. 2006;7(6):311–21. Epub 2007/01/11.

23 Genetics, Epigenetics and Precision Medicine

KEY POINTS

- Enormous progress has been made in identifying lifestyle-related risk factors for cardiovascular disease including abnormal lipids, high blood pressure, cigarette smoking, inactivity and poor nutrition.
- These advances have largely come from application of data across wide population groups.
- The emerging fields of genetics, epigenetics and precision medicine offer an opportunity to potentially apply lifestyle medicine techniques with even more precision for the future to lower the risk of cardiovascular disease.
- While most of the information from genetics, epigenetics and precision medicine is not currently available for clinical application, it is increasingly becoming more sophisticated and carries great potential for the future.
- The combination of lifestyle medicine modalities and genetics, epigenetics and precision medicine may culminate in dramatic advances in what the American Heart Association has called "primordial" prevention, which is lowering the likelihood of risk factors before they even develop. Lifestyle medicine will play an important role in fulfilling this vision.

23.1 INTRODUCTION

Despite decades of progress in areas of lifestyle medicine and their relationship to reducing risk factors for heart disease, cardiovascular disease (CVD) remains the leading cause of death in the United States and around the world. In the United States, over 37% of all mortality is caused by CVD (1), despite the fact that enormous progress has been made in linking dyslipidemia, hypertension, inactivity, obesity and cigarette smoking to increased risk of heart disease (2). While all of these risk factors are key components of the lifestyle medicine approach to CVD, it remains frustratingly true that CVD remains so prevalent in the United States (3).

Over the past 20 years, there have also been enormous advances in the area of genetics, epigenetics and precision prevention (4). While these issues may seem somewhat far from the practice of lifestyle medicine, in fact, lifestyle strategies are critically important as modalities related to genetics, epigenetics and precision prevention and are likely to become even more so in the next 20 years (5). For this reason, it is important that lifestyle medicine practitioners understand the current and emerging fields of genetics, epigenetics and precision medicine.

While these concepts are unlikely to dramatically influence the current practice of lifestyle medicine, they are increasingly likely to play a major role moving forward.

DOI: 10.1201/b23245-26

Lifestyle medicine practitioners need to understand these fields and how they interact both with CVD and the practice of lifestyle medicine. We already practice, at least to some degree, the concept of genetics when we think about the relationship of family history to risk of coronary heart disease (CHD) and some other forms of CVD (6). Significant advances in the area of high-speed computing and technologies for deciphering the human genome have made it likely that our sophistication of applying genetics, epigenetics and precision medicine to lowering the risk of CVD and, indeed, many other chronic diseases is destined to become more prominent and clinically relevant in the next two decades.

23.2   GENETICS AND CARDIOVASCULAR DISEASE

The Human Genome Project issued a draft sequence of the human genome in 2001 (7). This greatly expanded the understanding of potential genetic contributions of CVD. Before the Human Genome Project, there had been genes associated with Mendelian aspects of CVD. A good example of this is familial hypercholesterolemia (FH) (8). Conditions associated with Mendelian genetics represent a very small minority of clinical CVD. These conditions are basically the result of a mutation of a single gene and are, hence, called monogenetic. This is the basis of Mendelian disease (9).

There are other forms of Mendelian CVD such as hypertrophic cardiomyopathy, long QT syndrome and aortic aneurysms (9). In addition, there are recessive mutations that underlie forms of cardiovascular risk factors such as hypertension, hypercholesterolemia and type 2 diabetes mellitus (T2DM).

Mendelian diseases have led to important discoveries related to CVD. The classic example is the Nobel Prize–winning discovery that mutations in the LDL receptor caused hypocholesterolemia and early onset myocardial infarctions (8). This led to LDL cholesterol lowering therapies such as statins that have significantly reduced the risk of cardiovascular events. However, the vast majority of risk factors for CVD are polygenetic and have both heritable and environmental contributions (see subsequent section).

23.3   A BRIEF PRIMER ON HUMAN GENETICS

Human DNA is a molecule with two strands in a configuration known as the double helix. DNA comprises four different nucleotides: adenine (A), thymine (T), guanine (G), and cytosine (C), which are linked together in a nonrandom manner. For example, adenine on one strand is always paired with thymine on the other strand, and a cytosine on one strand is always paired with a guanine on the other strand (4,9).

Human DNA is organized into 23 pairs of chromosomes, and each of these chromosomes has millions of based pairs. Each chromosome has numerous genes. These are called "coding" DNA and are separated by long stretches of noncoating DNA.

The process of copying information from DNA is called "transcription." The information from DNA is encoded in a single strand of RNA, which is called messenger RNA (mRNA). Subsequently, the process of translation converts mRNA sequence into an amino acid sequence that makes up proteins that can serve a variety of roles.

The application of this process has been recently and famously utilized to generate mRNA-based vaccines for the COVID-19 virus, which code for the proteins making up the spikes on the COVID-19 molecule.

If a change occurs in the DNA sequence of the genome, it may result in abnormalities in the protein being coded by the gene, and this can carry significant consequences for what is called the "phenotype" of an organism. Phenotype refers to any observable characteristic in the human body. Genetic changes underlie most of the heritability of disease that have a genetic component.

23.4   EPIGENETICS

Epigenetics relate to phenotypic changes that are caused by external factors that influence the process of gene transcription (4). These factors can result in altered levels or types of RNA that are transcribed by the DNA; this, in turn, can result in altered levels of proteins. The most common epigenetic modification is methylation of cytosine bases, which typically results in reduced transcription or "silencing" of the gene. At this level of epigenetics, it is postulated that most lifestyle-related alterations manifestation of DNA occurs. Thus, epigenetics has become an important and widely studied area of the impact of lifestyle habits and practices on cardiovascular risk.

23.5   PRECISION MEDICINE

Precision medicine has been defined as an integrative approach to prevention and treatment that "considers an individual's genetics, lifestyle and exposures as determined by their cardiovascular health and disease phenotypes" (1). The basic idea behind precision medicine is to overcome the limitations of medicine that, in the past, have presumed that all patients who carry the same signs or manifestations of disease share a common "pathophenotype" and should be treated similarly (10). Precision medicine incorporates not only typical clinical and health record data but also advanced panomics (that is genomics, transcriptomics, epigenomics, proteomics, metabolomics). This allows deep investigation to uncover relationships between diseases and potentially select pharmacotherapeutics in a more sophisticated way than has been utilized in the past. Precision medicine is an attempt to make a deep dive into data utilizing advanced tools, which may result in improved CVD health. It should be noted that lifestyle medicine has played a key role in reducing the risk of CVD through adoptions of various practices such as increased physical activity, dietary and tobacco interventions, and so on. These behavioral approaches have assumed that individuals at risk for CVD share a common at-risk profile.

The concept behind precision medicine is to delve more deeply into the individual components of these lifestyle and other related factors. Precision medicine is based on advances in all the panomics already listed and includes advanced technologies and "big data." The goal of precision medicine is to identify optimal care for an individual based on their unique personal profile rather than the average population.

While precision medicine holds considerable promise, it should be noted that at the current time, many of these techniques are not available for clinicians. Nonetheless, precision medicine represents an important opportunity moving forward. One manifestation of this opportunity that can be seen is in recent attempts to define which patients benefit most from lipid lowering utilizing statins. In one study in this area, it was determined that individuals within the spectrum of elevated LDL benefited most if they were in the highest genetic risk category.

The ability to conduct genome-wide association studies (GWAS) on large cardiovascular populations offers the promise to blend genetic information with other sources of information that may lead to more precise treatments in the future (11). It should be noted that precision medicine is not the same as "personalized" medicine. Personalized medicine still applies to adopting therapies to an individual but does not utilize the broad-based genetic information that is increasingly becoming available.

23.6   MONOGENETIC VERSUS POLYGENETIC APPROACHES

When a single pathologic gene is discovered for a specific disorder, this is called a "monogenetic" approach (12). A classic example of this is the mutation of the low-density lipoprotein receptor (LDLR) that causes familial hypercholesterolemia and led to the development of statin medications. In contrast, atherosclerosis and myocardial infarction are multifaceted diseases with complex inheritance that cannot be explained by a single pathogenetic gene and are likely to be due to derangements of large and possibly phenotypically related genes and other environmental factors. This, of course, has been an underlying concept behind why various lifestyle-related factors have been studied to lower the risk of CVD.

23.7   NEW APPROACHES TO RISK FACTORS

Advances in genetic sequencing have expanded the understanding of genetic cases of CVD, in particular, and other human diseases, in general. Unfortunately, even though a great deal of information is available in this area, it quickly becomes extremely complicated. For example, there are greater than 150,000 disease-related genetic variants. Thus, there are relatively few therapies developed that can provide genetic maps to greater than 6,000 mendelian disorders. Unfortunately, even though this information is available, relatively few therapies are currently available to treat or cure these mendelian diseases. This information, however, has been used in some clinical studies to explore why some individuals who have genetic bases to increase their risk of CVD, nonetheless, do not develop these conditions. There are now some examples of how these concepts are being applied to lifestyle interventions. In one study, a healthy lifestyle, which was defined as regular physical activity, absence of obesity, no tobacco use and a healthy diet can modify genetic risk for CVD. In this study of over 55,000 individuals with a high genetic risk but who maintained a healthy lifestyle, a 46% reduction in the relative risk of coronary events was determined. Thus, one use of genetic information may be to emphasize to one group of individuals of high genetic risk the extreme importance of positive lifestyle changes.

23.8 CORONARY HEART DISEASE AND MYOCARDIAL INFARCTION

GWAS have identified 30 loci associated with MI and CHD. Subsequent studies of over 22,000 individuals with CHD also identified 13 new loci associated with CHD (13,14). Loci were associated with elevated levels of triglycerides and cholesterol subfractions. This points to the fact there is still a considerable distance to go before these types of data can be applied to individuals in a clinical setting.

23.9 PRIMORDIAL PREVENTION

In the 2020 Strategic Plan, the American Heart Association (AHA) articulated that one of its goals moving forward would be to emphasize "primordial" prevention (15). This concept involves preventing the development of risk factors in the first place rather than simply treating existing risk factors. This is an area where there are clear implications for genetics, epigenetics and precision medicine. If these techniques can be refined to the degree that they can be applied to individual clinical situations, this offers a window into the potential for lowering risk factors for heart disease before they even develop, particularly in genetically susceptible individuals. This is an area in which we in the lifestyle medicine and CVD communities will watch with great interest in the future.

23.10 BIG DATA AND COMPUTING POWER

To truly identify individuals within a broad range of the population for a particular application of genetic, epigenetic and precision prevention techniques, it will be necessary to employ enormous amounts of data (16). Fortunately, the computing power to do this, along with the advances in genetic sequencing, have become increasingly rapid and cost effective. This "big data" approach allows the potential to explore the kind of enormous database that will allow eventual application to individual clinical settings. Precision medicine will require the input and cooperation of multiple stakeholders since this is an application of rapidly changing datasets, including standard clinical imaging and laboratory testing as well as next-generation genetic sequencing and historic health record data. These data will need to be analyzed using advanced system biology and network analysis methods that may ultimately be sophisticated enough to use for prevention diagnosis and treatment of a broad range of CVD health factors, risk factors and diseases.

Precision medicine, thus, as it is applied to CVD, has the promise for improving health as well as revolutionizing prevention and treatment options. This is an area where there is enormous potential for lifestyle medicine and modalities to be applied in the future with even more sophistication than we have now when they are applied in a more general population sense. Good examples of this application involve such risk factors as blood pressure and cholesterol levels. Clearly within these broad categories, there are individuals who have abnormalities in either blood pressure or cholesterol but will not ultimately develop significant disease. Conversely, there are individuals who have normal values within the broad range of the population who may be more genetically susceptible to developing CVD.

23.11 APPLICATION OF GENETIC CONCEPTS IN PHARMACOLOGIC MANAGEMENT OF CARDIOVASCULAR DISEASE

Randomized clinical trials have been typically used to determine the efficacy of new therapeutics across large populations of individuals. However, there is still a great diversity of response to drugs (17,18). This remains a highly relevant and challenging situation where genetic rules can be applied. We are already seeing this type of application in a number of pharmacologic areas. For example, the P2Y12 clopidogrel, which is part of a typical dual antiplatelet regimen, has enormous individual variability (17). Some individuals are clopidogrel "nonresponders." There are certain genetic abnormalities that make this more likely to occur. At this juncture, however, even this information has not resulted in reductions in cardiovascular death, myocardial infarction or stent thrombosis.

Another example is that approximately 50% of patients taking statins stop these medications due to side effects or adverse events. There appears to be at least some genetic basis for these responses. Genetic determination may underlie which patients do not respond to statins or have adverse effects. Another example is warfarin, which is a commonly used anticoagulant that has a narrow therapeutic window, but a high interindividual variation. Some studies have demonstrated that there is a 10%–50% variability in dose requirements for warfarin depending on genotype. This is an area where the U.S. Food and Drug Administration has recognized the importance of genetic experience and updated drug packaging to include information on dosing based on specific genotypes.

23.12 USE OF GENETICS, EPIGENETICS AND PRECISION MEDICINE IN LIFESTYLE MEDICINE

While the field of genetics, epigenetics and precision prevention remains in its infancy, substantial progress has already been made and further progress is anticipated in the future. It is hoped that whole genome sequencing at birth may allow primordial prevention in individuals by assessing genetic determinants allowing for an individual's lifetime risk of CVD at birth to be assessed and the appropriate interventions including lifelong exercise and dietary habits offered. Thus, the combination of genetic advances coupled with the current available modalities of lifestyle medicine offer enormous potential for helping people throughout their life span lower their risk of the number one killer in the United States and enjoy maximum life free of CVD (19).

23.13 SUMMARY/CONCLUSIONS

The field of genetics, epigenetics and precision medicine is beginning to emerge as a potentially important way of applying lifestyle medicine principles from birth throughout the lifetime for individual patients. While at the current time the complexity of these fields has not offered many specific clinically applicable solutions, the potential is there to make a significant impact on lowering the risk of CVD. These techniques, along with advances in data accumulation and application, combined with available knowledge of lifestyle medicine modalities, offer enormous potential for lowering the risk of CVD.

Clinical Applications

- Current, powerful lifestyle medicine modalities such as increased physical activity, weight management, avoidance of tobacco products and proper nutrition have made an enormous impact on lowering the risk of CVD.
- The emerging field of genetics, epigenetics and precision medicine offer the potential in years to come to make further application of these lifestyle medicine modalities more individualized and powerful.

REFERENCES

1. Benjamin EJ, Muntner P, Alonso A, et al. Heart disease and stroke statistics—2019 update: A report from the American Heart Association. Circulation. 2019;139(10):e56–e528. Epub 2019/02/01.
2. Rippe JM. Lifestyle strategies for risk factor reduction, prevention, and treatment of cardiovascular disease. Am J Lifestyle Med. 2019;13(2):204–12. Epub 2019/02/26.
3. Tsao CW, Aday AW, Almarzooq ZI, et al. Heart disease and stroke statistics—2022 update: A report from the American Heart Association. Circulation. 2022;0(0):CIR. 0000000000001052.
4. Musunuru K, Kathiresan S. Principles of cardiovascular genetics. In Zipes, Libby, Bonow, Mann, Tomaselli, eds. Braunwald's Heart Disease. 11th ed. Philadelphia, PA: Elsevier; 2019.
5. Rippe JM. The future of lifestyle medicine. In Rippe JM, ed. Manual of Lifestyle Medicine. Boca Raton, FL: CRC Press; 2021.
6. Lloyd-Jones DM, Nam BH, D'Agostino RB, Sr., et al. Parental cardiovascular disease as a risk factor for cardiovascular disease in middle-aged adults: A prospective study of parents and offspring. JAMA. 2004;291(18):2204–11. Epub 2004/05/13.
7. Lander ES, Linton LM, Birren B, et al. Initial sequencing and analysis of the human genome. Nature. 2001;409(6822):860–921. Epub 2001/03/10.
8. Brown MS, Goldstein JL. A receptor-mediated pathway for cholesterol homeostasis. Science. 1986;232(4746):34–47. Epub 1986/04/04.
9. Nabel EG. Cardiovascular disease. N Engl J Med. 2003;349(1):60–72. Epub 2003/07/04.
10. Shah SH, Arnett D, Houser SR, et al. Opportunities for the cardiovascular community in the precision medicine initiative. Circulation. 2016;133(2):226–31. Epub 2016/03/31.
11. O'Donnell CJ, Nabel EG. Genomics of cardiovascular disease. N Engl J Med. 2011;365(22):2098–109. Epub 2011/12/02.
12. Lee DS, Pencina MJ, Benjamin EJ, et al. Association of parental heart failure with risk of heart failure in offspring. N Engl J Med. 2006;355(2):138–47. Epub 2006/07/14.
13. Myocardial Infarction Genetics Consortium, Kathiresan S, Voight BF, et al. Genome-wide association of early-onset myocardial infarction with single nucleotide polymorphisms and copy number variants. Nat Genet. 2009;41(3):334–41. Epub 2009/02/10.

14. Schunkert H, Konig IR, Kathiresan S, et al. Large-scale association analysis identifies 13 new susceptibility loci for coronary artery disease. Nat Genet. 2011;43(4):333–8. Epub 2011/03/08.

15. Lloyd-Jones DM, Hong Y, Labarthe D, et al. Defining and setting national goals for cardiovascular health promotion and disease reduction: The American Heart Association's strategic impact goal through 2020 and beyond. Circulation. 2010;121(4):586–613.

16. Antman EM, Harrington RA. Transforming clinical trials in cardiovascular disease: Mission critical for health and economic well-being. JAMA. 2012;308(17):1743–4. Epub 2012/11/03.

17. Mega JL, Close SL, Wiviott SD, et al. Cytochrome p-450 polymorphisms and response to clopidogrel. N Engl J Med. 2009;360(4):354–62. Epub 2008/12/25.

18. Simon T, Verstuyft C, Mary-Krause M, et al. Genetic determinants of response to clopidogrel and cardiovascular events. N Engl J Med. 2009;360(4):363–75. Epub 2008/12/25.

19. Leopold JA, Loscalzo J. Emerging role of precision medicine in cardiovascular disease. Circ Res. 2018;122(9):1302–15. Epub 2018/04/28.

24 Reversing Heart Disease

KEY POINTS

- Literature generated over the past few decades has shown that Intensive Therapeutic Lifestyle Change measures can result in angiographically demonstrated reversal of coronary heart disease (CHD).
- The area of Intensive Therapeutic Lifestyle Change (ITLC) involving very low-fat nutrition, regular physical activity and stress reduction as key components may lead to reversing heart disease.
- There is an increasing emphasis within all cardiovascular medicine for lowering risk factors.
- A number of secondary prevention studies have utilized components of lifestyle medicine to lower risk factors for heart disease.

24.1 INTRODUCTION

Over the past 20 years, a number of studies have demonstrated that lifestyle measures can be extremely effective in potentially reversing heart disease. These lifestyle factors include stringent control of the amount of fat in the diet, regular physical activity and stress reduction. It should be noted that in order for these factors to be effective in actually reversing heart disease, they typically need to be applied with a higher level of intensity than regular therapeutic lifestyle changes. This has given rise to a field that has been called "Intensive Therapeutic Lifestyle Change" (ITLC). Dr. John Kelly from the American College of Lifestyle Medicine has been a leader in developing techniques and applications for this ITLC (1).

It is also important to note that while we refer to this area as "reversing heart disease," in fact, the underlying process of atherosclerotic cardiovascular disease (ASCVD) is not completely altered by these techniques. Stringent applications of these techniques in the area of lifestyle medicine, however, have been clearly shown to reduce the size of plaque in coronary arteries and dramatically reduce cardiovascular risk factors.

The topic of reversing heart disease interacts with secondary prevention. Other lifestyle modalities may be combined with various cardioprotective medicines to further reduce the risk of recurrence cardiovascular disease (CVD). This chapter focuses on a number of studies that have been performed to show that the intense application of lifestyle medicine techniques can lead to some degree of reversal of heart disease. We also discuss some of the programs in the area of secondary prevention that have shown to at least stabilize CVD and its risk factors.

DOI: 10.1201/b23245-27

24.2   INTENSIVE HIGH-INTENSITY THERAPEUTIC LIFESTYLE CHANGE AND HEART DISEASE REVERSAL

The most compelling evidence for the effectiveness of changes in lifestyle habits and actions comes from studies that employ ITLC. TLC programs have been studied repeatedly with demonstrated reduction in risk factors for heart disease. Specific reversal of heart disease, however, has not been demonstrated for TLC programs. ITLC is particularly valuable for individuals who have severe ASCVD conditions where less intensive interventions may be inadequate or ineffective. For more details on high-intensity ITLC, refer to the chapter on this modality by Dr. John Kelly in the third edition of *Lifestyle Medicine* (1).

24.3   COMPARISON OF ITLC TO TLC

The major difference between ITLC and TLC is the depth of intensity. ITLC uses a total immersion approach to change rather than the more gradual incremental changes that are typically incorporated in many of the national guidelines and recommended by physicians. ITLC is particularly appropriate for individuals who already have significant risk factors for CVD or have a significant degree of already established CVD (typically coronary heart disease [CHD]). At the current time, few individuals are actually practicing ITLC, although there are some resident programs that provide this approach (see subsequent section), and an increasing number of lifestyle physicians are developing skills and interest in ITLC.

TLC provides less-intensive intervention and a more gradual approach to lifestyle change. This may be particularly appropriate for individuals who have a low number of risk factors or are asymptomatic. TLC typically would not be utilized or appropriate for individuals who have significant CVD, except for the desire to further reduce risk factors and prevent progression. In this regard, TLC is a component of secondary prevention.

It should also be noted that patients who have a significant amount of preexisting disease are also candidates for more intensive pharmacologic treatment such as a higher starting dose of a statin for individuals who have dyslipidemia or multiple drug therapy for individuals who have hypertension. It should be emphasized that even in these individuals, lifestyle modalities are particularly important and can be used in conjunction with pharmacologic therapy.

In the next two sections, we list some of the early landmark studies that established the basis for ITLC and its role in reversing heart disease. We follow this with a brief discussion of some of the secondary prevention trials that form the basis for many of the lifestyle-oriented risk factor reduction literature.

24.4   HEART DISEASE REVERSAL STUDIES

Perhaps the first notable study that demonstrated the role of intensive lifestyle modalities to reverse elements of heart disease was published in the *Lancet* in 1995 (by Ornish and colleagues). It was entitled the "Lifestyle Heart Trial" (LHT) (2,3). This trial randomized 28 subjects with existing CHD to experimental treatment using

ITLC and 20 subjects to usual care. The ITLC arm utilized a program developed by Dr. Dean Ornish which involved a very low-fat diet, regular physical exercise and stress reduction. The individuals in the usual care group followed the more modest lifestyle recommendations that came from the National Cholesterol Education Program (NCEP Step II).

The outcomes measured were CHD blockages and cardiac events. Blood lipids and medications were also tracked, as were levels of medication needed. At 1 year, the individuals in the ITLC program had a 37% reduction in LDL, a 91% reduction in angina and a 5.5% regression of stenoses (40% blockage on average reduced to 37.8%). The controls, in contrast, had a 6% reduction in LDL, a 165% increase in angina and an 8% regression of stenoses.

Findings at 5 years were confirmatory. Individuals in the ITLC arm had a 7.9% increase in stenoses, and controls had a 27.7% increase. Controls who were not taking statins had a 46.7% increase in stenoses. No experimental subjects took statins. It should be emphasized that statin therapy is a standard practice in secondary prevention and recommended for most individuals who have established CHD.

A second, larger trial entitled the "Lifestyle Modification Demonstration Project" (LMPD) was conducted at Brandeis University for Medicare (4). This trial was designed to evaluate both treatment effects and cost benefits of ITLC for Medicare beneficiaries with existing CHD. This program utilized the Ornish Program for Reversing Heart Disease and the Cardiac Wellness Program from the Benson-Henry Mind Body Institute (M/BMI). A total of 580 patients who had experienced acute myocardial infarction (MI), had undergone coronary artery bypass grafting or percutaneous coronary intervention or had documented stable angina pectoris were enrolled. At the end of 1 year, most cardiac risk factors improved significantly in both of the intervention programs. These changes as well as improved functional cardiac capacity were maintained or improved at 12–24 months' follow-up.

A third trial was conducted by Esselstyn and colleagues (5). In this study, the 5-year results on 22 subjects were reported in 1995, and 12-year results were reported in 1999 (6). Results from a study with a larger cohort (198 subjects) with an average of 3.7 years with the program developed by Esselstyn were published in 2014. Main outcome measures included lipids, medications, and angiographic studies of coronary blockages. The Esselstyn program emphasizes a strict plant-based diet with no more than 10% of energy from fat and no added oils or nuts.

In the first cohort of 22 subjects, 17% showed uniform improvement and somewhat more improvement at 5 years than at 12 years. Total mean cholesterol was 137 mg/dL at 5 years and 143 mg/dL at 12 years. Mean LDL cholesterol was 76 mg/dL at 5 years and 82 mg/dL at 12 years. Of the 11 individuals who underwent angiographic analysis at 5 years, none showed progression, and 8 of 11 (73%) showed regression. There were no adverse events even up through Year 12.

24.5   SECONDARY PREVENTION USING LIFESTYLE MEASURES

A variety of studies have shown reduction in risk factors for CHD based on lifestyle measures. The Lyon Diet Heart Study published in 1999 with a mean follow-up of 46 months compared a Mediterranean diet to a Prudent Western diet for the secondary prevention of heart disease (7). The individuals in the Mediterranean diet group dramatically reduced their risk of primary endpoints that were either noncardiac deaths or all-cause deaths as well as nonfatal myocardial infarction (MI). The study did not provide quantitative measures of CHD or stenoses. However, this study showed dramatic improvements based on diet alone in lowering endpoints to reduce manifestations of CHD.

The Dietary Approach to Systolic Hypertension (DASH) was a trial designed to explore how nutrition could impact systolic hypertension (8). The study enrolled 459 adults with systolic blood pressure between 140 and 160 mm Hg and diastolic blood pressure of 80–95 mm Hg. The DASH diet is rich in fruits and vegetables, low-fat dairy products and reduced saturated and total fat. Sodium intake and body weight were maintained at constant levels. After 8 weeks, this diet reduced systolic blood pressure by 5.5 mm Hg and diastolic blood pressure by 3.0 mm Hg.

The DASH-Sodium trial looked at the impact of sodium reduction on blood pressure comparing the American diet to the DASH diet (9). This trial showed that the lower the sodium intake, the lower was the blood pressure. This study showed systolic blood pressure was reduced by 7.1 mm Hg in participants without hypertension and 11.5 mm Hg lower in participants with hypertension. Unfortunately, subsequent studies have shown that only 20% of individuals with hypertension reduce the risk factor of sodium consumption by following the DASH-style diet.

The PREMIER trial utilized the DASH diet (10). This study compared a DASH diet with other lifestyle recommendations to a DASH diet alone and controls, who received advice only. This study demonstrated that individuals with above optimal blood pressure could both lower blood pressure and reduce CVD risk by following the DASH diet and other positive lifestyle behaviors utilizing the established lifestyle medicine recommendations.

The Complete Health Improvement Program (CHIP) was conducted both at a work site and in the community (11–13). This program demonstrated that multiple lifestyle modalities conducted in conjunction with each other, including low-fat nutrition and increased physical activity, achieved multiple risk factor reduction outcomes including lower body fat, blood pressure and cholesterol.

The Pritikin program utilized lifestyle modalities, including an aggressive diet and exercise program in conjunction with cholesterol-lowering drugs and showed dramatic reductions in total cholesterol and triglycerides (14–16). Total cholesterol dropped by 20% in the cholesterol-lowering medication arm alone, whereas adding lifestyle measures to this resulted in a further 19% reduction.

Several other secondary risk factor reduction programs were designed to look at specific aspects of diabetes and lifestyle measures. The Diabetes Prevention Program demonstrated that individuals who lost 5–7 pounds and followed regular moderate-intensity levels of exercise reduced the risk of prediabetes turning into diabetes by 58% (17). The Look AHEAD Trial utilized intensive lifestyle interventions and showed reduction in all CVD risk factors, except cholesterol (18). However, the endpoint of reduction in the risk of MI was not demonstrated. The Counterpoint Secondary Prevention Trial showed that lifestyle measures can be highly effective for lowering risk factors for CVD and diabetes (19).

While coronary angiography has not been performed in these trials, we know that lowering risk factors such as dyslipidemia, hypertension and obesity can all lower the risk of developing CHD.

24.6   LIPID MANAGEMENT IN SECONDARY PREVENTION

The major risk factor for CVD is low-density lipoprotein cholesterol (LDL-C). Reduction of LDL-C has clearly been demonstrated to lower the risk of both primary and secondary cardiovascular events. Statin treatment represents the cornerstone for pharmacologic therapy to lower LDL-C in patients who already have ASCVD. Statins reduce secondary events both by reducing LDL-C and decreasing inflammation.

A typical reduction of LDL-C to less than 70 mg/dL has been recommended by both the American Heart Association (AHA) and the American College of Cardiology (20) as an appropriate goal for high-risk patients. Lifestyle measures, in conjunction with statin therapy, including following a diet low in saturated fat, maintaining regular exercise and maintaining a proper weight through calorie control, are all important components of lipid management in high-risk patients. Typically, statin therapy, in addition to these modalities, will be required to achieve LDL-C <70 mg/dL.

24.7   LIFESTYLE MODALITIES IN COMBINATION
WITH CARDIOPROTECTIVE MEDICATIONS

Advances in pharmacotherapy have played a major role in management of CVD. However, cardioprotective medications, by themselves, are not adequate for many patients. Unhealthy lifestyles and behaviors are clearly associated with risk factors that lead to CVD. The INTERHEART study, which was a large multinational trial, found that lifestyle risk factors such as dyslipidemia, smoking, hypertension, diabetes, abdominal obesity, psychosocial factors, diet, alcohol and physical activity accounted for 90% of the population attributable risk (21). Clearly, there is a need to combine cardioprotective medications such as statins with "optimal medical therapy" to achieve high levels of risk reduction for CVD.

24.8   PRIMORDIAL PREVENTION

Although this chapter has focused on modalities, particularly in the area of lifestyle habits and actions on the potential lifestyle actions to reverse heart disease in individuals who have existing, severe ASCVD, it should be emphasized that the whole field of CVD prevention has moved dramatically forward. For example, the AHA has now focused attention on what the AHA has called "primordial prevention" (22). This means prevention of risk factors in the first place rather than treating risk factors. Certainly, the modalities from lifestyle medicine will continue to play a role in all levels of CVD prevention starting with primordial prevention and then moving on to risk factor reduction, secondary prevention and, ultimately, reversing heart disease.

24.9 IMPLICATIONS FOR LIFESTYLE MEDICINE PRACTITIONERS

The basic components of lifestyle medicine that we emphasize throughout this book are key modalities for reducing CVD at all levels. It is our hope that lifestyle medicine practitioners will continue to utilize these powerful techniques, sometimes in conjunction with pharmaceutical therapy, to reduce the risk of CVD at all levels. There will be some practitioners of lifestyle medicine who wish to take the next step to become practitioners of ITLC. This field is continuing to evolve. We believe this is somewhat analogous to the subspecialties of medicine. Practitioners of ITLC will increasingly be called upon by other physicians to implement the high levels of lifestyle medicine therapies that have been shown to result in such benefits as potentially reversing heart disease.

24.10 SUMMARY/CONCLUSIONS

The literature for reversing heart disease has grown dramatically in the last 20 years. Therapies that have been shown to result in some reversal of heart disease are typically practiced in individuals who have severe CVD. There is an overlap between those modalities and multiple interventions in secondary prevention, which are outlined in many chapters of this book. Lifestyle medicine remains a key modality at all levels of reducing the risk of CVD and potentially reversing heart disease when practiced at its highest level.

Clinical Applications

- TLC remains a mainstay of lifestyle medicine.
- ITLC presents the most advanced and strenuous form of lifestyle medicine and is typically applied to individuals who already have established ASCVD.
- ITLC may be practiced either by itself or in conjunction with pharmaceutical therapy.
- Low-fat nutrition, regular physical activity and stress reduction are all key components of ITLC.
- An increasing number of lifestyle medicine practitioners are becoming skillful in ITLC.

REFERENCES

1. Kelly J. High intensity therapeutic lifestyle change. In Lifestyle Medicine. 3rd ed. Boca Raton, FL: CRC Press; 2019, Ch 87 p. 1019.
2. Ornish D, et al. Can lifestyle changes reverse coronary atherosclerosis? The lifestyle heart trial. Lancet. 1990;336:129–33.
3. Ornish D, et al. Intensive lifestyle changes for reversal of coronary heart disease. JAMA. 1998;280:2001–7.
4. Shepard DS, et al. Executive Summary: Evaluation of Lifestyle Modification and Cardiac Rehabilitation in Medicare Beneficiaries. Schneider Institutes for Health Policy, Heller School, Brandeis University 2009 April 30.

5. Esselstyn CB Jr. A strategy to arrest and reverse coronary artery disease: A 5-year longitudinal study of a single physician's practice. J Fam Pract. 1995;41:560–8.

6. Esselstyn CB Jr. Updating a 12-year experience with arrest and reversal therapy for coronary heart disease (an overdue requiem for palliative cardiology). Am J Cardiol. 1999;84:339–41, A8.

7. deLorgeril M, et al. Mediterranean diet, traditional risk factors, and the rate of cardiovascular complications after myocardial infarction-final report of the lyon diet heart study. Circulation. 1999;99:779–85.

8. Appel LJ, et al. A clinical trial of the effects of dietary patterns on blood pressure. NEJM. 1997;336:1117–24.

9. Sacks FM, et al. Effects on blood pressure of reduced dietary sodium and the dietary approaches to stop hypertension (DASH) diet. NEJM. 2001 Jan;344:3–10.

10. Appel LJ, et al. Effects of comprehensive lifestyle modification on blood pressure control-main results of the PREMEIR clinical trial. JAMA. 2003;289:2083–93.

11. Diehl HA. Coronary risk reduction through intensive community-based lifestyle intervention: The Coronary Health Improvement Project (CHIP) experience. Am J Cardiol. 1998;82:83T–7T.

12. Aldana SG, et al. The effects of a worksite chronic disease prevention program. J Occup Environ Med. 2005;47:558–64.

13. Aldana SG, et al. Effects of an intensive diet and physical activity modification program on the health risks of adults. J Am Diet Assoc. 2005;105:371–81.

14. Barnard RJ, et al. Effects of intensive diet and exercise intervention in patients taking cholesterol-lowering drugs. Am J Cardiol. 1997;79:1112–14.

15. Barnard RJ. Effects of a life-style modification program on serum lipids. Arch Intern Med. 1991;151:1389–94.

16. Roberts CK, et al. Effects of exercise and diet on chronic disease. J Appl Physiol. 2005 Jan;98:3–30.

17. Knowler WC, et al. Reduction in the incidence of type 2 diabetes with lifestyle intervention or metformin. NEJM. 2002 Feb;346:393–403.

18. Look Ahead Research Group, Wadden TA, West DS, et al. The look AHEAD study: A description of the lifestyle intervention and the evidence supporting it. Obesity. 2006;14(5):737–52. Epub 2006/07/21.

19. Lim EL, et al. Reversal of type 2 diabetes: Normalisation of beta cell function in association with decreased pancreas and liver triacylglycerol. Diabetologia. 2011 Oct;54(10):2506–14.

20. Grundy SM, Stone NJ, Bailey AL, et al. 2018 AHA/ACC/AACVPR/AAPA/ABC/ACPM/ADA/AGS/APhA/ASPC/NLA/PCNA guideline on the management of blood cholesterol: A report of the American College of Cardiology/American Heart Association Task Force on Clinical Practice Guidelines. J Am Coll Cardiol. 2019;73(24):e285–e350. Epub 2018/11/14.

21. Rosengren A, Hawken S, Ounpuu S, et al. Association of psychosocial risk factors with risk of acute myocardial infarction in 11119 cases and 13648 controls from 52 countries (the INTERHEART study): Case-control study. Lancet. 2004;364(9438):953–62. Epub 2004/09/15.

22. Lloyd-Jones DM, Hong Y, Labarthe D, et al. Defining and setting national goals for cardiovascular health promotion and disease reduction: The American Heart Association's strategic Impact Goal through 2020 and beyond. Circulation. 2010;121(4):586–613.

25 The Future of Lifestyle Medicine and Cardiovascular Disease
Research and Applications

KEY POINTS

- Cardiovascular disease (CVD) remains the leading cause of mortality around the world.
- Great strides have been made in understanding risk factors for CVD, such as elevated blood pressure, dyslipidemia, inactivity, obesity and poor diet, and cigarette smoking.
- In the future, various technologies such as advanced computational techniques and genomic sequencing offer great potential for advancing the understanding of how to lower the risk of CVD.
- These technologies offer the potential to identify patients at birth who are highly susceptible to CVD and achieve the goal that has been articulated by the American Heart Association of "primordial" prevention.
- The field of genetics and epigenetics offers a particularly fruitful avenue of research for CVD prevention in the future.

25.1 INTRODUCTION

Despite enormous data linking positive lifestyle habits and practices to reduction of various chronic diseases including cardiovascular disease (CVD), CVD remains by far the largest source of mortality in the United States, resulting in over 37% of all mortality (1). Around the world, mortality from CVD has increased from 26% of all deaths to 32% of all deaths in the past 20 years (2).

Substantial progress has been made in identifying, on a population level and also on an individual level, risk factors for coronary heart disease (CHD) and CVD. Established risk factors include dyslipidemia, high blood pressure, an inactive lifestyle, cigarette smoking and obesity. Despite some progress in many of these areas, the prevalence of CVD remains frustratingly high.

Great advances have also occurred in a variety of technical areas such as genetics and computation science (3–5). While many of these technologies are not currently applicable to clinical medicine, they are increasingly becoming available and have the potential in the future to lead us to a more sophisticated understanding of not only the process of atherosclerosis, but also specific reasons why such lifestyle

DOI: 10.1201/b23245-28

modalities such as increased physical activity, healthy nutrition and weight management carry such profound benefits for lowering the risk for both CVD and type 2 diabetes mellitus (T2DM). In this chapter, we enumerate some of the more promising technologies that are likely to become increasingly relevant to the practice of cardiovascular medicine, in general, and particularly the interface between CVD and lifestyle medicine.

25.2 EPIGENETICS

As discussed in some detail in the previous chapter, the science of epigenetics deals with how mRNA and proteins may be modified after transcription and translation cytokine. There is emerging evidence that diet and level of physical activity can modify both DNA and its products. Some research suggests that methylation cyst (6) within the DNA can cause some genes to be turned off. This process of methylation of cytosine appears to be more prevalent in individuals who follow a high-fat diet as opposed to a plant-based diet. Moreover, some of the changes in DNA may lead to increases in inflammation and changes in leukocytes and macrophages, both of which are components of the atherosclerotic process (see Chapter 11).

25.3 GENETIC RISK AND LIFESTYLE MODALITIES

Several studies have suggested that intensive therapy such as increasing physical activity and lowering dietary fat may significantly change the expression of genes and pathways that are relevant to vascular function. In one study examining peripheral-blood gene expression profiling, 63 participants were compared to 63 match controls. When dietary fat was substantially reduced (minus 61%) and physical fitness was increased (plus 34%), 26 genes after 12 weeks and 143 genes after 62 weeks were differentially expressed from baseline in subjects who underwent these changes (7). In contrast, controls showed no change in CVD risk factors for gene expression. Specifically, lifestyle modification reduced expression of pro-inflammatory disease genes associated with neutrophil activation and a variety of molecular pathways important to vascular function, including cytokine production, carbohydrate metabolism and steroid hormones. The study also concluded that lifestyle changes could lead to successful and sustained modulation of gene expression and carry beneficial effects to the vascular system, which are not apparent in traditional risk factors. Interestingly, adoption of rigorous lifestyle modalities helped restore homeostasis in genes that are important to the pathogenesis of atherosclerosis.

In another study that combined four cohorts involving 65,685 patients, genetic and lifestyle factors were independently associated with susceptibility to coronary artery disease (8). Among individuals at high genetic risk, a favorable lifestyle was associated with nearly 50% lower relative risk of coronary artery disease than compared to an unfavorable lifestyle (9). Favorable lifestyle was defined as four lifestyle factors at strategic goals from the American Heart Association (AHA), namely, no current smoking, no obesity (body mass index less than 30), physical activity of at least once weekly, a healthy dietary pattern involving the recommended increased amounts of fruits, nuts, vegetables, whole grains, fish and dairy products, and reduced amounts of refined grains, unprocessed red meat, sugar-sweetened beverages and trans-fat, as well as sodium. These studies suggest that in addition to healthy lifestyle factors impacting mRNA and proteins, healthy lifestyle practices also impact the likelihood of the expression of various genes relevant to atherosclerosis being either turned on or turned off. These findings provide intriguing evidence about the underlying mechanisms for the known efficacy of positive lifestyle factors to reduce the risk of CVD.

25.4   TECHNOLOGY

Advances in a variety of technologies have also opened opportunities to advance understandings of the underlying processes of atherosclerosis. These include advances in the speed of determining whole-body genetics as well as a variety of advances in computational science and handling of enormous amounts of data ("big data"). These technologies open the door for computer modeling of vast amounts of data (so called *in silico* modeling) that has contributed to artificial intelligence (AI). AI involves a computer's ability to make decisions based on data analysis, which allows large amounts of data to be increasingly used in the area of lifestyle medicine, particularly in the area of epidemiology. These approaches are based on computer algorithms to generate statistically grounded models of various correlations within data with the hope of discovering hidden or nonintuitive associations for predicting risk of CVD. Advances in this area have also led to a discussion of the application of machine learning in medicine. Machine learning is currently in its infancy but holds great promise for the future in all areas of medicine, particularly in reduction of risk of CVD.

25.5   PRECISION MEDICINE

As outlined in Chapter 23, advances in technology and computation have opened the door for the emerging field that has been called "precision medicine" (10). This represents an evolving strategy utilizing the tools to make disease prevention and tailor treatment more precisely both for populations and for individuals by incorporating individual genetic, environmental and experiential variability. In order for precision medicine to accomplish these goals, tools will be required for describing cardiovascular health status in individuals and populations including patient-generated data and an array of data from electronic medical records. This process will require overcoming barriers to incorporate a range of technical and genetic issues and will require multiple stakeholders to contribute accurate data and participate actively in shared decision-making. Rethinking previously defined diseases that may have underlying common mechanisms (such as inflammation) will be required. This approach offers great potential, but it is currently not available for clinical application, although it is likely to become more prominent moving forward.

25.6   INFLAMMATION

Inflammatory processes have increasingly been identified as key components of CVD, in general, and atherosclerosis, in particular (see also Chapter 11).

Inflammation appears to be a key component of underlying risk factors for CVD, including obesity and diabetes. Multiple theories have been postulated for why inflammation plays such a persistent and prominent role in these chronic diseases. It has been argued that the microbiome creates a "leaky gut" that stimulates the inflammatory process. It has been argued that nutritional practices in the Western diet may promote and perpetuate inflammatory processes. As indicated in a previous section, in one study, a rigorous CVD reduction program involving significant decreases in dietary fat and increases in physical activity effectively reduced expression of pro-inflammatory disease genes associated with neutrophil activation (7). Because neutrophils and macrophages are key components of the atherosclerotic process, this represents another example of how lifestyle medicine modalities can play a critically important role in reducing CVD. Both a plant-based diet and regular physical activity have been shown to have anti-inflammatory attributes.

Inflammation serves as one of the underlying links to atherosclerosis. Atherosclerosis appears to be a result of oxidative damage to the endothelial cells that line the vascular system (see also Chapter 11). Oxidation of LDL contributes to its ability to penetrate the endothelial layer and, ultimately, to the subsequent development of atherosclerotic plaque. The rupture of these plaques may cause myocardial infarction and potentially sudden death.

25.7 MICROBIOTA

Billions of bacteria inhabit the colon. Several research studies have demonstrated that dietary components consumed by the majority of populations in Western countries may promote CVD by directly affecting the gut microbiota. Red meats, for example, are high in L-carnitine, which elevates some levels of trimethylamine oxide (TMAO) (11). Reducing red meat results in decreased TMAO and downregulates macrophage uptake and oxidation of LDL. A lifestyle program incorporating whole plant-based diets may significantly alter the microbiota and help slow or even reverse CVD. Several large epidemiologic studies have reported that the plant-based diet may decrease the risk of CVD development by almost 25%.

25.8 STRESS, ANXIETY AND DEPRESSION

It is hoped that in the future more research will be available providing specific links between stress, anxiety and depression and CVD risk. Depression is a recognized risk factor for the development of CVD and a prognostic indicator of poor outcomes for those who already have CVD. Stress is difficult to measure scientifically, but it is thought to be very common within the population. Some evidence exists that the gut microbiota may be involved, at least to some degree, in emotional resilience affecting anxiety and depression. There are data to suggest that regular physical activity also reduces anxiety and depression. Future research in this area should focus on gut microbiota as well as genetic and epigenetic responses to anxiety and depression.

25.9 FUTURE RESEARCH IN BEHAVIORAL MEDICINE

By far the largest problem when it comes to lifestyle medicine modalities and the reduction of risk of CVD resides in finding ways to help people incorporate such issues as regular physical activity, proper diet and weight management into their daily lives. There is an enormous gap between what physicians recommend and the public understands and what the public is actually doing. Future research should be focused on how to encourage people to actually incorporate lifestyle medicine modalities into their daily lives.

25.10 INTEGRATION OF LIFESTYLE MEDICINE INTO MAINSTREAM MEDICINE

Some steps have already been launched to incorporate the concept of lifestyle medicine into mainstream cardiovascular medicine. For example, one Clinical Council of the American Heart Association (AHA) has changed its name from the "Council on Nutrition and Metabolism" to the "Council on Lifestyle and Cardiometabolic Health" (12). Furthermore, the most recent guidelines for both cholesterol (13) and blood pressure management (14) from the AHA and the American College of Cardiology (ACC) have both focused on the fundamental importance of altering lifestyle and indicated that by name. The practice guidelines from the AHA/ACC entitled the "2013 AHA/ACC Guideline on Lifestyle Management to Reduce Cardiovascular Risk" underscore this trend (15). Unfortunately, a distinct minority of medical schools incorporate routine education in the areas of physical activity and nutrition and their role in lowering the risk of CVD. For example, in one survey of 51 internal medicine residents, only 25% demonstrated adequate knowledge of physical activity that could be applied to their patient population (16). In a survey of 175 primary care physicians, only 12% were aware of the recommendations from the American College of Sports Medicine (ACSM) for physical activity (17). In order to convey the benefits of these lifestyle measures to our patient population, we need to do a better job of incorporating these modalities into standard medical education. This is an area of great importance for the future of lifestyle medicine as applied to cardiovascular disease.

25.11 INCORPORATION OF LIFESTYLE MEDICINE INTO CORPORATE AMERICA

Since CVD is a high-cost area, many companies have recently mandated that healthcare providers incorporate lifestyle medicine modalities in the prevention of disease. Future research in this area demonstrating how lifestyle medicine programs can be incorporated into Corporate America will be important and could yield important cost reductions and health benefits.

25.12 INTERNATIONAL INITIATIVES

Since CVD is the largest single source of mortality around the world, it is incumbent upon medical associations worldwide to incorporate cost-effective ways of reducing the risk of CVD. This is one of the underlying principles behind the World

Health Organization initiative to combat noncommunicable diseases (18). Already some evidence has occurred in the field of cardiovascular medicine that lifestyle medicine is being increasingly considered as an important component of overall cardiac care. For example, the Fuwai Hospital in Beijing, China, which is one of the largest cardiovascular treatment centers in China, has recently established the Center for Healthy Lifestyle Medicine and has sponsored an annual conference on healthy lifestyle medicine. The first of these conferences, which was held in 2020, attracted over 600,000 participants. In the future, we hope that there will be more international efforts to incorporate lifestyle medicine in the prevention and treatment of CVD.

25.13   FRAMEWORK FOR RESEARCH

Traditional evidence in CVD prevention and treatment has focused on randomized controlled trials. Such trials may not be appropriate when utilized to assess multiple components of lifestyle medicine (19). Advances in computational techniques and genomic assays may allow different models of research to be undertaken in the future, which could greatly benefit the field of CVD prevention and treatment (20).

25.14   SUMMARY/CONCLUSIONS

Great progress has been achieved in the last 20 years with regard to lowering risk factors for CVD. However, CVD remains the leading cause of mortality in the United States and around the world. For this reason, future research and its application will play a very important role in helping to reduce the burden of CVD in the United States and around the world. Fortunately, computational advancements and advancements in technology such as genetic sequencing offer the potential to continue to drive down the leading cause of mortality around the world, namely, CVD. Many of these technologies are not currently available for clinical application. The future for advancements in this area is indeed bright.

Clinical Applications

- There is no longer any serious doubt that positive lifestyle measures can significantly lower the risk of all forms of CVD.
- Advances in a variety of technologies such as computational science and AI may pave the way for an even more robust application of lifestyle medicine to lower the risk of CVD at the earliest stages.
- Advances in genetics and epigenetics are providing some intriguing insights into why lifestyle medicine modalities significantly reduce risk factors for CVD.
- Advances in technologies also may herald the way toward precision medicine, more accurately and specifically defining therapeutic modalities, including lifestyle medicine, for each individual patient.
- While these technologies are not currently clinically available, they may play a much more prominent role in the future.

- Lifestyle medicine practitioners should keep abreast of advances in technology and genetic understanding to more effectively promote daily habits and actions and their profound impact not only on CVD but on other chronic diseases.

REFERENCES

1. Virani SS, Alonso A, Aparicio HJ, et al. Heart disease and stroke statistics—2021 update: A report from the American Heart Association. Circulation. 2021;143(8):e254–e743. Epub 2021/01/28.
2. Global Burden of Disease Study 2013. Age-Sex Specific All-Cause and Cause-Specific Mortality, 1990–2013. Seattle, WA: Institute for Health Metrics and Evaluations; 2014.
3. Lourida I, Hannon E, Littlejohns TJ, et al. Association of lifestyle and genetic risk with incidence of dementia. JAMA. 2019;322(5):430–7. Epub 2019/07/16.
4. O'Donnell CJ, Nabel EG. Genomics of cardiovascular disease. N Engl J Med. 2011;365(22):2098–109. Epub 2011/12/02.
5. Khera AV, Emdin CA, Drake I, et al. Genetic risk, adherence to a healthy lifestyle, and coronary disease. N Engl J Med. 2016;375(24):2349–58. Epub 2016/12/14.
6. Hernandez-Saavedra D, Moody L, Xu GB, et al. Epigenetic regulation of metabolism and inflammation by calorie restriction. Adv Nutr. 2019;10(3):520–36. Epub 2019/03/28.
7. Ellsworth DL, Croft DT, Jr., Weyandt J, et al. Intensive cardiovascular risk reduction induces sustainable changes in expression of genes and pathways important to vascular function. Circ Cardiovasc Genet. 2014;7(2):151–60. Epub 2014/02/25.
8. Samani NJ, Erdmann J, Hall AS, et al. Genomewide association analysis of coronary artery disease. N Engl J Med. 2007;357(5):443–53. Epub 2007/07/20.
9. Tada H, Melander O, Louie JZ, et al. Risk prediction by genetic risk scores for coronary heart disease is independent of self-reported family history. Eur Heart J. 2016;37(6):561–7. Epub 2015/09/24.
10. Antman EM, Loscalzo J. Precision medicine in cardiology. Nat Rev Cardiol. 2016;13(10):591–602. Epub 2016/07/01.
11. Koeth RA, Wang Z, Levison BS, et al. Intestinal microbiota metabolism of L-carnitine, a nutrient in red meat, promotes atherosclerosis. Nat Med. 2013;19(5):576–85. Epub 2013/04/09.
12. American Heart Association. Council on Lifestyle and Cardiometabolic Health. https://professional.heart.org/professional/MembershipCouncils/ScientificCouncils/UCM_322856_Council-on-Lifestyle-and-Cardiometabolic-Health.jsp. Accessed April 14, 2022.
13. Grundy SM, Stone NJ, Bailey AL, et al. 2018 AHA/ACC/AACVPR/AAPA/ABC/ACPM/ADA/AGS/APhA/ASPC/NLA/PCNA guideline on the management of blood cholesterol: A report of the American College of Cardiology/American Heart Association Task Force on Clinical Practice Guidelines. J Am Coll Cardiol. 2019;73(24):e285–e350. Epub 2018/11/14.
14. Whelton PK, Carey RM, Aronow WS, et al. 2017 ACC/AHA/AAPA/ABC/ACPM/AGS/APhA/ASH/ASPC/NMA/PCNA guideline for the prevention, detection, evaluation, and management of high blood pressure in adults: Executive summary: A report of the American College of Cardiology/American Heart Association Task Force on Clinical Practice Guidelines. Hypertension. 2018;71(6):1269–324. Epub 2017/11/15.
15. Eckel RH, Jakicic JM, Ard JD, et al. 2013 AHA/ACC guideline on lifestyle management to reduce cardiovascular risk: A report of the American College of Cardiology/

American Heart Association Task Force on Practice Guidelines. Circulation. 2014;129(25 Suppl 2):S76–99. Epub 2013/11/14.

16. Walsh JM, Swangard DM, Davis T, et al. Exercise counseling by primary care physicians in the era of managed care. Am J Prev Med. 1999;16(4):307–13. Epub 1999/09/24.

17. Rogers LQ, Gutin B, Humphries MC, et al. Evaluation of internal medicine residents as exercise role models and associations with self-reported counseling behavior, confidence, and perceived success. Teach Learn Medicine. 2006;18(3):215–21. Epub 2006/06/17.

18. World Health Organization. Noncommunicable Diseases. Noncommunicable Diseases. who.int. Accessed April 14, 2022.

19. Katz DL, Karlsen MC, Chung M, et al. Hierarchies of evidence applied to lifestyle Medicine (HEALM): Introduction of a strength-of-evidence approach based on a methodological systematic review. BMC Med Res Methodol. 2019;19(1):178. Epub 2019/08/21.

20. Vodovotz Y, Barnard N, Hu FB, et al. Prioritized research for the prevention, treatment, and reversal of chronic disease: Recommendations from the lifestyle medicine research summit. Front Med. 2020;7:585744. Epub 2021/01/09.

Index

Page numbers in *italics* indicate a figure and page numbers in **bold** indicate a table on the corresponding page.